Critical Care Medicine
at a Glance

Dedication

To Clare, Helen, Marc and Niall

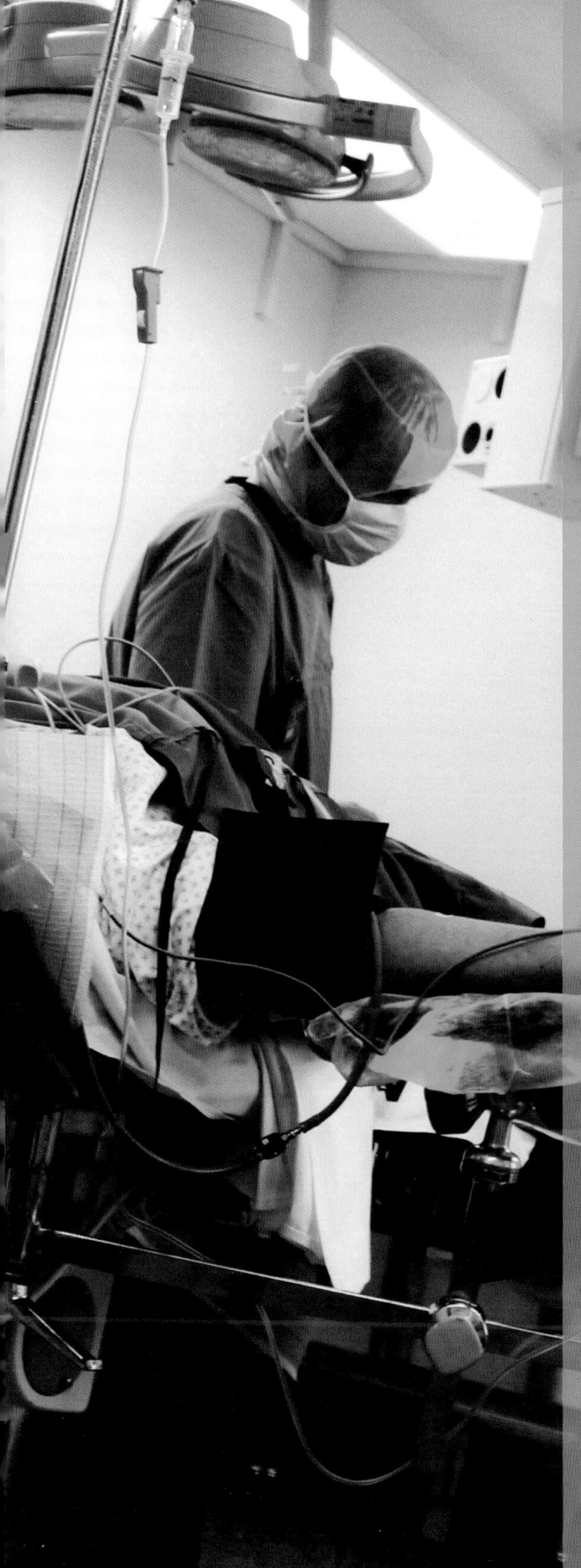

Critical Care Medicine
at a Glance

Third Edition

Richard Leach

MD, FRCP
Clinical Director for Acute Medicine
Directorates of Acute and Critical Care Medicine
Guy's and St Thomas' Hospital Trust and King's
College, London

WILEY Blackwell

This edition first published 2014 © John Wiley & Sons Ltd

Registered Office
John Wiley & Sons Ltd, The Atrium, Southern Gate, Chichester, West Sussex, PO19 8SQ, UK

Editorial Offices
350 Main Street, Malden, MA 02148-5020, USA
9600 Garsington Road, Oxford, OX4 2DQ, UK
The Atrium, Southern Gate, Chichester, West Sussex, PO19 8SQ, UK

For details of our global editorial offices, for customer services, and for information about how to apply for permission to reuse the copyright material in this book please see our website at www.wiley.com/wiley-blackwell.

The right of Richard Leach to be identified as the author of this work has been asserted in accordance with the UK Copyright, Designs and Patents Act 1988.

Library of Congress Cataloging-in-Publication Data

Leach, Richard M. (Haematologist), author.
  Critical care medicine at a glance / Richard Leach. – 3rd edition.
       p. ; cm. – (At a glance series)
  Preceded by: Acute and critical care medicine at a glance / Richard Leach. Second edition. 2009.
  Includes bibliographical references and index.
  ISBN 978-1-118-30276-7 (pbk. : alk. paper)
  I. Title. II. Series: At a glance series (Oxford, England).
  [DNLM: 1. Critical Care–methods–Handbooks. WX 39]
  RC86.8
  616.02'8–dc23
                        2014005311

A catalogue record for this book is available from the British Library.

Cover image: Reproduced from iStock © davidbuehn
Cover design by Meaden Creative

Set in 9.5/11.5 pt Minion Pro by Toppan Best-set Premedia Limited
Printed and bound in Singapore by Markono Print Media Pte Ltd

Contents

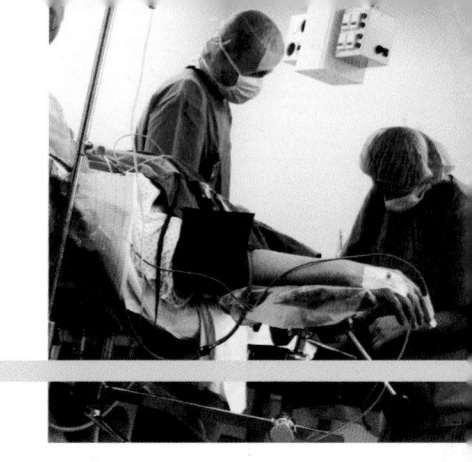

Part 1 General 1

Part 2 Medical 59

Cardiac

Part 3

Surgical 139

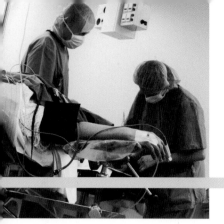

Preface

Critical care medicine encompasses the clinical, diagnostic and therapeutic skills required to manage critically ill patients in a variety of settings including intensive care, high dependency, surgical recovery and coronary care units. These disciplines have developed rapidly over the past 30 years and are an integral part of most medical, anaesthetic and surgical specialties. Medical students, junior doctors, nursing and paramedical staff are increasingly expected to develop the skills necessary to recognize and manage critically ill patients, and most will be familiar with the apprehension that precedes such training. Unfortunately, most current texts relating to critical care medicine are unavoidably extensive. It is the aim of *Critical Care Medicine at a Glance* to provide a brief, rapidly informative text, easily assimilated before starting a new job, that will prepare the newcomer for those aspects of these specialties with which they may not be familiar. These include assessment of the acutely unwell patient, monitoring, emergency resuscitation, oxygenation, circulatory support, methods of ventilation and management of a wide variety of medical and surgical emergencies.

As with other volumes in the 'At a Glance' series, this book is based around a two-page spread for each main topic, with figures and text complementing each other to give an overview of a topic at a glance. Although primarily designed as an introduction to critical care medicine, it should also be a useful undergraduate revision aid. However, such a brief text cannot hope to provide a complete guide to clinical practice and postgraduate students are advised that additional reference to more detailed textbooks will aid deeper and wider understanding of the subject. On the advice of our readers, the third edition includes new chapters on fluid management, arrhythmias, infection, stroke, jaundice, intestinal obstruction, ascites and imaging; and previous chapters have been extensively updated to include recent guidelines and innovations. As with many new specialties, certain aspects of critical care medicine remain controversial. When controversy exists, I have attempted to highlight the differences of opinion and, with the help of many colleagues and reviewers, to provide a balanced perspective, although on occasions this has proven difficult. Nevertheless, errors and omissions may have occurred and these are entirely our responsibility.

Many colleagues, junior doctors and medical students have advised and commented on the content of *Critical Care Medicine at a Glance*. I would particularly like to thank my medical colleagues on the acute medical, high dependency and intensive care units at Guy's, St Thomas' and Johns Hopkins Hospitals, and the Anaesthetic Department at St Thomas' Hospital. Special thanks are due to the senior nurses at Guy's and St Thomas' Hospitals and to Mrs Clare Leach for their advice on the many aspects of nursing care so essential in critical care medicine. Finally, I would like to thank all the staff at Wiley-Blackwell, especially Karen Moore and Katrina Rimmer, for all their help and support in producing this text.

Richard Leach

Acknowledgements

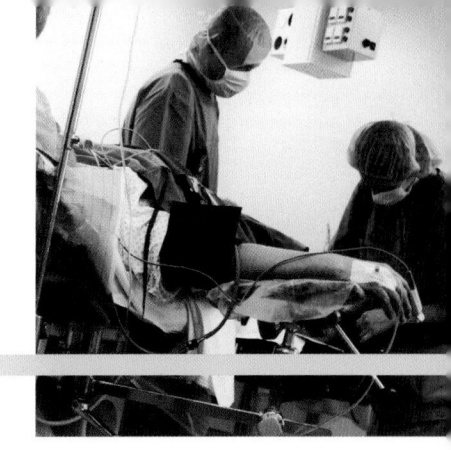

List of contributors

Ms Clare Meadows, Ms Janet Nicholls, Ms Helen Dickie, Mr Tony Convery, Senior Nursing Staff on the High Dependency and Intensive Care Units, Guy's and St Thomas' Hospital Trust, London

Dr David Treacher: Oxygen transport and shock
Dr Michael Gilles: Cardiopulmonary resuscitation
Dr Duncan Wyncoll: Fluid management, acute pancreatitis and overdose
Dr Rosalind Tilley: Airways management and endotracheal intubation
Dr Angela McLuckie: SIRS, sepsis, severe sepsis and septic shock
Dr Chris Langrish: ARDS, Mechanical ventilation
Dr Nicholas Barrett: ARDS, Mechanical ventilation
Consultant Intensivists, Guy's and St Thomas' Hospital Trust, London

Dr Marlies Ostermann: Acute kidney injury
Consultant Renal Physician and Intensivist,
Guy's and St Thomas' Hospital Trust, London

Professor Richard Beale: Enteral and parenteral nutrition
Clinical Director of Perioperative, Critical Care and Pain Services,
Guy's and St Thomas' Hospital Trust, London

Dr Nicholas Hart: Non-invasive ventilation and respiratory management
Consultant Respiratory Physician, Lane Fox Unit,
Guy's and St Thomas' Hospital Trust, London

Dr Craig Davidson: Oxygenation and oxygen therapy
Consultant Respiratory Physician and Director, Lane Fox Unit,
Guy's and St Thomas' Hospital Trust, London

Mr Jonathan Lucas: Trauma and chest trauma
Consultant Orthopaedic and Spinal Surgeon
Guy's and St Thomas' Hospital Trust, London

Professor Jeremy Ward: Acute coronary syndromes, arterial blood gases, deep venous thrombosis and pulmonary embolism
Head of Department of Physiology and Professor of Respiratory Cell Physiology, Kings College, London

Professor James T. Sylvester: Asthma
Professor of Pulmonary and Critical Care Medicine
The Johns Hopkins Medical Institutions, Baltimore, MD: USA

Professor Charles M. Wiener: Asthma and COPD
Professor of Medicine and Physiology
Johns Hopkins School of Medicine, Baltimore, MD: USA

Ms Catherine McKenzie, Senior Pharmacist, Guy's and St Thomas' Hospital Trust, London

Mr Neil Morton MBiochem (Oxon): Arterial blood gases and acid–base balance
Barts and the London, Queen Mary's School of Medicine and Dentistry

Figures

Some figures in this book are taken from:
Norwitz, E. and Schorge, J. (2006) *Obstetrics and Gynecology at a Glance*, 2nd edition. Blackwell Publishing Ltd, Oxford.
O'Callaghan, C. (2006) *The Renal System at a Glance*, 2nd edition. Blackwell Publishing Ltd, Oxford.
Ward, J.P.T. *et al.* (2006) *The Respiratory System at a Glance*, 2nd edition. Blackwell Publishing Ltd, Oxford.

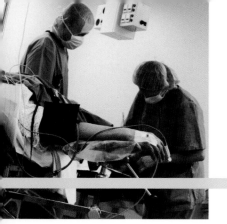

Units, symbols and abbreviations

Units

The medical profession and scientific community generally use SI (Système International) units.

Pressure conversion. SI unit of pressure: 1 pascal (Pa) = $1\,N/m^2$. Because this is small, in medicine the kPa (= $10^3\,Pa$) is more commonly used. Note that millimetres of mercury (mmHg) are still the most common unit for expressing arterial and venous blood pressures, and low pressures – e.g. central venous pressure and intrapleural pressure – are sometimes expressed as centimetres of H_2O (cmH_2O). Blood gas partial pressures are reported by some laboratories in kPa and by some in mmHg, so you need to be familiar with both systems.

$1\,kPa = 7.5\,mmHg = 10.2\,cmH_2O$
$1\,mmHg = 1\,torr = 0.133\,kPa = 1.36\,cmH_2O$
$1\,cmH_2O = 0.098\,kPa = 0.74\,mmHg$
1 standard atmosphere ($\approx$ 1 bar) = $101.3\,kPa = 760\,mmHg = 1033\,cmH_2O$

Contents are still commonly expressed per 100 mL (dL^{-1}), and these need to be multiplied by 10 to give the more standard SI unit per litre. Contents are also increasingly being expressed as mmol/L.
For haemoglobin: $1\,g/dL = 10\,g/L = 0.062\,mmol/L$
For ideal gases (including oxygen and nitrogen): 1 mmol = 22.4 mL standard temperature and pressure dry (STPD)
For non-ideal gases, such as nitrous oxide and carbon dioxide: 1 mmol = 22.25 mL STPD

Symbols

Symbols used in respiratory and cardiovascular physiology are shown in Table 1.

Typical inspired, alveolar and blood gas values in healthy young adults are shown in Table 2. Ranges are given for arterial blood gas values. Mean arterial Po_2 falls with age, and by 60 years is about 11 kPa/82 mmHg. Typical values for lung volumes and other lung function tests are given in Table 3 and Ward *et al.* (2006). Ranges for many values are affected by age, sex and height, as well as by the method of measurement; hence it is necessary to refer to appropriate nomograms.

Table 1 Standard respiratory symbols

Primary symbols
C = content of a gas in blood
F = fractional concentration of gas
V = volume of a gas
P = pressure or partial pressure
S = saturation of haemoglobin with oxygen
Q = volume of blood
A dot over a letter means a time derivative, e.g. $\dot{V}$ = ventilation (L/min) $\dot{Q}$ = blood flow (L/min)

Secondary symbols
Gas
I = inspired gas
E = expired gas
A = alveolar gas
D = dead space gas
T = tidal
B = barometric
ET = end-tidal
Blood
a = arterial
v = venous
c = capillary
A dash means mixed or mean, e.g. $\bar{v}$ = mixed venous
A' after a symbol means end, e.g. c' = end-capillary

Tertiary symbols
O_2 = oxygen
CO_2 = carbon dioxide
CO = carbon monoxide

Examples
Vo_2 = oxygen consumption
P_Aco_2 = alveolar partial pressure of carbon dioxide

Table 2 Inspired, alveolar and blood gas values

Inspired P_{O_2} (dry, sea level)	21 kPa	159 mmHg
Alveolar P_{O_2}	13.3 kPa	100 mmHg
Arterial P_{O_2}	12.5 (11.2–13.9) kPa	94 (84–104) mmHg
A–a P_{O_2} gradient	<2 kPa	<15 mmHg (greater in elderly)
Oxygen saturation	>97%	
Oxygen content	20 mL/dL	
Inspired P_{CO_2}	0.03 kPa	0.2 mmHg
Alveolar P_{CO_2}	5.3 (4.7–6.1) kPa	40 (35–45) mmHg
Arterial P_{CO_2}	5.3 (4.7–6.1) kPa	40 (35–45) mmHg
Arterial CO_2 content	48 ml/dL	
Arterial $[H^+]$/pH	36–44 nmol/L/7.44–7.36	
Resting mixed venous P_{O_2}	5.3 kPa	40 mmHg
Resting mixed venous O_2 content	15 mL/dL	
Resting mixed venous O_2 saturation	75%	
Resting mixed venous P_{CO_2}	6.1 kPa	46 mmHg
Resting mixed venous CO_2 content	52 mL/dL	
Arterial $[HCO_3^-]$	24 (21–27) mM	

Table 3 Typical lung volumes for an adult male

Tidal volume (V_T) (at rest)	500 mL
Vital capacity (VC)	5500 mL
Inspiratory capacity (IC)	3800 mL
Expiratory reserve volume (ERV)	1200 mL
Total lung capacity (TLC)	6000 mL
Functional residual capacity (FRC)	2200 mL
Residual volume (RV)	1000 mL

Abbreviations

±	with or without
>	greater than
<	less than
~	about
A-a gradient	$P_{(A-a)}O_2$ gradient, the difference between alveolar and arterial P_{O_2}
AA	amino acids
ABC	airways, breathing, circulation
ABG	arterial blood gas
ABI	acute bowel ischaemia
ABPA	allergic bronchopulmonary aspergillosis
AC	activated charcoal
AbC	abnormal conduction
ACE	angiotensin-converting enzyme
ACh	acetylcholine
AChR	acetylcholine receptor
ACS	acute coronary syndrome
ACT	activated clotting time
ACTH	adrenocorticotrophic hormone
ADH	antidiuretic hormone
AE	acute exacerbation
AF	atrial flutter; atrial fibrillation
AFE	amniotic fluid embolism
AG	anion gap
AIDS	acquired immunodeficiency syndrome
AKI	acute kidney injury
ALF	acute liver failure
ALI	acute lung injury
ALP	alkaline phosphatase
ALS	advanced life support
ALT	alanine transaminase
ANA	antinuclear antibodies
ANCA	antineutrophil cytoplasmic antibodies
APo	action potential
AP	anteroposterior
APACHE	acute physiology and chronic health evaluation
APH	antepartum haemorrhage
APTT	activated partial thromboplastin time
ARDS	acute respiratory distress syndrome
ARF	acute renal failure
ASD	atrial septal defect
AST	aspartate transaminase
AT	atrial tachycardia
ATLS	advanced trauma life support
ATN	acute tubular necrosis
ATP	adenosine triphosphate
ATS	American Thoracic Society
AV	atrioventricular
AVM	arteriovenous malformation
AVN	atrioventricular node
AXR	Abdominal radiograph
BE	base excess
BIPAP	bilevel positive pressure ventilation
BIPAP-APRV	BIPAP airways pressure release ventilation
BBB	bundle branch block
BLS	basic life support
BMI	body mass index
BMR	basal metabolic rate
BNP	serum b-type natriuretic peptide
BP	blood pressure
BPF	bronchopleural fistula

BS	blood sugar
BSA	body surface area
BSD	brainstem death
BSFT	brainstem function test
BTS	British Thoracic Society
CoA	coronary artery
CA	cardiac arrest
cAMP	cyclic adenosine monophosphate
C_aO_2	Arterial oxygen content
CAP	community-acquired pneumonia
CBF	cerebral blood flow
CBV	cerebral blood volume
CCA	calcium channel antagonist
CCB	calcium channel blocker
CCF	congestive cardiac failure
CCM	critical care medicine
CE	cardiac enzyme
CHF	chronic heart failure
CIDP	chronic inflammatory demyelinating polyneuropathy
CKD	chronic kidney disease
CK-MB	creatine kinase-MB
CLD	chronic liver disease
CMV	controlled mechanical ventilation
CMV	cytomegalovirus
CN	cyanide
CNS	central nervous system
CO	cardiac output
CO	carbon monoxide
CO_2	carbon dioxide
CO-Hb	carboxyhaemoglobin
COPD	chronic obstructive pulmonary disease
COX	cyclo-oxygenase
CPA	cardiopulmonary arrest
CPAP	continuous positive airways pressure
CPB	cardiopulmonary bypass
CPD	central pontine demyelinolysis
CPD-A	citrate, phosphate, dextrose-adenine
CPP	cerebral perfusion pressure
CPR	cardiopulmonary resuscitation
CRF	chronic renal failure
CRP	C-reactive protein
CS	caesarian section
CSF	cerebrospinal fluid
CUS	carotid artery ultrasonography
CT	computed tomography
CTn	cardiac troponin
CTD	connective tissue disease
CTT	cardiac troponin T
CVA	cerebrovascular accident
CVC	central venous catheter
CVT	cerebral venous sinus thrombosis
C_vO_2	oxygen content in venous blood
CVP	central venous pressure
CVS	cardiovascular system
CXR	chest radiograph/y
D5%	5% dextrose
DBP	diastolic blood pressure
DC	direct current
DCT	distal convoluted tube
DD	diastolic dysfunction
DDAVP	desmopressin acetate or arginine vasopressin
DI	diabetes inspidus
DIC	disseminated intravascular coagulation
DKA	diabetic ketoacidosis
DM	diabetes mellitus
Do_2	global oxygen delivery
DPG	2,3 diphosphoglycerate
DVT	deep venous thrombosis
EBV	Epstein–Barr virus
ECF	extracellular fluid
ECG	electrocardiogram
ECM	external cardiac massage
ECMO	extracorporeal membrane oxygenation
EDV	end-diastolic volume
EEG	electroencephalogram
EF	ejection fraction
EMD	electromechanical dissociation
EMS	emergency medical services
EN	enteral nutrition
EPAP	expiratory positive airways pressures
ER	emergency room
ERCP	endoscopic retrograde choledochopancreatography
ERF	established renal failure
ESR	erythrocyte sedimentation rate
ETI	endotracheal intubation
ETT	endotracheal tube
EUS	endoscopic ultrasound
f	frequency
FDG	fluorinated analogue of glucose
FDP	fibrinogen degradation product
FEV_1	forced expiratory volume in 1 second
FID	failed intubation drill
FFP	fresh frozen plasma
F_iO_2	fraction of inspired oxygen
FRC	functional residual capacity
FVC	forced vital capacity
FWB	fresh whole blood
GBS	Guillain–Barré syndrome
GCS	Glasgow Coma Score
GDP	gross domestic product
GFR	glomerular filtration rate
GH	growth hormone
GI	gastrointestinal
GL	gastric lavage
H_2O	water
HAP	hospital-acquired pneumonia
HASU	hyperacute stroke unit
Hb	haemoglobin
HB	heart block
HCA	hyperchloraemic acidosis
HCAP	healthcare-associated pneumonia
HCRF	hypercapnic respiratory failure
HDU	high dependency unit
HE	hypertensive emergency
HF	heart failure

PCWP	pulmonary capillary wedge pressure	**SAN**	sinoatrial node
PD	potential difference	S_aO_2	saturation of oxygen in arterial blood
PE	pulmonary embolism	**SAPS**	simplified acute physiology score
PEA	pulseless electrical activity	**SBO**	small bowel obstruction
PEEP	positive end-expiratory pressure	**SBP**	spontaneous bacterial peritonitis
PEEP$_i$	intrinsic or auto-PEEP	**SCr**	serum creatinine
PEFR	peak expiratory flow rate	**SDB**	second-degree burn
PET	positron emission tomography	**SDH**	subdural haemorrhage/haematoma
pH	logarithmic hydrogen ion concentration in arterial blood	**SE**	subcutaneous emphysema
		SEMI	subendocardial myocardial infarction
PHT	pulmonary hypertension	**SEp**	status epilepticus
PiCCO	pulsion continuous cardiac output monitor	**SIADH**	syndrome of inappropriate antidiuretic hormone
PIH	pregnancy-induced hypertension		
P_iO_2	partial pressure of inspired oxygen	**SIMV**	synchronized intermittent mandatory ventilation
PIP	peak inspiratory pressure		
pK_A	log of the dissociation constant K_A	**SIRS**	systemic inflammatory response syndrome
Po_2	partial pressure of oxygen	S_jO_2	cerebral oxygen saturation
POD	paracetamol overdose	**SK**	streptokinase
POP	plasma oncotic (colloid) pressure	**SLE**	systemic lupus erythematosus
PP	placenta praevia	**SMA**	superior mesenteric artery
PPH	postpartum haemorrhage	**SMR**	standard mortality ratio (observed mortality : predicted mortality)
PPI	proton pump inhibitor		
PPV	positive pressure ventilation	**SNPA**	soft nasopharyngeal airway
P_{plat}	plateau pressure	So_2	haemoglobin saturation
PRC	packed red cells	**SOH**	Severe obstetric haemorrhage
PrHT	portal hypertension	**SOL**	space-occupying lesion
PS	pressure support	**SP**	secondary pneumothorax
PSP	primary spontaneous pneumothorax	**SR**	sinus rhythm
PSV	pressure support ventilation	**SRI**	serotonin reuptake inhibitor
PT	prothrombin time	**SS**	scoring system(s)
PTCA	percutaneous coronary angioplasty	**ST**	surgical tracheostomy
PTH	parathyroid hormone	**SV**	spontaneous ventilation
PVC	peripheral venous catheter	**SV**	stroke volume
PVD	peripheral vascular disease	S_vO_2	mixed venous oxygen saturation
PVS	persistent vegetative state	**SVR**	systemic vascular resistance
QOL	quality of life	**SVT**	supraventricular tachycardia
Qs/Qt	shunt fraction	**SVT/AC**	supraventricular tachycardia with abnormal conduction
Q_T	cardiac output		
RA	right atrial; right atrium	**T3**	triiodothyronine
RAAS`	renin-angiotensin-aldosterone system	**T4**	thyroxine
RAD	right axis deviation	**TB**	tuberculosis
RAP	right atrial pressure	**TBW**	total body water
RBBB	right bundle branch block	**TC**	time constant
RBF	renal blood flow	**TCA**	tricyclic antidepressant
RES	reticuloendothelial system	**TDB**	third-degree burn
RF	respiratory failure	**TE**	thromboembolic
RFCA	radiofrequency catheter ablation	**TF**	thromboplastin/tissue factor
RPC	retained products of conception	**TIA**	transient ischaemic attack
RR	respiratory rate	**TID**	tubulointerstitial disease
RRT	renal replacement therapy	**TII**	toxic inhalational injury
RSI	rapid sequence induction	**TIPS**	transjugular intrahepatic portal stent
RUQ	right upper quadrant	**TISS**	therapeutic intervention scoring system
RV	right ventricular; right ventricle	**TLC**	total lung capacity
RV	residual volume	**TNF**	tumour necrosis factor
RVF	right ventricular failure	**TP**	traumatic pneumothorax
SA	stable angina	**tPA**	tissue plasminogen activator
SAG-M	saline, adenine, glucose-mannitol	**TPN**	total parenteral nutrition
SAH	subarachnoid haemorrhage	**TS**	trauma score
SAI	secondary adrenal insufficiency	**TSH**	thyroid-stimulating hormone

TT	thrombolytic therapy
TTP	thrombotic thrombocytopenic purpura
Tv	tidal ventilation
UA	unstable angina
UAO	upper airways obstruction
UC	ulcerative colitis
UFH	unfractionated heparin
UO	urine output
USS	ultrasound scan
UTI	urinary tract infection
VAP	ventilator-associated pneumonia
VC	vital capacity
VCV	volume-controlled ventilation
VF	ventricular fibrillation
VMA	vanillyl mandelic acid
Vo_2	global oxygen consumption
V/Q	ventilation/perfusion

VSD	ventricular septal defect
V_T	respiratory tidal volume *or* tidal ventilation
VT	ventricular tachycardia
VTE	venous thromboembolism
VWD	Von Willebrand's disease
WC	wide QRS complex
WCC	white cell count
WoB	work of breathing
WOT	withdrawal of treatment
WPW	Wolff–Parkinson–White
Na^+	sodium
K^+	potassium
Ca^{2+}	calcium
Mg^{2+}	magnesium
Cl^-	chloride
HCO_3^-	bicarbonate

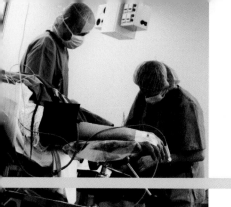

How to use your textbook

Features contained within your textbook

Each topic is presented in a double-page spread with clear, easy-to-follow diagrams supported by succinct explanatory text.

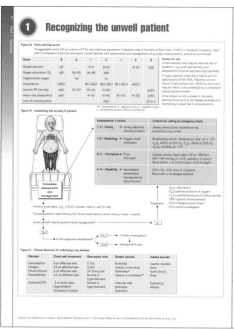

Clinical pearl boxes give inside information on a topic.

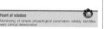

Pearl of wisdom

Hypocalcaemia (due to the effects of the citrate used in blood storage) may cause persisting hypotension during massive transfusion, despite adequate fluid replacement, unless corrected with supplemental calcium

Dilution of clotting factors and platelets may potentiate bleeding after massive transfusion unless actively supplemented with fresh frozen plasma (FFP) and platelet transfusions

Your textbook is full of **photographs, illustrations and tables.**

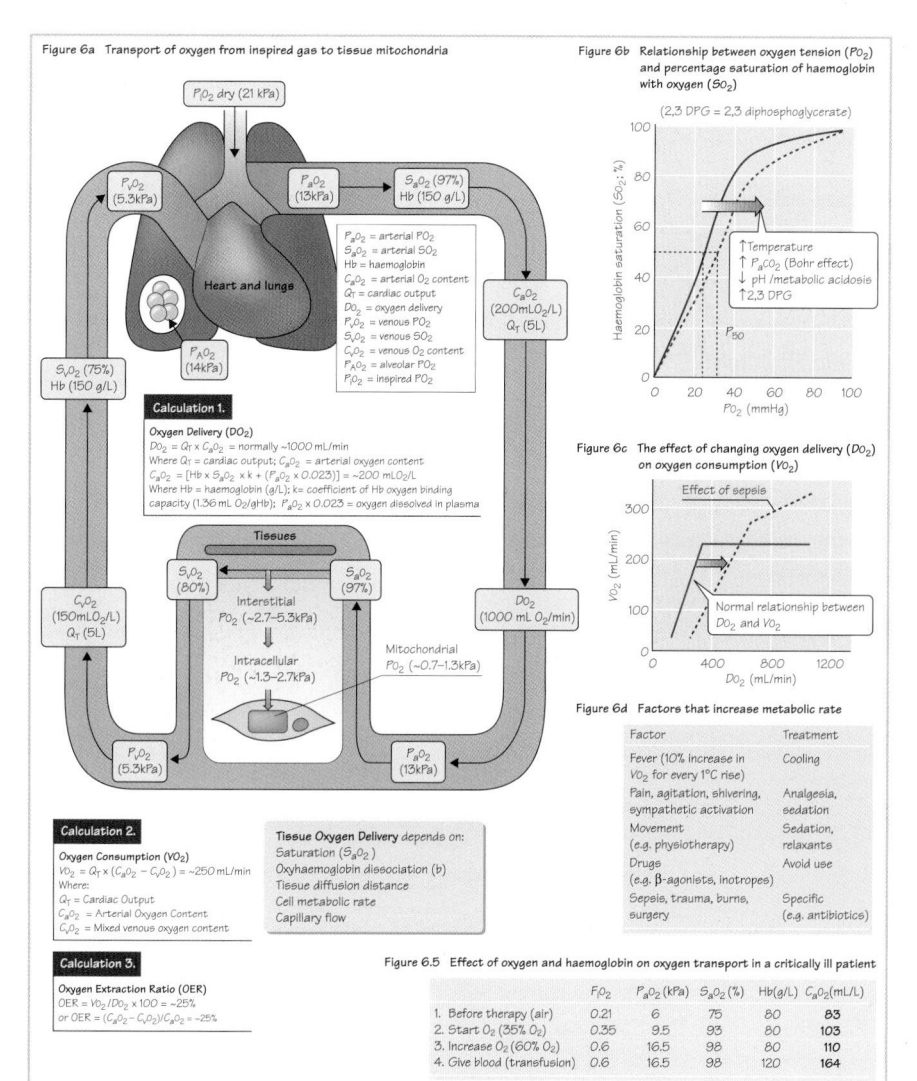

Figure 6a Transport of oxygen from inspired gas to tissue mitochondria

P_IO_2 dry (21 kPa)

P_vO_2 (5.3kPa)

P_aO_2 (13kPa)

S_aO_2 (97%) Hb (150 g/L)

Heart and lungs

P_AO_2 (14kPa)

S_vO_2 (75%) Hb (150 g/L)

C_aO_2 (200mLO_2/L) Q_T (5L)

P_aO_2 = arterial PO_2
S_aO_2 = arterial SO_2
Hb = haemoglobin
C_aO_2 = arterial O_2 content
Q_T = cardiac output
DO_2 = oxygen delivery
P_vO_2 = venous PO_2
S_vO_2 = venous SO_2
C_vO_2 = venous O_2 content
P_AO_2 = alveolar PO_2
P_IO_2 = inspired PO_2

Calculation 1.

Oxygen Delivery (DO_2)
$DO_2 = Q_T \times C_aO_2$ = normally ~1000 mL/min
Where Q_T = cardiac output; C_aO_2 = arterial oxygen content
$C_aO_2 = [Hb \times S_aO_2 \times k + (P_aO_2 \times 0.023)]$ = ~200 mLO_2/L
Where Hb = haemoglobin (g/L); k= coefficient of Hb oxygen binding capacity (1.36 mL O_2/gHb); $P_aO_2 \times 0.023$ = oxygen dissolved in plasma

Tissues

C_vO_2 (150mLO_2/L) Q_T (5L)

S_vO_2 (80%) Interstitial PO_2 (~2.7–5.3kPa)

S_aO_2 (97%)

Intracellular PO_2 (~1.3–2.7kPa)

Mitochondrial PO_2 (~0.7–1.3kPa)

DO_2 (1000 mL O_2/min)

P_vO_2 (5.3kPa)

P_aO_2 (13kPa)

Calculation 2.

Oxygen Consumption (VO_2)
$VO_2 = Q_T \times (C_aO_2 - C_vO_2)$ = ~250 mL/min
Where:
Q_T = Cardiac Output
C_aO_2 = Arterial Oxygen Content
C_vO_2 = Mixed venous oxygen content

Tissue Oxygen Delivery depends on:
Saturation (S_aO_2)
Oxyhaemoglobin dissociation (b)
Tissue diffusion distance
Cell metabolic rate
Capillary flow

Calculation 3.

Oxygen Extraction Ratio (OER)
OER = $VO_2/DO_2 \times 100$ = ~25%
or OER = $(C_aO_2 - C_vO_2)/C_aO_2$ = ~25%

Figure 6b Relationship between oxygen tension (PO_2) and percentage saturation of haemoglobin with oxygen (SO_2)

(2,3 DPG = 2,3 diphosphoglycerate)

↑Temperature
↑ P_aCO_2 (Bohr effect)
↓ pH /metabolic acidosis
↑2,3 DPG

P_{50}

PO_2 (mmHg)

Haemoglobin saturation (SO_2; %)

Figure 6c The effect of changing oxygen delivery (DO_2) on oxygen consumption (VO_2)

Effect of sepsis

Normal relationship between DO_2 and VO_2

VO_2 (mL/min)

DO_2 (mL/min)

Figure 6d Factors that increase metabolic rate

Factor	Treatment
Fever (10% increase in VO_2 for every 1°C rise)	Cooling
Pain, agitation, shivering, sympathetic activation	Analgesia, sedation
Movement (e.g. physiotherapy)	Sedation, relaxants
Drugs (e.g. β-agonists, inotropes)	Avoid use
Sepsis, trauma, burns, surgery	Specific (e.g. antibiotics)

Figure 6.5 Effect of oxygen and haemoglobin on oxygen transport in a critically ill patient

	F_IO_2	P_aO_2 (kPa)	S_aO_2 (%)	Hb(g/L)	C_aO_2(mL/L)
1. Before therapy (air)	0.21	6	75	80	83
2. Start O_2 (35% O_2)	0.35	9.5	93	80	103
3. Increase O_2 (60% O_2)	0.6	16.5	98	80	110
4. Give blood (transfusion)	0.6	16.5	98	120	164

Case studies and questions help you revise.

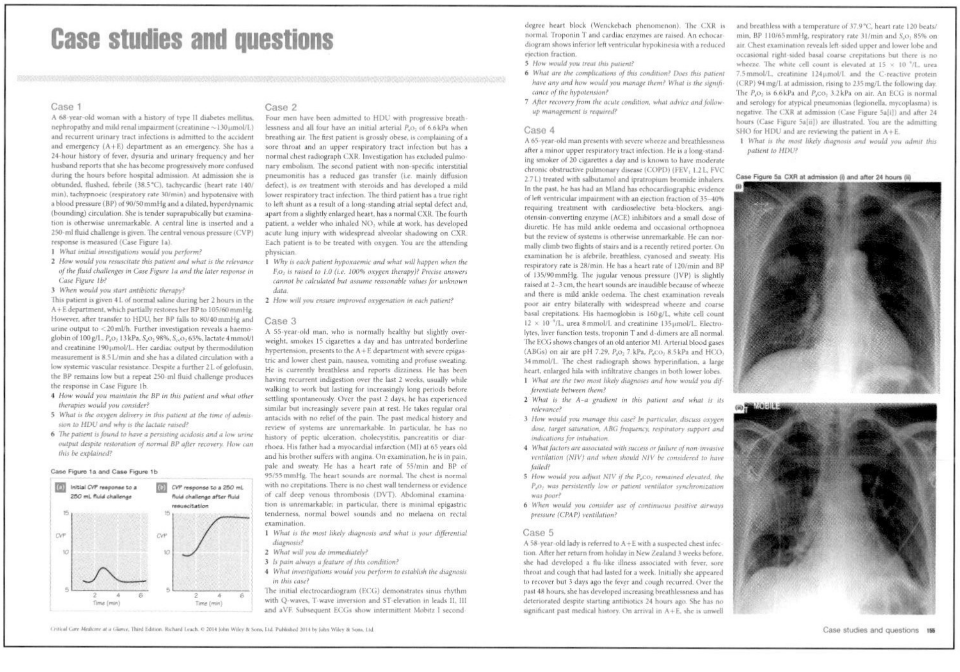

Case studies and questions

Case 1

A 68-year-old woman with a history of type II diabetes mellitus, nephropathy and mild renal impairment (creatinine ~130μmol/L) and recurrent urinary tract infections is admitted to the accident and emergency (A+E) department as an emergency. She has a 24-hour history of fever, dysuria and urinary frequency and her husband reports that she has become progressively more confused during the hours before hospital admission. At admission she is obtunded, flushed, febrile (38.5°C), tachycardic (heart rate 140/min), tachypnoeic (respiratory rate 30/min) and hypotensive with a blood pressure (BP) of 90/50 mmHg and a dilated, hyperdynamic (bounding) circulation. She is tender suprapubically but examination is otherwise unremarkable. A central line is inserted and a 250-ml fluid challenge is given. The central venous pressure (CVP) response is measured (Case Figure 1a).

1 *What initial investigations would you perform?*
2 *How would you resuscitate this patient and what is the relevance of the fluid challenges in Case Figure 1a and the later response in Case Figure 1b?*
3 *When would you start antibiotic therapy?*

This patient is given 4L of normal saline during her 2 hours in the A+E department, which partially restores her BP to 105/60 mmHg. However, after transfer to HDU, her BP falls to 80/40 mmHg and urine output to <20 ml/h. Further investigation reveals a haemoglobin of 100 g/L, P_aO_2 13 kPa, S_aO_2 98%, S_vO_2 65%, lactate 4 mmol/l and creatinine 190 μmol/L. Her cardiac output by thermodilution measurement is 8.5 L/min and she has a dilated circulation with a low systemic vascular resistance. Despite a further 2L of gelofusin, the BP remains low but a repeat 250 ml fluid challenge produces the response in Case Figure 1b.

4 *How would you maintain the BP in this patient and what other therapies would you consider?*
5 *What is the oxygen delivery in this patient at the time of admission to HDU and why is the lactate raised?*
6 *The patient is found to have a persisting acidosis and a low urine output despite restoration of normal BP after recovery. How can this be explained?*

Case Figure 1a and Case Figure 1b

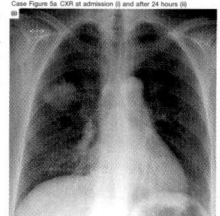

(a) Initial CVP response to a 250 mL fluid challenge

(b) CVP response to a 250 mL fluid challenge after fluid resuscitation

Case 2

Four men have been admitted to HDU with progressive breathlessness and all four have an initial arterial P_aO_2 of 6.6 kPa when breathing air. The first patient is grossly obese, is complaining of a sore throat and an upper respiratory tract infection but has a normal chest radiograph CXR. Investigation has excluded pulmonary embolism. The second patient with non-specific interstitial pneumonitis has a reduced gas transfer (i.e. mainly diffusion defect), is on treatment with steroids and has developed a mild lower respiratory tract infection. The third patient has a true right to left shunt as a result of a long-standing atrial septal defect and, apart from a slightly enlarged heart, has a normal CXR. The fourth patient, a welder who inhaled NO_x while at work, has developed acute lung injury with widespread alveolar shadowing on CXR. Each patient is to be treated with oxygen. You are the attending physician.

1 *Why is each patient hypoxaemic and what will happen when the F_IO_2 is raised to 1.0 (i.e. 100% oxygen therapy)? Precise answers cannot be calculated but assume reasonable values for unknown data.*
2 *How will you ensure improved oxygenation in each patient?*

Case 3

A 55-year-old man, who is normally healthy but slightly overweight, smokes 15 cigarettes a day and has untreated borderline hypertension, presents to the A+E department with severe epigastric and lower chest pain, nausea, vomiting and profuse sweating. He is currently breathless and reports dizziness. He has been having recurrent indigestion over the last 2 weeks, usually while walking to work but lasting for increasingly long periods before settling spontaneously. Over the past 2 days, he has experienced similar but increasingly severe pain at rest. He takes regular oral antacids with no relief of the pain. The past medical history and review of systems are unremarkable. In particular, he has no history of peptic ulceration, cholecystitis, pancreatitis or diarrhoea. His father had a myocardial infarction (MI) at 65 years old and his brother suffers with angina. On examination, he is in pain, pale and sweaty. He has a heart rate of 55/min and BP of 95/55 mmHg. The heart sounds are normal. The chest is normal with no crepitations. There is no chest wall tenderness or evidence of calf deep venous thrombosis (DVT). Abdominal examination is unremarkable; in particular, there is minimal epigastric tenderness, normal bowel sounds and no melaena on rectal examination.

1 *What is the most likely diagnosis and what is your differential diagnosis?*
2 *What will you do immediately?*
3 *Is pain always a feature of this condition?*
4 *What investigations would you perform to establish the diagnosis in this case?*

The initial electrocardiogram (ECG) demonstrates sinus rhythm with Q-waves, T-wave inversion and ST-elevation in leads II, III and aVF. Subsequent ECGs show intermittent Mobitz 1 second-degree heart block (Wenckebach phenomenon). The CXR is normal. Troponin T and cardiac enzymes are raised. An echocardiogram shows inferior left ventricular hypokinesia with a reduced ejection fraction.

5 *How would you treat this patient?*
6 *What are the complications of this condition? Does this patient have any and how would you manage them? What is the significance of the hypotension?*
7 *After recovery from the acute condition, what advice and follow-up management is required?*

Case 4

A 65-year-old man presents with severe wheeze and breathlessness after a minor upper respiratory tract infection. He is a long-standing smoker of 20 cigarettes a day and is known to have moderate chronic obstructive pulmonary disease (COPD) (FEV₁ 1.2 L, FVC 2.7 L) treated with salbutamol and ipratropium bromide inhalers. In the past, he has had an Mland has echocardiographic evidence of left ventricular impairment with an ejection fraction of 35–40% requiring treatment with cardioselective beta-blockers, angiotensin-converting enzyme (ACE) inhibitors and a small dose of diuretic. He has mild ankle oedema and occasional orthopnoea but the review of systems is otherwise unremarkable. He can normally climb two flights of stairs and is a recently retired porter. On examination he is afebrile, breathless, cyanosed and sweaty. His respiratory rate is 28/min. He has a heart rate of 120/min and BP of 135/90 mmHg. The jugular venous pressure (JVP) is slightly raised at 2–3 cm, the heart sounds are inaudible because of wheeze and there is mild ankle oedema. The chest examination reveals poor air entry bilaterally with widespread wheeze. Investigations: His haemoglobin is 160 g/L, white cell count 12 × 10⁻⁹/L, urea 8 mmol/L and creatinine 135μmol/L. Electrolytes, liver function tests, troponin T and d-dimers are all normal. The ECG shows changes of an old anterior MI. Arterial blood gases (ABGs) on air are pH 7.29, P_aO_2 7.2 kPa, P_aCO_2 8.5 kPa and HCO_3 34 mmol/L. The chest radiograph shows hyperinflation, a large heart, enlarged hila with infiltrative changes in both lower lobes.

1 *What are the two most likely diagnoses and how would you differentiate between them?*
2 *What is the A–a gradient in this patient and what is its relevance?*
3 *How would you manage this patient? In particular, discuss oxygen dose, target saturation, ABG frequency, respiratory support and indications for intubation.*
4 *What factors are associated with success or failure of non-invasive ventilation (NIV) and when should NIV be considered to have failed?*
5 *How would you adjust NIV if the P_aCO_2 remained elevated, the P_aO_2 was persistently low or patient ventilator synchronization was poor?*
6 *When would you consider use of continuous positive airways pressure (CPAP) ventilation?*

Case 5

A 58-year-old lady is referred to A+E with a suspected chest infection. After her return from holiday in New Zealand 3 weeks before, she had developed a flu-like illness associated with fever, sore throat and cough that had lasted for a week. Initially she appeared to recover 3 days ago the fever and cough recurred. Over the past 48 hours, she has developed increasing breathlessness and has deteriorated despite starting antibiotics 24 hours ago. She has no significant past medical history. On arrival in A+E, she is unwell and breathless with a temperature of 37.9°C, heart rate 120 beats/min, BP 110/65 mmHg, respiratory rate 31/min and S_aO_2 85% on air. Chest examination reveals left-sided upper and lower lobe and occasional right-sided basal coarse crepitations but there is no wheeze. The white cell count is elevated at 15 × 10⁻⁹/L, area 7.5 mmol/L, creatinine 124μmol/L and the C-reactive protein (CRP) 94 mg/L at admission, rising to 235 mg/L the following day. The P_aO_2 is 6.6 kPa and P_aCO_2 3.2 kPa on air. An ECG is normal and serology for atypical pneumonias (legionella, mycoplasma) is negative. The CXR at admission (Case Figure 5a(i)) and after 24 hours (Case Figure 5a(ii)) are illustrated. You are the admitting SHO for HDU and are reviewing the patient in A+E.

1 *What is the most likely diagnosis and would you admit this patient to HDU?*

Case Figure 5a CXR at admission (i) and after 24 hours (ii)

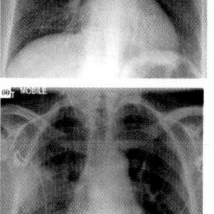

Critical Care Medicine at a Glance, Third Edition. Richard Leach. © 2014 John Wiley & Sons, Ltd. Published 2014 by John Wiley & Sons, Ltd.

Case studies and questions

The anytime, anywhere textbook

Wiley E-Text

Your book is also available to purchase as a **Wiley E-Text: Powered by VitalSource** version – a digital, interactive version of this book which you own as soon as you download it.

Your **Wiley E-Text** allows you to:

Search: Save time by finding terms and topics instantly in your book, your notes, even your whole library (once you've downloaded more textbooks)

Note and Highlight: Colour code, highlight and make digital notes right in the text so you can find them quickly and easily

Organize: Keep books, notes and class materials organized in folders inside the application

Share: Exchange notes and highlights with friends, classmates and study groups

Upgrade: Your textbook can be transferred when you need to change or upgrade computers

The **Wiley E-Text** version will also allow you to copy and paste any photograph or illustration into assignments, presentations and your own notes.

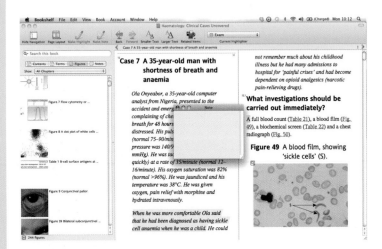

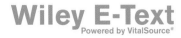

To access your Wiley E-Text:

- Visit **www.vitalsource.com/software/bookshelf/downloads** to download the Bookshelf application to your computer, laptop, tablet or mobile device.
- Open the Bookshelf application on your computer and register for an account.
- Follow the registration process.

CourseSmart

CourseSmart gives you instant access (via computer or mobile device) to this Wiley-Blackwell e-book and its extra electronic functionality, at 40% off the recommended retail print price. See all the benefits at: **www.coursesmart.com/students**

Instructors ... receive your own digital desk copies!

CourseSmart also offers instructors an immediate, efficient, and environmentally friendly way to review this book for your course.

For more information visit **www.coursesmart.com/instructors**.

With CourseSmart, you can create lecture notes quickly with copy and paste, and share pages and notes with your students. Access your **CourseSmart** digital book from your computer or mobile device instantly for evaluation, class preparation, and as a teaching tool in the classroom.

Simply sign in at **http://instructors.coursesmart.com/bookshelf** to download your Bookshelf and get started. To request your desk copy, hit 'Request Online Copy' on your search results or book product page.

We hope you enjoy using your new book. Good luck with your studies!

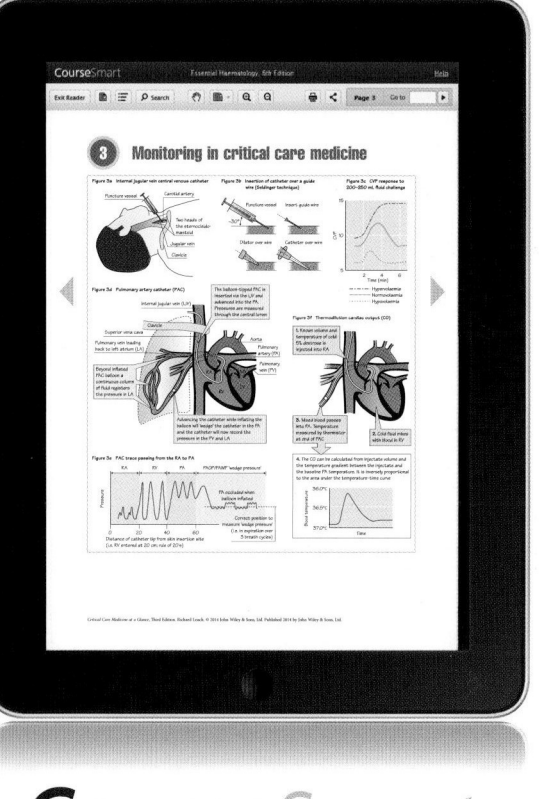

CourseSmart
Learn Smart. Choose Smart.

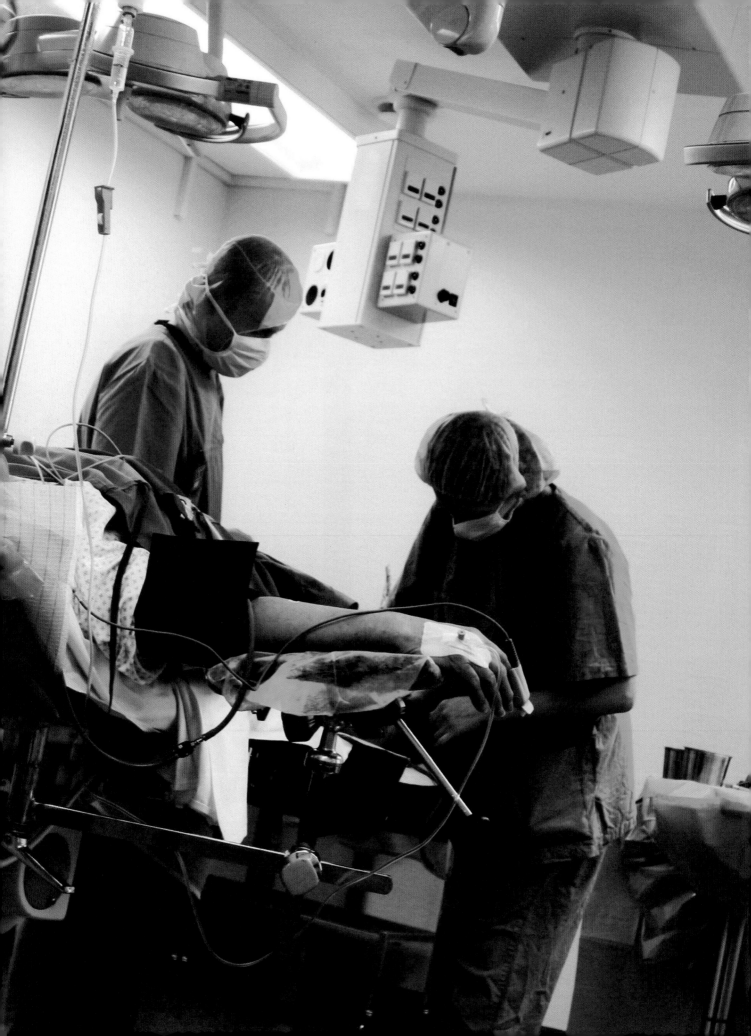

General

Part 1

Chapters

1 # Recognizing the unwell patient

Figure 1a Early warning score

An aggregate score ≥5 (or a score of 3 for any individual parameter) indicates that a 'Patient at Risk Team' (PART) or 'Medical Emergency Team' (MET) composed of doctors and senior nurses familiar with assessment and management of acutely unwell patients, should be summoned.

Score	3	2	1	0	1	2	3
Breath rate/min	≤8		9–11	12–20		21–24	≤25
Oxygen saturation (%)	≤91	92–93	94–95	≥96			
Supplemental oxygen		Yes		No			
Temperature	≤35.0		35.1–36.0	36.1–38.0	38.1–39.0	≥39.0	
Systolic BP (mmHg)	≤90	91–100	101–110	111–219			≥220
Heart rate (beats/min)	≤40		41–50	51–90	91–100	111–130	≥130
Level of consciousness				Alert			V,P or U

BP = blood pressure, V = response to voice, P = response to pain,
U = unresponsive to voice or pain (or unconscious)

Notes for use

Consciousness level may be reduced due to sedation, (e.g. post-operatively) and assessment must be adjusted appropriately.

In hypercapnoeic respiratory failure aim for saturations of 88–92%. Patients will still 'score' if saturations are <92% but the score may be 'reset' (+documented) by a competent clinical decision-maker.

Urine output is not included in the early warning score as it is not always available but monitoring is essential in some patients.

Figure 1b Assessing the acutely ill patient

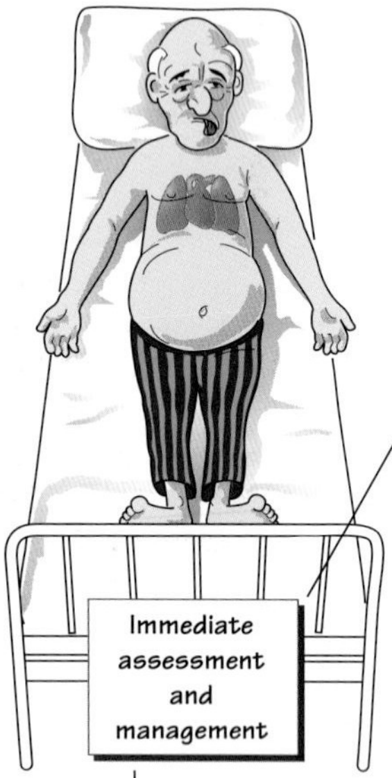

Assessment + Action		Criteria for calling an emergency team
1. A – Airway	→ Airway adjuncts recovery position	Airway obstruction, impaired airway protection (e.g. coma)
1. B – Breathing	→ Oxygen, mask ventilation	Respiratory arrest, Respiratory rate <8 or >20 S_aO_2 ≤90% on 50% O_2, P_aO_2 <8kPa on 50% O_2 P_aCO_2 >6.5kPa, pH <7.3
3. C – Circulation	→ Fluid Inotropes	Cardiac arrest, Heart rate <40 or >130/min SBP <90 mmHg, pH <7.3, Lactate >2 mmoL/l Base deficit >−4, Urine output <0.5 mL/kg/hr
4. D – Disability	→ Neurological assessment Hypoglycaemia Injury/trauma	GCS <12, GCS drop of >2 points Recurrent or prolonged seizures

Immediate assessment and management

Monitor vital signs, S_aO_2 ± ECG; consider need to call for help

Full assessment; take history, full clinical examination, review charts, notes + results

Is the patient improving with initial management? ——————→ No

Yes

Is the diagnosis established? → No → Further investigation

→ Yes → Management plan

Reassess

S_aO_2 = saturation
P_aO_2 = partial pressure of oxygen
P_aCO_2 = partial pressure of carbon dioxide
SBP = systolic blood pressure
GCS = Glasgow Coma Scale
ECG = electrocardiogram

Figure 1c Clinical features of underlying lung disease

Disorder	Chest wall movement	Percussion note	Breath sounds	Added sounds
Consolidation	↓ on affected side	↓ Dull	Bronchial	Coarse crackles
Collapse	↓↓ on affected side	↓ Dull	Absent or bronchial	None
Pleural effusion	↓ on affected side	↓↓ Stony dull	Diminished	None (±rub)
Pneumothorax	↓↓ on affected side	Normal or hyperresonant	Absent or diminished	None
Asthma/COPD	↓ on both sides Hyperinflation Accessory muscles	Normal or hyperresonant	Vesicular with prolonged expiration	Expiratory wheeze

Critical Care Medicine at a Glance, Third Edition. Richard Leach. © 2014 John Wiley & Sons, Ltd. Published 2014 by John Wiley & Sons, Ltd.

In the acutely unwell patient, assessment of deranged physiology and immediate resuscitation precedes diagnostic considerations because incomplete history, cursory examination and limited investigation often preclude classification by primary organ dysfunction. It is this initial diagnostic uncertainty and the need for immediate physiological support that defines critical care medicine.

Recognizing the acutely unwell patient

Early recognition that a patient's condition is deteriorating is essential and should initiate immediate action to correct abnormal physiology and prevent vital organ damage (e.g. brain). Clinical severity may be obvious from the end of the bed: as in sudden, catastrophic events (e.g. pulmonary embolism); presentation with established severe illness (e.g. emergency room); or in advanced, previously unrecognized, deterioration on the ward. In these cases, organ damage may have already occurred but immediate action prevents further injury. It is the failure to recognize progressive deterioration (e.g. worsening physiological variables), and to initiate preventative action, that is a common and unacceptable cause of harm.

Identification of 'at-risk' patients (e.g. post-operative) allows complications to be anticipated and prevented. 'At-risk' patients must be monitored, deterioration recognized and appropriate action initiated. Simple physiological parameters including temperature, blood pressure (BP), heart rate, respiratory rate, urine output and conscious level correlate with mortality. One, two or three abnormalities correlate with 30-day mortalities of 4.4%, 9.2% and 21.3% respectively. Early warning scoring systems based on these parameters (Figure 1a) promote early detection and trigger interventions aimed at preventing cardiac arrests and critical care admissions.

Assessment of the acutely ill patient

A normal response to the question 'Are you alright?' indicates that a patient's airway is patent and that they are breathing, conscious and orientated. No response (e.g. coma) or difficulty responding (e.g. breathlessness) suggests serious illness. Immediate assessment and management of these acutely ill patients are summarized in Figure 1b. They aim to ensure patient safety and survival rather than to establish a diagnosis. Assessment starts with detection and simultaneous treatment of life-threatening emergencies. It uses the **ABC system: A** – Airway, **B** – Breathing, **C** – Circulation, in this order, because airways obstruction causes death faster than disordered breathing, which in turn causes death faster than circulatory collapse. Appropriate life-saving procedures or investigations are performed (e.g. airway clearance, tension pneumothorax decompression) during examination (i.e. before the next step). Simple monitors (e.g. saturation, BP) are used to assist assessment when safely possible.

Airway (Chapters 5, 11) Obstruction is a medical emergency and unless rapidly corrected leads to hypoxia, coma and death within minutes. Causes include aspiration (e.g. food, coins, teeth, vomit), laryngeal oedema (e.g. allergy, burns), bronchospasm and pharyngeal obstruction by the tongue when reduced tone causes it to fall backwards in obtunded patients.

• **Complete obstruction** is characterized by absent airflow (feel over the patient's mouth), accessory muscle use, intercostal recession on inspiration, paradoxical abdominal movement and absent breath sounds on chest auscultation.

• **Partial obstruction** reduces airflow despite increased respiratory effort. Breathing is often noisy, with 'stridor' suggesting laryngeal and 'snoring' nasopharyngeal obstruction.

Simple measures correct most airway obstruction. Suction removes blood, vomit and foreign bodies. Obstruction by the tongue (i.e. during coma) can usually be prevented by chin lift manoeuvres or insertion of an oropharyngeal (Guedel) airway. Occasionally endotracheal intubation or, rarely, emergency cricothyroidectomy are required.

Breathing (Chapters 5, 11) The most useful early sign that breathing is compromised is a respiratory rate ≤ 8 or ≥ 20/min, whereas central cyanosis is usually a late sign. Examine depth and pattern of breathing, accessory muscle use, abdominal breathing and chest wall expansion. Abnormal expansion, altered percussion note (e.g. hyper-resonance), airway noise (e.g. stridor) and breath sounds may determine the cause of underlying lung disease (Figure 1c). Saturation (S_aO_2), measured by pulse oximetry, and inspired oxygen concentration (F_iO_2) should be recorded. Arterial blood gases (ABGs) provide information about ventilation as well as oxygenation (i.e. normal S_aO_2 with high P_aCO_2 due to poor ventilation). The S_aO_2 should be >90% in all critically ill patients. Respiratory acidosis (pH < 7.3, P_aCO_2 > 6.7 kPa) or hypoxaemia despite high flow oxygen therapy (S_aO_2 < 90%, P_aO_2 < 8 kPa) requires urgent intervention. Treatment depends on cause (e.g. chronic obstructive pulmonary disease [COPD]) and is discussed in later chapters.

Circulation (Chapters 5, 8) Assessment includes central and peripheral pulses (i.e. rate, rhythm, equality), BP, peripheral perfusion (e.g. limb temperature), urine output and conscious level. Initially BP is maintained by compensatory mechanisms (e.g. increased peripheral resistance). Cardiac output (CO) has to fall by >20% (i.e. equivalent to 1 L of rapid blood loss) before BP falls. Thready, fast pulses indicate poor CO, whereas bounding pulses suggest sepsis. Capillary refill time is usually <2 secs and prolongation suggests poor tissue perfusion. Metabolic acidosis (base excess >−4) and raised lactate (>2 mmol/L) on ABG may be due to tissue hypoxia. Hypovolaemia should be considered the primary cause of shock, unless there is obvious heart failure (i.e. resuscitate hypotensive patients with cool peripheries and tachycardia with intravenous fluids [Chapters 9, 11]).

Disability Neurological status is rapidly determined by pupil examination and assessment of conscious level using simple systems (Figure 1a) or the Glasgow Coma Scale (Chapters 3, 72). Exclude hypoglycaemia, ischemia and injury (e.g. hip fracture) in every patient.

Full patient assessment When stability has been achieved and assistance summoned, a thorough history and examination is required. Review the patient's notes, treatment, investigations and charts. Trends in physiological parameters are often more useful than isolated values. If a diagnosis has not been established, arrange further investigations as appropriate. Document and communicate a clear management plan.

Management of the acutely unwell patient often involves several teams (e.g. medicine, surgery, critical care) but should be a 'seamless' process in which co-operation, communication and patient interests are foremost. Treatment should occur in clinical areas where staffing and technical support are matched to patient needs.

Pearl of wisdom

Monitoring of simple physiological parameters reliably identifies early clinical deterioration

② Managing the critically ill patient

1. Regular review of monitored trends and response to therapy
Followed by clinical examination, reassessment of the care plan (with written instructions) and adjustment of prescribing. Clearly communicate the revised plan to other caregivers

Drug chart
- Antibiotics
- Inotropes
- Sedatives etc.

Written care plan

8. Typical Doctors daily checklist
F = Feeding
L = Line care
A = Aperients
T = Thrombo-prophylaxis
H = Hydration
U = Ulcer prophylaxis
G = Glucose

10. Infection Control
HAND WASHING is vital to prevent transmission of organisms between patients DISPOSABLE APRONS are recommended STERILE TECHNIQUE (e.g. gloves, masks, gowns, sterile field) for all invasive procedures (e.g. line insertion). ISOLATION (±negative pressure ventilation) for transmissable infections THOROUGH CLEANING OF BED SPACES (e.g. routine, post discharge)

2. Respiratory care
Altered ventilation, poor secretion clearance, impaired muscle function and lung collapse (atelectasis) occur in the supine position. Respiratory care includes assisted coughing, deep breathing and alveolar recruitment techniques (e.g. CPAP), chest percussion, postural drainage, positioning (e.g. sitting up), bronchodilators, tracheal toilette, suctioning and tracheostomy care

7. Communication with the patient
Use of amnesic drugs makes repeated explanations and reassurance essential. Assist interaction with appropriate communication aids

11. Skin care, general hygiene + mouthcare
Pressure sores are due to local pressure (e.g. bony prominences), friction, malnutrition, oedema, ischaemia and damage related to moist or soiled skin. Turn patients every two hours and protect susceptible areas. Special beds relieve pressure and assist turning. Mouthcare and general hygiene are essential

3. Cardiovascular care
Prolonged immobility impairs autonomic vasomotor responses to sitting and standing causing profound postural hypotension. Tilt tables may be beneficial prior to mobilization

12. Fluid, electrolyte and glucose balance
Regularly assess fluid + electrolyte balance Insulin resistance + hyperglycaemia are common but maintaining normoglycaemia improves outcome

13. Dressing and wound care
Replace wound dressings as necessary. Change arterial and central venous catheter dressings every 48–72h

4. Gastrointestinal (GI) / nutritional care
The supine position predisposes to gastro-oesophageal reflux and aspiration pneumonia. Nursing patients 30° head-up prevents this. Early enteral feeding reduces infection, peptic ulceration and GI bleeding. Immobility is associated with gastric stasis and constipation; gastric stimulants and laxatives are essential

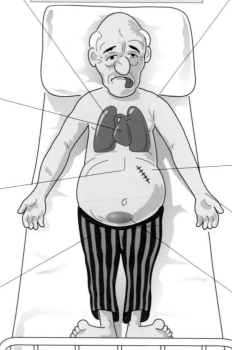

14. Line care
Lines must be inspected daily. Peripheral lines should be changed every 72–96hrs. Central and arterial lines are not changed routinely but risk infection after >5 days

15. Bladder care
Urinary catheters can cause painful urethral ulcers and must be stabilised. Early removal reduces urinary tract infections

5. Neuromuscular
Immobility (± prolonged neuro-muscular blockade) and sedation promote muscle atrophy, joint contractures and foot drop. Physiotherapy and splints may be required

Guiding principles
- Delivery of optimal and appropriate care
- Relief of distress
- Compassion and support
- Dignity
- Information
- Care and support of relatives and care-givers

16. Visiting hours
Opinions differ with regard to relatives visiting hours. Some units restrict visits (e.g. 2 periods/day), others have almost unrestricted hours

6. Comfort and reassurance
Anxiety, discomfort and pain must be recognized and relieved with reassurance, physical measures, analgesics and sedatives. In particular, endotracheal or nasogastric tubes, bladder or bowel distention, inflamed line sites, painful joints and urinary catheters often cause discomfort and may be overlooked. Fan use is controversial as dust-borne microorganisms may be disseminated. Visible clocks help patients maintain circadian rhythms (i.e. day/night patterns)

9. Venous thrombosis prophylaxis
Trauma, sepsis, surgery and immobility predispose to lower limb thrombosis. Mechanical and pharmacological prophylaxis prevent potentially life-threatening pulmonary embolism

17. Communication with relatives
Family members receive information from many caregivers with different perspectives and knowledge. Critical care-teams must aim to be consistent in their assessments and honest about uncertainties. One or two physicians should act as primary contacts. All conversations must be documented. Compassionate care of relatives is always appreciated, avoids anger and is one of the best indicators of good care

Critical Care Medicine at a Glance, Third Edition. Richard Leach. © 2014 John Wiley & Sons, Ltd. Published 2014 by John Wiley & Sons, Ltd.

Organization

Critical care wards provide monitoring and treatment for patients with potentially reversible, life-threatening conditions that are not available on general wards. Patients should be managed and moved between areas where staffing and technical support match their severity of illness and clinical needs. Five types of ward area are described: (a) level 3: intensive care units (ICUs); (b) level 2: medical/surgical high dependency units (HDUs), post-operative recovery areas, emergency resuscitation rooms; (c) level 1: acute admission wards, coronary care units; (d) general wards (e) self-care wards.

Critical care medicine (CCM) encompasses the initial resuscitation, monitoring, investigation and treatment of critically ill patients in level 2–3 wards. These patients usually require a high degree of monitoring and nursing support. Level 3 patients are often mechanically ventilated or have multi-organ failure. Level 2 patients may need invasive monitoring (i.e. arterial line), non-invasive ventilation, inotropic support or renal replacement therapy. Level 1 patients usually require non-invasive monitoring (e.g. electrocardiogram [ECG], saturation, blood pressure [BP]) and close observation. There is considerable overlap between level 1 and 2 patients. Provision of level 2 and 3 care varies from ~2–5% of hospital beds in the UK to >5–10% in the USA.

Admission and discharge guidelines

Aggressive hospital treatment may be inappropriate in advanced disease and patients must be allocated to a ward appropriate to their needs and prognosis. Resuscitation status should always be documented. Admission and discharge guidelines for ICU/HDU facilitate appropriate use of resources and prevent unnecessary suffering in patients who have no prospect of recovery. Factors determining ICU/HDU admission include the primary diagnosis, severity, likely outcome, co-morbid illness, life expectancy, post-discharge quality of life and patient's or relative's wishes. Age alone is not a contraindication to admission and each case must be judged on its merit. If there is uncertainty, the patient should be given the benefit of the doubt and active treatment continued until further information is available.

Discharge occurs when the patient is physiologically stable and relatively independent of monitoring and support. Avoid out-of-hours and weekend discharges and ensure a detailed handover. After family consultation, withdrawal of therapy may be appropriate in patients with no realistic hope of recovery. When feasible, organ donation should be tactfully discussed. Management must always remain positive to ensure death with dignity (Chapter 29).

General supportive care

Optimal care is delivered by a multi-skilled team of doctors, nurses, physiotherapists, technicians and other care-givers. Figure 2 illustrates important aspects of general management. Prolonged bed rest predisposes to respiratory (e.g. atelectasis), cardiovascular (e.g. autonomic failure), neurological (e.g. muscle wasting) and endocrine (e.g. glucose intolerance) problems. Fluid and electrolyte imbalance (e.g. Na^+, K^+, Ca^{2+} depletion), constipation, infection, venous thrombosis and pressure sores also occur. The importance of skilled nursing in the care of these patients cannot be over-emphasised. Assessment, continuous monitoring ($\pm$intervention),

drug administration, comfort (e.g. analgesia, toilette), reassurance and psychological support, assistance with communication, advocacy, skin care, positioning (e.g. to prevent aspiration, atelectasis, pressure sores), feeding and early detection of clinical complications (e.g. line infection) are all vital nursing roles that have a profound effect on outcome. Nurses also provide essential support for relatives, doctors, physiotherapists and other care-givers (e.g. technicians).

Severity of Illness Scoring Systems

Severity of Illness Scoring Systems (SISS) predict outcome and evaluate care in ICUs and HDUs. Two have been validated and are widely used:
- **APACHE II** (Acute Physiology and Chronic Health Evaluation) measures case-mix and predicts outcome in ICU patients **as a group**. It should not be used to predict individual outcomes. Scoring is based on the primary disease process, physiological reserve including age, chronic health history (e.g. chronic liver, cardiovascular, respiratory, renal and immune conditions) and the severity of illness determined from the worst value in the first 24 hours of 12 acute physiological variables including rectal temperature, mean BP, heart rate, respiratory rate (RR), arterial P_aO_2 and pH, serum sodium, potassium and creatinine, haemocrit, white cell count and Glasgow Coma Score (GCS; Chapter 72). Predicted mortality, by diagnosis, has been calculated from large databases, which allows individual units to evaluate their performance against reference ICUs by calculating standard mortality ratio (SMR = observed mortality ÷ predicted mortality) for each diagnostic group. A high SMR (>1.5) should prompt investigation and management changes for specific conditions.
- **SAPS** (Simplified Acute Physiology Score) is similar to APACHE II with equivalent accuracy.

Pathology Specific Scoring Systems (PSSS) can be used in CCM.
- **Trauma Score (TS)** assesses triage status based on RR, respiratory effort, systolic BP, capillary refill and GCS. TS is related to survival in blunt and penetrating injuries. A high score prompts transfer to a trauma centre. **Revised TS:** uses only GCS, RR and systolic BP. It is less suitable for triage but improves prognostic reliability.
- **Abbreviated Injury Scale** assesses multiple injuries and correlates with morbidity and mortality.
- **Other PSSS:** include the paediatric trauma score, neonatal Apgar score and GCS (Chapter 72).

Cost of critical care medicine

Measuring costs is complex. In ICU/HDU, the most widely used system is the **Therapeutic Intervention Scoring System** (TISS), which scores the overall requirements for care, by measuring nursing activity and interventions. TISS correlates well with staff, equipment and drug costs and can also be used as an index of nurse dependency. Most (>50%) ICU expenditure is on labour costs (e.g. constant bedside nursing). Drugs, imaging, laboratory tests and supplies account for ~40% of spending. Current estimates of daily ('basic') ICU costs vary from £800 to £1600 in the UK. HDU costs are ~50% and general ward care ~20% of ICU costs. The USA spends ~14%, and the UK ~9% of gross domestic product (GDP) on healthcare with ICU/HDU costs of ~7% and 4–5% respectively.

3 Monitoring in critical care medicine

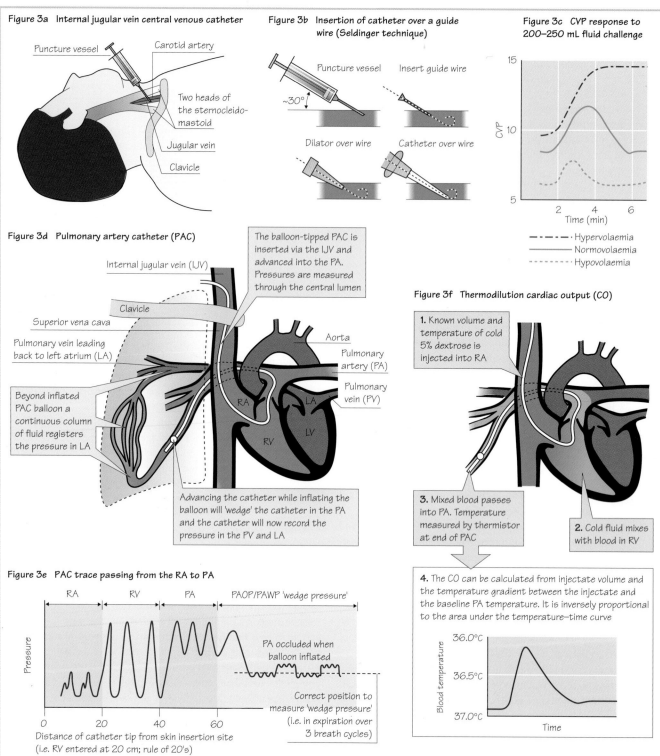

Figure 3a Internal jugular vein central venous catheter

Puncture vessel
Carotid artery
Two heads of the sternocleido-mastoid
Jugular vein
Clavicle

Figure 3b Insertion of catheter over a guide wire (Seldinger technique)

Puncture vessel
~30°
Insert guide wire
Dilator over wire
Catheter over wire

Figure 3c CVP response to 200–250 mL fluid challenge

— · — · — Hypervolaemia
———— Normovolaemia
· · · · · · Hypovolaemia

Figure 3d Pulmonary artery catheter (PAC)

Internal jugular vein (IJV)
Clavicle
Superior vena cava
Pulmonary vein leading back to left atrium (LA)
Aorta
Pulmonary artery (PA)
Pulmonary vein (PV)
RA
LA
RV
LV

The balloon-tipped PAC is inserted via the IJV and advanced into the PA. Pressures are measured through the central lumen

Beyond inflated PAC balloon a continuous column of fluid registers the pressure in LA

Advancing the catheter while inflating the balloon will 'wedge' the catheter in the PA and the catheter will now record the pressure in the PV and LA

Figure 3f Thermodilution cardiac output (CO)

1. Known volume and temperature of cold 5% dextrose is injected into RA

3. Mixed blood passes into PA. Temperature measured by thermistor at end of PAC

2. Cold fluid mixes with blood in RV

4. The CO can be calculated from injectate volume and the temperature gradient between the injectate and the baseline PA temperature. It is inversely proportional to the area under the temperature–time curve

Figure 3e PAC trace passing from the RA to PA

RA | RV | PA | PAOP/PAWP 'wedge pressure'

PA occluded when balloon inflated

Correct position to measure 'wedge pressure' (i.e. in expiration over 3 breath cycles)

Distance of catheter tip from skin insertion site (i.e. RV entered at 20 cm; rule of 20's)

Critical Care Medicine at a Glance, Third Edition. Richard Leach. © 2014 John Wiley & Sons, Ltd. Published 2014 by John Wiley & Sons, Ltd.

Continuous monitoring ensures early detection of change in clinical parameters and aids assessment of progress and response to therapy. However, the following principles apply:
- **Regular clinical examination** remains essential. Simple physical signs like appearance (e.g. pallor), peripheral perfusion and conscious level are as important as parameters displayed on a monitor. When clinical signs disagree with monitored parameters, *assume that clinical assessment is correct* until potential errors from monitored variables have been excluded (e.g. incorrect calibration). **Trends** are usually more reliable than single readings.
- **Use non-invasive techniques when possible** because invasive monitoring is associated with risks (e.g. line infection) and complications (e.g. pneumothorax). Review 'invasive monitoring' regularly and replace as soon as possible. **Alarms** are crucial safety features (e.g. ventilator disconnection), set to physiological safe limits, and should never be disconnected.

Haemodynamic monitoring

Blood pressure (BP) is often measured intermittently using an automated sphygmomanometer. In severely ill patients, continuous intra-arterial monitoring is preferred. It should be appreciated that BP does not reflect cardiac output (CO). Thus, BP can be normal/high but CO low if peripheral vasoconstriction raises systemic vascular resistance (SVR). Conversely, vasodilated, 'septic' patients with low SVR may be hypotensive despite a high CO (Chapters 8, 25).

Central venous pressure (CVP) reflects right atrial pressure (RAP) and is measured using internal jugular (Figures 3a and 3b) or subclavian vein catheters. It is a relatively useful means of assessing circulating blood volume and determining the rate at which fluid should be administered. However, increased venous tone can act to maintain CVP and mask volume depletion during hypovolaemia or haemorrhage. Consequently, CVP may not be as important as **the response to a fluid challenge** (Figure 3c). A high CVP indicates 'fluid overload', impaired myocardial contractility or high right ventricular afterload. Management depends on the cause (Chapters 7, 8, 34).

Pulmonary artery wedge/occlusion pressure (PAWP/PAOP) reflects left atrial pressure (LAP). Normally LAP is $\sim$5–7 mmHg greater than RAP, but in ischaemic heart disease (IHD) or severe illness there is often 'disparity' between left and right ventricular function. Thus, in left ventricular (LV) dysfunction, LAP may be high despite a low RAP, and a small RAP increase may cause a large rise in LAP with associated pulmonary oedema (Chapter 34). PAWP (i.e. LAP) can be monitored with a pulmonary artery (PAr) catheter (Figures 3d and 3e). PAWP is normally 6–12 mmHg, but may be >25–35 mmHg in LV failure (LVF). If pulmonary capillary membranes are intact (i.e. not 'leaky'), a PAWP of $\sim$15–20 mmHg ensures good LV filling and optimal function without risking pulmonary oedema. PAr catheters also measure CO, mixed venous saturation and right ventricular ejection fraction (see later).

Cardiac output Thermodilution techniques for CO measurement (Figure 3f; e.g. PAr catheter, pulsion continuous cardiac output monitor [PiCCO]) are considered the 'gold standard', but error is at least 10%. Non- (or less) invasive techniques of CO monitoring utilize dye/lithium dilution, trans-oesophageal doppler ultrasonography, echocardiography or impedance methods.

Electrocardiogram (ECG) Rate and rhythm are displayed by standard single-lead ECG monitors. ST segment changes can be monitored in patients with IHD.

Respiratory monitoring

Arterial blood gases monitor P_aO_2, P_aCO_2 and acid–base balance. Measurement aids diagnosis and allows adjustment of ventilation to achieve optimum gas exchange (Chapters 13, 18, 20).

Arterial oxygen saturation (S_aO_2) is determined by spectrophotometric analysis of the ratio of saturated to desaturated haemoglobin. Oxygenation is usually adequate if S_aO_2 is >90%. Finger and earlobe probes may be unreliable if peripheral perfusion is poor.

Mixed venous oxygen saturation (S_vO_2) is measured using fibreoptic PAr catheters or PAr/right atrial blood sampling and co-oximetry. It is normally >65–70%. A low S_vO_2 (<55–60%) may indicate inadequate tissue O_2 delivery even if S_aO_2 or P_aO_2 are normal (e.g. anaemia).

Lung function Alveolar–arterial Po_2 gradient and P_aO_2/F_iO_2 ratio measure gas exchange. Arterial and end-tidal CO_2 (see later) reflect alveolar ventilation (V_A) and P_aCO_2 is inversely proportional to V_A ($P_aCO_2 \propto 1/V_A$). Peak expiratory flow rate (PEFR) and spirometry (e.g. FEV_1, vital capacity) are used to monitor airways obstruction and lung volumes in self-ventilating patients (Chapters 40, 41). In intubated patients, maximum inspiratory pressure (MIP) is normally $\sim$100 cmH$_2$O. An MIP < 25 cmH$_2$O indicates respiratory muscle weakness and that extubation is unlikely to be successful.

Lung compliance (LC) reflects lung 'stiffness' or ease of inflation and is reduced in damaged lungs. It is calculated by dividing tidal ventilation (Tv; ml) by the pressure (cm/H$_2$O) required to achieve Tv. High airways pressures during ventilation indicate reduced LC.

Capnography Inspired air contains virtually no CO_2. At the end of expiration, end-tidal CO_2 concentration mirrors arterial P_aCO_2 and reflects V_A if the distribution of ventilation is uniform.

Organ and tissue oxygenation

Global measures (e.g. S_vO_2, lactate) reflect total tissue perfusion but can be normal despite severe regional perfusion abnormalities. Raised serial lactate levels and metabolic acidosis suggest anaerobic metabolism and inadequate tissue oxygenation, although lactate may increase in the absence of hypoxia (e.g. liver failure). An S_vO_2 <55% indicates global tissue hypoxia.

Organ specific measures include:
- **Urine flow**, a sensitive measure of renal perfusion (Chapter 45) if the kidneys are not damaged or affected by drugs (e.g. diuretics). Hourly urine output is normally $\sim$1 ml/kg.
- **Core-peripheral temperature**, the gradient between peripheral (e.g. skin temperature over the dorsum of the foot) and core temperature (e.g. rectal) may be used as an index of peripheral perfusion.
- **Gastric tonometry**, occasionally used to detect splanchnic ischaemia by measuring gastric luminal Pco_2 and a derived mucosal pH.
- **Neurological monitoring**, using Glasgow Coma Scores, intracranial pressure measurements and jugular venous bulb saturations (Chapter 72).

Pearl of wisdom

If clinical and monitored variables disagree, clinical assessment is correct, until monitored errors have been excluded

4 The electrocardiogram

Figure 4a Limb leads and vectors

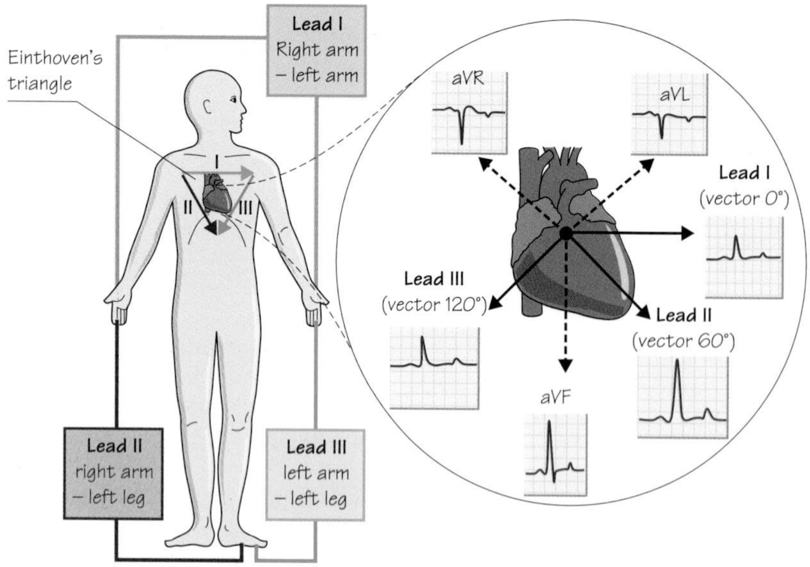

Einthoven's triangle

Lead I
Right arm
– left arm

aVR

aVL

Lead I
(vector 0°)

Lead III
(vector 120°)

Lead II
(vector 60°)

aVF

Lead II
right arm
– left leg

Lead III
left arm
– left leg

Figure 4b Precordial (chest) leads

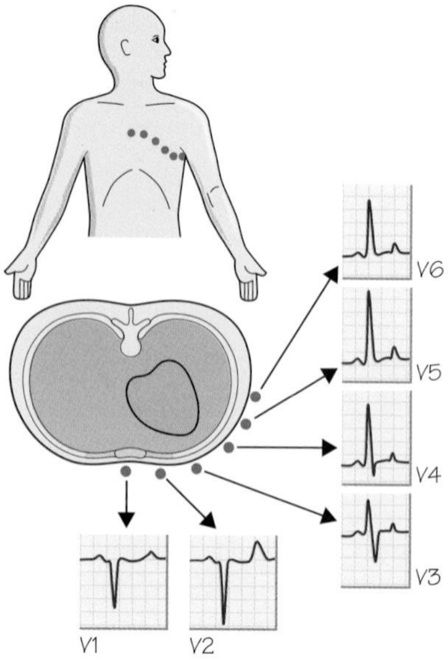

V6

V5

V4

V3

V1   V2

Figure 4c Relationship between depolarization and the ECG complex

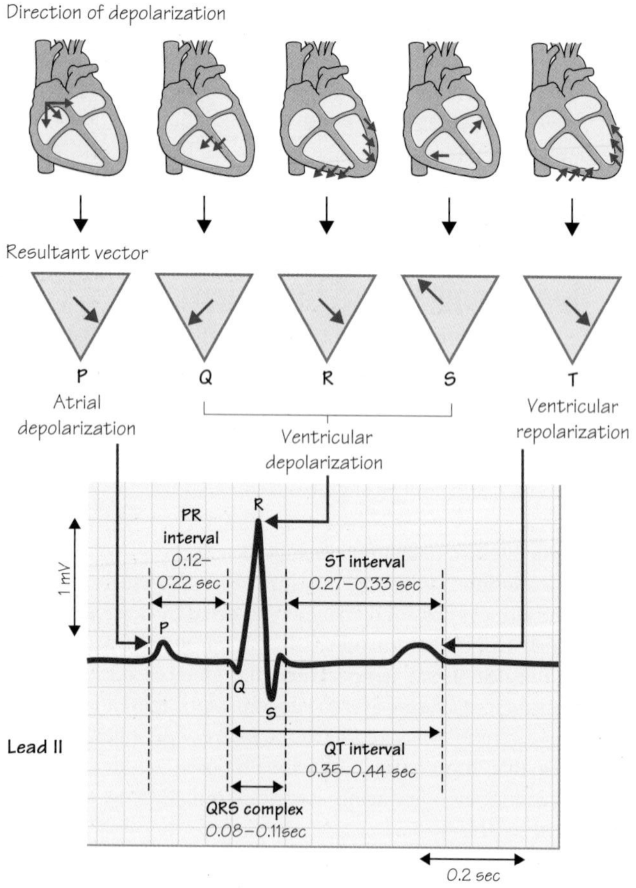

Direction of depolarization

Resultant vector

P
Atrial
depolarization

Q   R   S
Ventricular
depolarization

T
Ventricular
repolarization

PR interval
0.12–0.22 sec

R

ST interval
0.27–0.33 sec

1 mV

P

Q
S

QT interval
0.35–0.44 sec

Lead II

QRS complex
0.08–0.11sec

0.2 sec

Figure 4d Assessing mean frontal QRS axis

Use leads I, II and III (triaxial reference system). Decide which has the largest deflection (positive or negative). The QRS axis is closest to this lead. If the deflection in 2 leads is equally large the QRS axis is midway between them

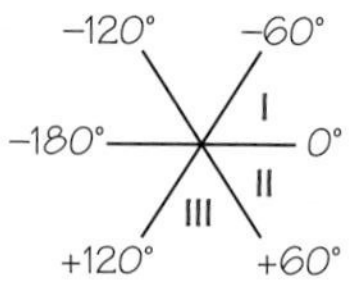

−120°   −60°

−180°   0°

+120°   +60°

Examples

I   II   III

(a)   =   Vector 0°

(b)   =   Vector +30°

(c)   =   Vector −30°

(d)   =   Vector +120°

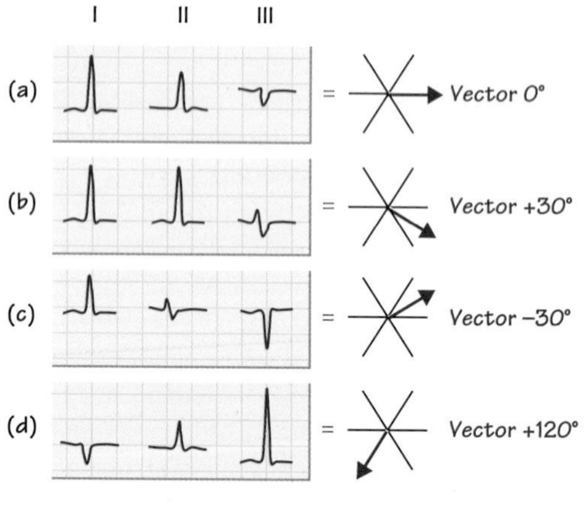

Pearl of wisdom
Apparent ischaemic ST segment elevation or depression is actually due to a change in the ECG baseline

Critical Care Medicine at a Glance, Third Edition. Richard Leach. © 2014 John Wiley & Sons, Ltd. Published 2014 by John Wiley & Sons, Ltd.

When cardiac muscle depolarizes, extracellular currents between depolarized and resting cells cause potentials that can be measured at the body surface as an electrocardiogram (ECG). The ECG uses the concept of *Einthoven's equilateral triangle* with the heart as the current source at the centre (Figure 4a). The corners of the triangle approximate to the limb leads connected to the right arm, left arm and left leg. The potential difference (PD) between two leads depends on amplitude (i.e. muscle mass) and current direction, which determines the *vector* (Figure 4b). By convention a positive voltage is recorded as an upward deflection.

- **Bipolar leads** record the PD across the sides of Einthoven's triangle (i.e. lead I, right and left arms; lead II, right arm and left leg; lead III, left leg and right arm). Lead II normally has the largest deflection (voltage) because it is best aligned to the direction of ventricular depolarization.
- **Unipolar leads** use a single sensing electrode and measure the PD between this and an estimate of zero potential, achieved by connecting the limb leads via a resistor. *Precordial (chest) leads* use a sensing lead placed at six points across the anterior chest wall (Figure 4c). *Augmented (limb) leads* use a single limb lead as a sensing electrode (right arm aVR; left arm aVL; left leg aVF) with the remaining two limb leads connected to estimate zero potential. The six limb leads view electrical activity every 30° (Figure 4d).

Electrocardiogram features

The ECG has 3 main components that are related to the amplitude and direction (i.e. vector) of the wave of depolarization (Figure 4b). The normal PR and ST segments are isoelectric (i.e. no current is flowing; zero PD) because the tissue is either all at rest or all depolarized.

- **P wave**: the initial, small positive deflection due to atrial depolarization.
- **QRS complex**: reflects ventricular depolarization. It is the largest amplitude due to the large ventricular mass with a duration of $\sim$0.08 secs. In lead II the Q wave is a small downward (negative) deflection due to left to right depolarization of the interventricular septum. The R wave is a strong positive deflection due to depolarization of the main mass of the ventricles. The S wave is a small downward deflection due to depolarization at the base of the ventricle. The Q, R and S components vary between leads depending on heart orientation.
- **T wave**: corresponds to ventricular repolarization. A negative deflection (i.e. repolarization of the positive QRS complex) might be expected in lead II but is positive because the cardiac action potential (APo) is shorter at the base of the heart and epicardium so that these areas repolarize first. Consequently, the wave of repolarization normally moves towards the heart apex resulting in a positive deflection. During ischaemia or heart diseases that prolong APo or slow conduction, repolarization at the base may be delayed until after that at the apex and in these circumstances the T wave will be inverted.
- **PR interval**: reflects the delay between depolarization of atria and ventricles due to the slow conduction through the atrioventricular node (AVN). Duration ranges from 0.12–0.2 secs and shortens with increased heart rate. Normally, the AVN is the only electrical connection between the atria and ventricles, because the non-conducting *annulus fibrosus* between these chambers prevents current flow at other sites.

- **ST segment**: represents the plateau of the ventricular APo and lasts 0.25 secs. During ischaemia or cardiac injury, baseline partial depolarization of some cells creates injury currents with undamaged tissue causing elevation or depression of the ECG baseline. However, during the ST segment, all cells are completely depolarized, which gives rise to an apparent elevation/depression of the ST segment, although it is actually the baseline that has changed.

Electrocardiogram interpretation

The ECG is recorded on standard paper and a 10 mm deflection represents 1 mV. The recording rate should be 25 mm/secs (1 mm square = 0.04 secs, 5 mm square = 0.2 secs). Interpreting ECGs requires an understanding of the considerable variation in normal ECGs. Some changes are always abnormal (e.g. left bundle branch block [LBBB]); others (e.g. right bundle branch block [RBBB]) may be normal.

A systematic approach should be followed:
- **Rate**: the normal resting heart rate is 60–100/min.
- **Rhythm**: determine regularity and additional beats.
- **Electrical axis**: the angle of the ECG vector at its maximum amplitude (i.e. current). The frontal plane axis can be calculated from the three bipolar leads and normally lies closest to lead II (range −30° and +90°). Normal QRS complexes should be largely positive in leads I and II. Left axis deviation (LAD) occurs when the axis is more negative than −30° (e.g. inferior myocardial infarction [MI], left anterior hemiblock, left ventricular hypertrophy (LVH)). Right axis deviation occurs when the axis is more positive than +90° (e.g. right ventricular hypertrophy, pulmonary embolism, cor pulmonale, left posterior hemiblock, lateral MI).
- **P waves** are normally upright in II and V_{4-6} and may be biphasic in V_1. A tall peaked P wave reflects right atrial hypertrophy; a widened bifid P wave suggests left atrial hypertrophy. P waves are absent in atrial fibrillation.
- **PR interval**: a short interval indicates rapid conduction between the atria and ventricles and implies an accessory pathway (e.g. Wolff–Parkinson–White [WPW] syndrome). A prolonged interval occurs in first degree heart-block. In second degree heart-block, only a proportion of P waves are followed by a QRS complex and in complete heart block there is no association between P waves and QRS complexes (Chapter 33).
- **Q waves**: can be normal in III, aVR and V_1. Q waves in I, II, aVF and aVL are abnormal if >50% of the height of the subsequent R wave (e.g. suggesting ischaemia).
- **QRS complex width and amplitude**: when prolonged indicates delayed intraventricular conduction and may be due to RBBB (RsR^1 in V_1), LBBB (QS in V_1, RsR^1 in V_6), tricyclic antidepressant overdose or ventricular tachyarrhythmia. The total QRS voltage can indicate LVH (i.e. S in V_2 + R in V_5 = >35 mm).
- **ST segment**: elevation occurs in acute MI (concave down), pericarditis (concave up), ventricular aneurysm, LVH and hypertrophic cardiomyopathy. ST depression occurs with myocardial ischaemia, digoxin and LVH with strain.
- **QT interval**: should be corrected for the heart rate ($QTc = QT/\sqrt{R\text{-}R} = \sim$0.39 secs). At rates of 60–100/min the QT should be <50% of the R-R interval. A prolonged QT interval predisposes to 'torsades de pointes' and occurs during hypothermia, hypocalcaemia, acute MI, sleep and drugs (e.g. quinidine, tricyclic antidepressants). A short QT interval may be secondary to hypercalcaemia or digoxin.
- **T waves**: abnormal if inverted in V_{4-6}. Peaked T waves occur in acute MI and hyperkalaemia. Flattened T waves (sometimes with prominent U waves) occur in hypokalaemia.

Cardiopulmonary resuscitation

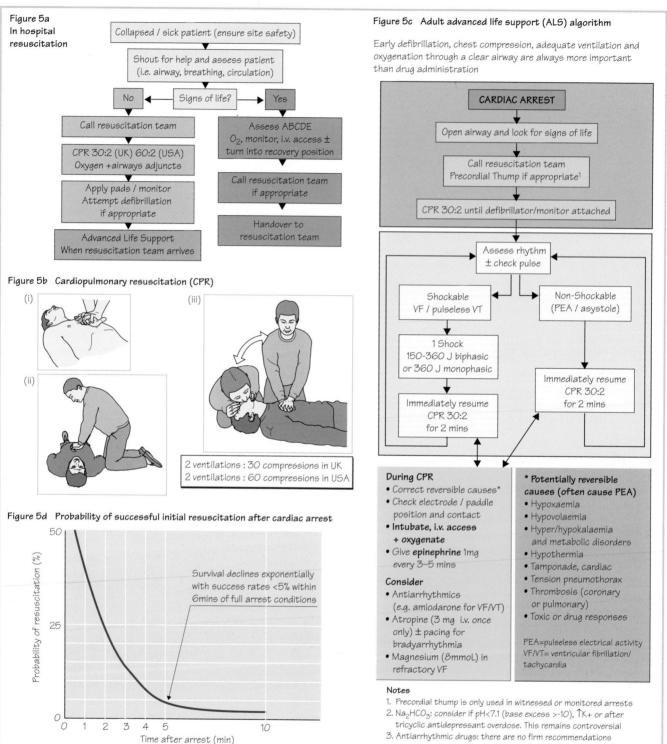

Figure 5a In hospital resuscitation

Collapsed / sick patient (ensure site safety)

Shout for help and assess patient (i.e. airway, breathing, circulation)

Signs of life?

No → Call resuscitation team

CPR 30:2 (UK) 60:2 (USA) Oxygen +airways adjuncts

Apply pads / monitor Attempt defibrillation if appropriate

Advanced Life Support When resuscitation team arrives

Yes → Assess ABCDE O₂, monitor, i.v. access ± turn into recovery position

Call resuscitation team if appropriate

Handover to resuscitation team

Figure 5b Cardiopulmonary resuscitation (CPR)

(i) (ii) (iii)

2 ventilations : 30 compressions in UK
2 ventilations : 60 compressions in USA

Figure 5d Probability of successful initial resuscitation after cardiac arrest

Survival declines exponentially with success rates <5% within 6mins of full arrest conditions

Figure 5c Adult advanced life support (ALS) algorithm

Early defibrillation, chest compression, adequate ventilation and oxygenation through a clear airway are always more important than drug administration

CARDIAC ARREST

Open airway and look for signs of life

Call resuscitation team Precordial Thump if appropriate¹

CPR 30:2 until defibrillator/monitor attached

Assess rhythm ± check pulse

Shockable VF / pulseless VT

1 Shock 150-360 J biphasic or 360 J monophasic

Immediately resume CPR 30:2 for 2 mins

Non-Shockable (PEA / asystole)

Immediately resume CPR 30:2 for 2 mins

During CPR
- Correct reversible causes*
- Check electrode / paddle position and contact
- **Intubate, i.v. access + oxygenate**
- Give **epinephrine** 1mg every 3–5 mins

Consider
- Antiarrhythmics (e.g. amiodarone for VF/VT)
- Atropine (3 mg i.v. once only) ± pacing for bradyarrhythmia
- Magnesium (8mmoL) in refractory VF

* Potentially reversible causes (often cause PEA)
- Hypoxaemia
- Hypovolaemia
- Hyper/hypokalaemia and metabolic disorders
- Hypothermia
- Tamponade, cardiac
- Tension pneumothorax
- Thrombosis (coronary or pulmonary)
- Toxic or drug responses

PEA=pulseless electrical activity
VF/VT= ventricular fibrillation/ tachycardia

Notes
1. Precordial thump is only used in witnessed or monitored arrests
2. Na₂HCO₃: consider if pH<7.1 (base excess >-10), ↑K+ or after tricyclic antidepressant overdose. This remains controversial
3. Antiarrhythmic drugs: there are no firm recommendations

Cardiac arrest (CA) occurs when clinically detectable cardiac output ceases. The main cause (~80%) is ischaemic heart disease (IHD). Most patients die and even in successfully resuscitated patients mortality is high (~70%). Overall survival to hospital discharge is ~10% but higher (~20%) in those with ventricular fibrillation or tachycardia (VF/VT).

- **Out-of-hospital arrests** (OHAs) are usually due to IHD-induced VF (~80%). Electrical defibrillation is the only effective treatment for VF. Delay reduces the chance of successful defibrillation by ~7–10% per minute.
- **In-hospital arrests** (IHAs) are mainly due to pulseless electrical activity (PEA) or asystole (~60–70%) and the outcome is usually

Critical Care Medicine at a Glance, Third Edition. Richard Leach. © 2014 John Wiley & Sons, Ltd. Published 2014 by John Wiley & Sons, Ltd.

poor. Progressive physiological deterioration often precedes IHA and about half present with hypoxaemic bradycardia due to a respiratory cause (e.g. pulmonary embolism [PE]).

Early recognition of patients at risk may prevent CA and has led to the development of 'Patient at Risk' and 'Medical Emergency' Teams (PART, MET).

Cardiopulmonary resuscitation

Effective cardiopulmonary resuscitation (CPR) maintains oxygen supply to vital organs (e.g. brain) while awaiting definitive medical treatment. It is started as soon as CA is established; interruptions should be minimized and defibrillation attempted as soon as possible for VF/VT.

Figure 5a shows the IHA management algorithm. Immediately summon help (i.e. CA/MET team at IHA or emergency medical services [EMS] at OHA) and exclude potential danger at the scene. Initial assessment of a collapsed or sick patient (Chapter 1) should include airway, breathing, circulation, neurological disability and exposure of the patient (**ABCDE**). Turn the patient onto their back. Open the airway using head tilt and chin lift, except after potential cervical injuries, when a 'jaw-thrust' manoeuvre is employed (Chapter 15). Clear the oropharynx of foreign bodies and vomitus. Then, while keeping the airway open, 'look, listen and feel' for breathing (i.e. place your cheek and ear over the patient's nose/mouth and observe chest movement) for ≤10 secs. At the same time feel for the carotid pulse.

Start CPR (Figure 5b) if no signs of life are detected (i.e. movement, pulse, breathing). Deliver chest compressions and lung ventilation in a ratio of 30:2 (UK) or ≥60:2 (USA).

• **Chest compressions** are performed at a rate of ~100/min. The correct hand position is found by placing the heel of one hand on the centre of the chest with the other hand on top. The compression depth is 4–5 cm and the chest should be allowed to recoil completely after each compression.

• **Ventilation** is performed with whatever equipment is available. A '**bag-valve mask**' and oropharyngeal airway should be available during IHA (Chapter 15). Endotracheal intubation (ETI) should only be performed by individuals with the requisite training (Chapter 17). After ETI, chest compressions and ventilation continue uninterrupted (i.e. no break for ventilation) at a breath rate of 10/min and tidal volume of ~500 ml. Avoid hyperventilation because this reduces cerebral blood flow. In OHA, chest compressions continue uninterrupted until the EMS arrive unless a pocket mask is available or 'mouth-to-mouth' ventilation (M-MV) is feasible/acceptable. To perform M-MV, pinch the nose while performing 'chin lift', maintain slight neck extension by gentle pressure on the forehead, take a breath and place your lips around the patient's mouth creating an airtight seal. Breath out slowly observing chest movement. Allow sufficient time for deflation between breaths.

Advanced life support

Figure 5c illustrates the adult advanced life support (ALS) algorithm. It is divided into management of '**shockable**' (VF/VT) and '**non-shockable**' (non-VF/VT, PEA, asystolic) rhythms. Only CPR and defibrillation improve outcome. Therefore, interruptions to CPR should be minimal (i.e. for intubation, pulse checks) and

defibrillation is attempted as soon as possible in VF/VT. A **precordial thump**, which generates a small electrical shock, may be given in witnessed and/or monitored VF/VT arrests if a defibrillator is not immediately available. Central venous access is best but peripherally injected drugs can be flushed with saline. If venous access is impossible, some drugs (e.g. epinephrine [adrenaline], atropine) can be administered endobronchially using double doses. During CPR administer:

• **Epinephrine** 1 mg every 3–5 min (i.e. every second loop of the algorithm).

• **Atropine** 3 mg once in asystole or PEA with a heart rate <60/min.

• **Amiodarone** after a third unsuccessful defibrillation in VF/VT.

ETI is the ideal means of securing the airway during CPR but pre-hospital ETI by unskilled personnel has no benefit and may cause harm. Supraglottic airway devices (e.g. laryngeal mask airway) are a useful alternative for those unskilled in ETI. **Reversible causes** (Figure 5c) must be detected and treated, including hypovolaemia, haemorrhage, PE, electrolyte disturbance, tension pneumothorax and cardiac tamponade.

Post-resuscitation care

Immediate post-CPR care involves stabilization, monitoring, reassessment (i.e. ABCDE) and transfer to a critical care area. Circulatory support is often required (e.g. fluids ± inotropes). A clear airway and appropriate ventilation prevent hypoxia and hypercapnia, which may exacerbate brain injury and predispose to further CAs. Neurological assessment is necessary and sedation may be needed to facilitate ongoing ventilation. Therapeutic mild hypothermia (32–34°C) for 12–24 hours is recommended in comatose patients following out-of-hospital VF/VT arrests (±consider after other forms of CA).

Investigations include routine blood tests, arterial blood gases, cardiac enzymes and an electrocardiogram (ECG) to exclude myocardial ischaemia. Chest radiography (CXR) excludes pneumothorax and checks line (± endotracheal tube) position. Echocardiography is often helpful.

Prognosis

Poor prognostic factors include initial rhythms of asystole/PEA, CA location (e.g. OHA), delayed CPR (i.e. >5 min) or defibrillation, myoclonic jerks, poor preceding health, peri-arrest hyperglycaemia, sepsis or renal injury and prolonged CPR. Age alone does not predict outcome. Most successful CPR requires <2–3 min; after >6 min success rates are <5% (Figure 5d) with the exceptions of hypothermia and near-drowning when survival may follow prolonged CPR. Absence of pupillary reflexes or motor responses to pain after 3 days predicts poor outcome with high specificity.

Neurological damage causes ~50% of deaths in CPR survivors. A third of comatose survivors develop seizure activity in the first 24 hours and permanent neurological damage affects ~50% of conscious survivors. Recovery of consciousness is greatest in the first 24 hours and then declines exponentially.

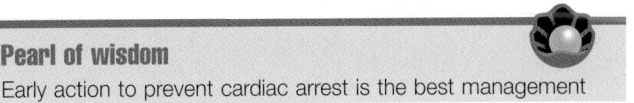

Pearl of wisdom
Early action to prevent cardiac arrest is the best management

6 Oxygen transport

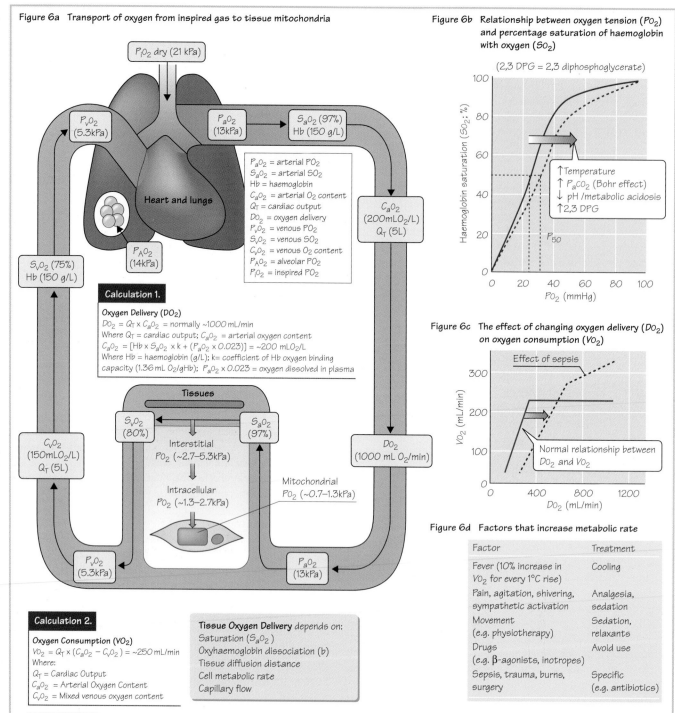

Figure 6a Transport of oxygen from inspired gas to tissue mitochondria

P_iO_2 dry (21 kPa)

P_vO_2 (5.3kPa)

P_aO_2 (13kPa) → S_aO_2 (97%) Hb (150 g/L)

Heart and lungs

P_AO_2 (14kPa)

S_vO_2 (75%) Hb (150 g/L)

P_aO_2 = arterial PO_2
S_aO_2 = arterial SO_2
Hb = haemoglobin
C_aO_2 = arterial O_2 content
Q_T = cardiac output
DO_2 = oxygen delivery
P_vO_2 = venous PO_2
S_vO_2 = venous SO_2
C_vO_2 = venous O_2 content
P_AO_2 = alveolar PO_2
P_iO_2 = inspired PO_2

C_aO_2 (200mLO₂/L) Q_T (5L)

Calculation 1.

Oxygen Delivery (DO_2)
$DO_2 = Q_T \times C_aO_2$ = normally ~1000 mL/min
Where Q_T = cardiac output; C_aO_2 = arterial oxygen content
$C_aO_2 = [Hb \times S_aO_2 \times k + (P_aO_2 \times 0.023)]$ = ~200 mLO₂/L
Where Hb = haemoglobin (g/L); k= coefficient of Hb oxygen binding capacity (1.36 mL O_2/gHb); $P_aO_2 \times 0.023$ = oxygen dissolved in plasma

Tissues

S_vO_2 (80%) S_aO_2 (97%)

Interstitial PO_2 (~2.7–5.3kPa)

Intracellular PO_2 (~1.3–2.7kPa)

Mitochondrial PO_2 (~0.7–1.3kPa)

C_vO_2 (150mLO₂/L) Q_T (5L)

DO_2 (1000 mL O_2/min)

P_vO_2 (5.3kPa) P_aO_2 (13kPa)

Figure 6b Relationship between oxygen tension (PO_2) and percentage saturation of haemoglobin with oxygen (SO_2)

(2,3 DPG = 2,3 diphosphoglycerate)

Haemoglobin saturation (SO_2; %)

↑Temperature
↑ P_aCO_2 (Bohr effect)
↓ pH /metabolic acidosis
↑2,3 DPG

P_{50}

PO_2 (mmHg)

Figure 6c The effect of changing oxygen delivery (DO_2) on oxygen consumption (VO_2)

Effect of sepsis

VO_2 (mL/min)

Normal relationship between DO_2 and VO_2

DO_2 (mL/min)

Figure 6d Factors that increase metabolic rate

Factor	Treatment
Fever (10% increase in VO_2 for every 1°C rise)	Cooling
Pain, agitation, shivering, sympathetic activation	Analgesia, sedation
Movement (e.g. physiotherapy)	Sedation, relaxants
Drugs (e.g. β-agonists, inotropes)	Avoid use
Sepsis, trauma, burns, surgery	Specific (e.g. antibiotics)

Calculation 2.

Oxygen Consumption (VO_2)
$VO_2 = Q_T \times (C_aO_2 - C_vO_2)$ = ~250 mL/min
Where:
Q_T = Cardiac Output
C_aO_2 = Arterial Oxygen Content
C_vO_2 = Mixed venous oxygen content

Tissue Oxygen Delivery depends on:
Saturation (S_aO_2)
Oxyhaemoglobin dissociation (b)
Tissue diffusion distance
Cell metabolic rate
Capillary flow

Calculation 3.

Oxygen Extraction Ratio (OER)
OER = $VO_2/DO_2 \times 100$ = ~25%
or OER = $(C_aO_2 - C_vO_2)/C_aO_2$ = ~25%

Figure 6e Effect of oxygen and haemoglobin on oxygen transport in a critically ill patient

	F_iO_2	P_aO_2 (kPa)	S_aO_2 (%)	Hb(g/L)	C_aO_2(mL/L)
1. Before therapy (air)	0.21	6	75	80	83
2. Start O_2 (35% O_2)	0.35	9.5	93	80	103
3. Increase O_2 (60% O_2)	0.6	16.5	98	80	110
4. Give blood (transfusion)	0.6	16.5	98	120	164

Critical Care Medicine at a Glance, Third Edition. Richard Leach. © 2014 John Wiley & Sons, Ltd. Published 2014 by John Wiley & Sons, Ltd.

The major function of the heart, lungs and circulation is to deliver oxygen and other nutrients to body tissues and remove carbon dioxide and other waste products of metabolism.

Oxygen transport is determined by:

1 Oxygen uptake by blood in the lung, which depends on blood haemoglobin (Hb) content, alveolar oxygen (P_AO_2), oxygen–haemoglobin uptake and the efficiency of lung gas exchange. It is measured as the arterial oxygen content (C_aO_2).

2 Convective oxygen transport from the lung to the tissues, which is determined (after oxygen loading in the lungs) by the magnitude and regional distribution of cardiac output (Q_T).

3 Diffusion of oxygen from the capillary blood to tissue mitochondria, governed by the capillary–mitochondrial Po_2 gradient, capillary surface area and diffusion distance.

Oxygen delivery

Figure 6a illustrates the transport of oxygen from inspired air to tissue mitochondria.

- **Global oxygen delivery (Do_2)** is determined from Q_T and C_aO_2 (Figure 6a; Calculation 1). Most oxygen carried in blood is attached to Hb. Only a small amount is dissolved in plasma. Arterial oxygen saturation (S_aO_2) and Hb concentration are the major determinants of C_aO_2. Figure 6e illustrates the relative effects of increasing oxygen and Hb on Do_2. Although transfusion rapidly increases Do_2, the optimum Hb level in critical illness is $\sim$70–100 g/L (7–10 g/dL) and is a balance between optimizing C_aO_2 and avoiding microcirculatory problem due to viscosity. Fluid administration and inotropes are used to increase Q_T and Do_2 (Chapter 9). However, increasing Do_2 is of limited benefit in organ ischaemia due to arterial obstruction (e.g. embolus, thrombus), whereas removal of the obstruction (e.g. embolectomy, thrombolysis) may be life-saving.

- **Tissue oxygen delivery** requires appropriate regional and microcirculatory distribution of Q_T, which is determined by a complex interaction of endothelial, receptor, metabolic and pharmacological factors. During stress or critical illness, blood flow is directed to vital organs (e.g. brain) and away from less essential tissue beds (e.g. splanchnic, skin), which are damaged if this effect persists. For example, prolonged splanchnic ischaemia compromises bowel wall integrity causing translocation of bacteria into the circulation. Therapeutically, receptor properties of certain vasoactive agents can be used to improve individual organ oxygen delivery (i.e. dopexamine may increase splanchnic blood flow).

- **Tissue factors** influence cellular oxygen status. Oxygen diffuses from the capillary to the cell and is dependent on capillary blood flow and surface area (i.e. reduced by capillary thrombosis), oxygen gradient and diffusion distance. However, increasing Do_2 cannot compensate for cellular metabolic failure (i.e. mitochondrial dysfunction during sepsis) and some tissues (e.g. brain, kidney) are more susceptible to, and rapidly damaged by, sustained hypoxia.

The oxyhaemoglobin dissociation curve

Figure 6b illustrates the relationship between the partial pressure of oxygen (Po_2) in the blood and haemoglobin saturation (So_2).

The position of the dissociation curve is affected by temperature, pH, P_ACO_2 and 2,3 diphosphoglycerate (DPG), and is expressed as the Po_2 at which haemoglobin is 50% saturated (P_{50}). This is normally 3.5 kPa (26 mmHg). Left or right shifts of the curve will alter uptake and release of oxygen by the Hb molecule. If the curve moves to the right, the S_aO_2 will be lower for a given Po_2 (i.e. less oxygen is taken up in the lungs but more is released in the tissues). Thus, as capillary P_aCO_2 increases (i.e. rightward shift of the curve), oxygen is released from Hb, a phenomenon known as the Bohr effect.

Oxygen consumption

- **Global oxygen consumption (Vo_2)** is the sum of the oxygen consumed by individual organs and tissues and is $\sim$250 ml/min for a 70 kg adult. It can be calculated from Q_T, S_aO_2 and S_vO_2 (Figure 6a; Calculation 2) or from the inspired and mixed expired oxygen and CO_2 concentrations. The oxygen extraction ratio (OER; Figure 6a; Calculation 3) determines the amount of oxygen used (Vo_2) as a percentage of that delivered (Do_2) and is normally $\sim$25%.

- **Metabolic rate** is increased by the factors listed in Figure 6d. It should be recognized that drugs used to increase Do_2 (e.g. inotropes) may also increase Vo_2. Simple measures including cooling, analgesia, sedation, prevention of shivering and muscle relaxation substantially reduce Vo_2 and subsequent Do_2 requirements.

Relationship between oxygen delivery and oxygen consumption

Figure 6c illustrates the effect of changing Do_2 on Vo_2 in normal and septic patients. Normally, oxygen extraction from capillary blood increases as tissue Vo_2 rises or blood supply decreases. The maximum OER is about 70%. Any further increase in tissue Vo_2 or fall in oxygen supply will result in hypoxia, anaerobic metabolism and lactic acid production. In this situation, Do_2 must be improved by increasing oxygenated blood flow or relieving obstruction (e.g. thrombolysis in myocardial infarction).

In sepsis, cellular dysfunction reduces the ability of tissues to extract oxygen. This alters the relationship between Do_2 and Vo_2 (Figure 6c). In particular, Vo_2 continues to increase even at 'supranormal' levels of Do_2. This observation encouraged the use of aggressive fluid loading and inotropic support to achieve a high Do_2 ($>$600 ml/min/m^2), in the belief that this strategy, sometimes termed **goal-directed therapy**, would relieve hypoxia and prevent tissue damage. However, this is probably not the case; microcirculatory impairment (i.e. capillary thrombi), failure of regional distribution and metabolic dysfunction are more likely than inadequate Do_2 to cause cellular toxicity in late sepsis.

Venous blood saturation varies according to the metabolic requirements of each tissue (i.e. hepatic 30–40%, renal $\sim$80%). In the pulmonary artery, the **mixed venous oxygen saturation** ($S_vO_2 > 6$ 5–70%) represents oxygen not used in the tissues (Do_2–Vo_2). It is influenced by both Do_2 and Vo_2 and, provided regional blood flow and cellular oxygen utilization are normal, reflects whether global Do_2 adequately matches global Vo_2 (Chapter 3).

7 Shock

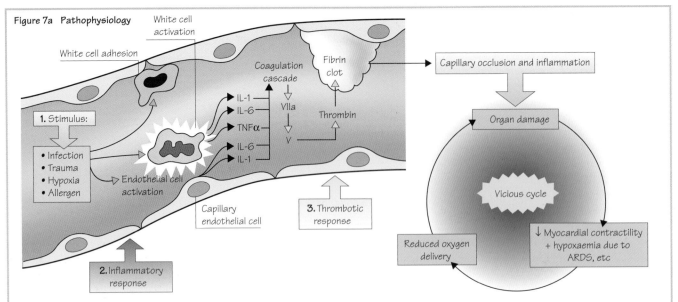

Figure 7a Pathophysiology

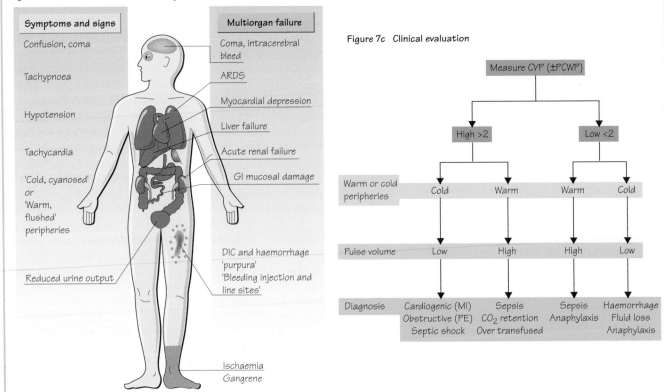

Figure 7b Clinical features and consequences of shock

Figure 7c Clinical evaluation

Definition and causes

Shock describes the clinical syndrome that occurs when acute circulatory failure with inadequate or inappropriately distributed perfusion results in failure to meet tissue metabolic demands causing generalized cellular hypoxia (±lactic acidosis).

Shock can be classified into six categories but more than one form of shock may occur in an individual patient (e.g. myocardial depression may occur in late sepsis).

- **Hypovolaemic:** due to major reductions in circulating blood volume caused by haemorrhage, plasma loss (e.g. burns, pancreatitis) or extracellular fluid loss (e.g. diabetic ketoacidosis, trauma).
- **Cardiogenic:** due to severe heart failure (e.g. myocardial infarction, acute mitral regurgitation).
- **Obstructive:** caused by circulatory obstruction (e.g. pulmonary embolism [PE], cardiac tamponade).
- **Septic/distributive:** with infection or septicaemia. Vasodilation, arteriovenous shunting and capillary damage (Figure 7a) cause hypotension and maldistribution of flow.

Critical Care Medicine at a Glance, Third Edition. Richard Leach. © 2014 John Wiley & Sons, Ltd. Published 2014 by John Wiley & Sons, Ltd.

- **Anaphylactic:** due to allergen-induced vasodilation (e.g. bee sting, peanut and food allergies).
- **Neurogenic (spinal):** follows traumatic spinal cord lesions above T6. Interruption of sympathetic outflow causes vasodilation, hypothermia and bradycardia, which may be severe if vagal stimulation (e.g. pain, hypoxia) is unopposed.

Clinical features

Depend on the underlying cause (Chapters 34, 36, 71) and severity. General features include hypotension (systolic BP <100 mmHg), tachycardia (>100 beats/min), rapid respiration (>30 min), oliguria (urine output <30 ml/h) and drowsiness, confusion or agitation (Figure 7b). Shock is either:
- **'Cold, clammy' shock** (e.g. hypovolaemic, cardiogenic, obstructive, late septic) with cold peripheries (skin vasoconstriction), weak pulses and evidence of low cardiac output (e.g. oliguria, peripheral cyanosis, confusion).
- **'Warm, dilated' shock** (e.g. early septic, anaphylactic) with warm peripheries (skin vasodilation), bounding pulses and a high cardiac output (i.e. flushed)

Investigations and monitoring

Investigations include routine blood tests, blood gases, lactic acid measurement, cardiac enzymes, amylase, electrocardiogram (ECG) and blood crossmatching if haemorrhage is suspected. **Imaging** should include a chest radiograph (CXR). **Microbiology:** examine blood, sputum, cerebrospinal fluid (CSF) and urine samples. **Monitor vital signs:** temperature, respiratory rate, $S_a o_2$, conscious level and urine output. **Haemodynamic assessment** often requires intra-arterial blood pressure (BP) measurement, echocardiography, central venous pressure (CVP) and ECG monitoring. Additional measurements (Chapter 3) are occasionally necessary (e.g. cardiac output [CO], sysemic vascular resistance [SVR], pulmonary capillary wedge pressure [PCWP], $S_v o_2$).

Assessment

Clinical features, CVP and SVR define the cause of shock (Figure 7c). Measurement of CVP, PCWP and SVR are useful when clinical signs are difficult to interpret. For example:
- CVP is: (i) **reduced** in hypovolaemic and anaphylactic shock; (ii) **elevated** in cardiogenic and obstructive shock; (iii) **low, normal or high** in septic shock.
- SVR is: (i) **high** in cardiogenic shock with sympathetic-mediated vasoconstriction ($\rightarrow$ 'cold, clammy' patient); or (ii) **low** in septic vasodilation due to release of inflammatory mediators ($\rightarrow$ 'warm, dilated' patient)

Consequently, simple haemodynamic patterns may aid diagnosis:
- Hypovolaemic shock $\rightarrow$ low CVP/PCWP + low CO + high SVR.
- Cardiogenic shock $\rightarrow$ high CVP/PCWP + low CO + high SVR.
- Septic shock $\rightarrow$ low CVP/PCWP + high CO + low SVR.

Complications

Circulatory failure and tissue hypoxia result in multi-organ failure including acute respiratory distress syndrome (ARDS), acute renal failure and mucosal (e.g. peptic) ulceration (Figures 7a and 7b). A cycle of increasing 'oxygen debt' and 'shock-induced' tissue damage develops as decreased myocardial contractility and hypoxaemia further impair oxygen delivery and tissue oxygenation (Figure 7a). Ischaemic damage to the intestinal mucosa causes bacterial and toxin translocation into the splanchnic circulation with further organ impairment. Eventually, 'refractory' shock develops with irreversible tissue damage and death.

Management

Early diagnosis and treatment are vital because mortality, which is high with all causes, increases if shock lasts >1 hour ('the golden hour'). Management aims to correct the cause, reverse 'tissue oxygen debt' and inhibit the cycle of progressive organ damage. Treatment of cardiogenic, obstructive and septic shock is discussed in later chapters. However, features common to all forms of shock are:
- **Identification and treatment of the cause** (e.g. sepsis).
- **Support:** patients should be managed in a critical care area with appropriate monitoring and good vascular access. Correct hypoxaemia, which can occur in the absence of lung disease due to ventilation–perfusion mismatch, low $S_v o_2$ or reduced pulmonary blood flow, with supplemental oxygen. **Ventilatory support** improves cardiac function, increases tissue oxygen delivery and reduces work of breathing, which is increased tenfold in shock (Chapters 16, 18). Indications include hypoxaemia ($P_a o_2$ < 8 kPa on >40% O_2), hypercapnia ($P_a co_2$ > 7.5 kPa), respiratory rate >35/min, reduced conscious level or exhaustion (Chapter 13).
- **Fluid resuscitation** is, with the exception of cardiogenic shock, essential in most forms of shock (e.g. haemorrhage, sepsis). Fluid is given rapidly following assessment of intravascular volume status (e.g. BP, CVP, PCWP) including the response to a fluid challenge (Chapters 7, 8). The merits of specific fluids (e.g. crystalloid, colloid) are discussed in Chapter 9 and depend on the cause of shock (Chapters 25, 71, 76). Thus, blood or blood products are most appropriate following haemorrhage or trauma. Cardiogenic shock, identified by raised CVP and PCWP, requires fluid restriction (although fluid administration may be required in right ventricular infarction!). Time course is also important; in early septic shock fluid administration is essential, but in late sepsis with ARDS, fluid restriction prevents pulmonary oedema.
- **Inotropic support** (Chapter 12) is indicated when *hypotension* (i.e. MAP < 60 mmHg) *or tissue hypoxaemia* (e.g. oliguria) persist despite adequate fluid replacement or when fluid resuscitation is contraindicated (e.g. cardiogenic shock). The type of inotropic support depends on the cause of shock. **In septic shock** ('warm, dilated' patient), CO is high but vasodilation and the associated low SVR cause hypotension, inadequate tissue perfusion and organ hypoxia (e.g. oliguria, confusion). In this scenario, norepinephrine, a peripheral vasoconstrictor, increases SVR, restoring BP and tissue perfusion. **In cardiogenic shock** ('cold, clammy' patient), CO is low due to poor myocardial contractility and SVR is high due to sympathetic vasoconstriction. Treatment with dobutamine increases myocardial contractility and CO and reduces SVR.
- **Renal replacement therapy** (e.g. haemofiltration) may be required for anuria, hyperkalaemia, persistent acidosis or fluid overload (Chapter 46).
- **Specific treatments** include thrombolysis (e.g. for PE), drainage of cardiac tamponade/pneumothorax and balloon pumps (e.g. cardiogenic shock).

8 Circulatory assessment

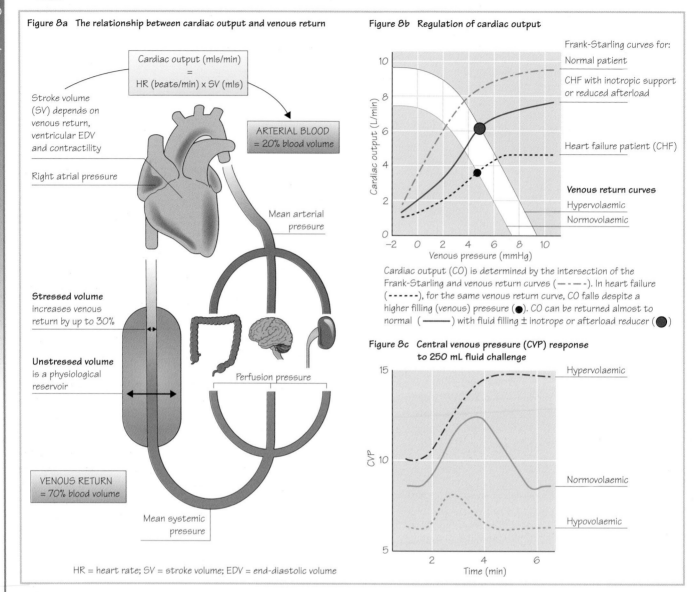

Figure 8a The relationship between cardiac output and venous return

Figure 8b Regulation of cardiac output

Cardiac output (CO) is determined by the intersection of the Frank-Starling and venous return curves (— · — · —). In heart failure (· · · · · ·), for the same venous return curve, CO falls despite a higher filling (venous) pressure (●). CO can be returned almost to normal (———) with fluid filling ± inotrope or afterload reducer (●)

Figure 8c Central venous pressure (CVP) response to 250 mL fluid challenge

HR = heart rate; SV = stroke volume; EDV = end-diastolic volume

Circulatory assessment is an essential clinical skill and when performed well is the hallmark of a good clinician. It can be particularly difficult during critical illness and depends on evaluation of both cardiac function and circuit factors (Figure 8a). The main aims of circulatory management are to maintain cardiac output (CO) and blood pressure (BP) and ensure adequate tissue blood supply to satisfy metabolic demands.

Circulatory assessment should address:

1 Cardiac function

This includes evaluation of CO and exclusion of heart failure. CO is the product of **heart rate (HR)** and **stroke volume (SV)** [CO (ml/min) = HR (beats/min) × SV (ml)], where SV is determined by:

a. **Preload**, which depends on ventricular end-diastolic volume (EDV) and is governed by the volume and pressure of blood returning to the heart (Figure 8b). Haemorrhage (i.e loss of intravascular volume), sepsis, anaphylaxis and raised intrathoracic pressures (e.g. severe asthma) are common causes of inadequate ventricular preload.

b. **Afterload:** the resistance, load or 'impedence' against which the ventricle has to work. Valve stenosis, hypertension, high systemic vascular resistance (SVR), low intrathoracic pressures and ventricular dilation increase afterload.

c. **Myocardial contractility**, or the heart's ability to perform work independently of preload or afterload. Failure is either due to:
  • **Systolic dysfunction** (i.e. inadequate systolic ejection) as a result of reduced contractility (e.g. ischaemia, cardiomyopathy,

Critical Care Medicine at a Glance, Third Edition. Richard Leach. © 2014 John Wiley & Sons, Ltd. Published 2014 by John Wiley & Sons, Ltd.

sepsis) or increased impedance (e.g. hypertension, aortic stenosis). Increasing ventricular EDV (i.e. heart volume) will maintain SV (Frank–Starling relationship) provided myocardial reserve is adequate (Figure 8b); otherwise SV and CO will fall and inotropic agents will be needed to maintain CO and BP.

• **Diastolic dysfunction:** characterized by reduced ventricular compliance with impaired diastolic filling (i.e. a stiff ventricle). It may be caused by mechanical factors (e.g. restrictive cardiomyopathy) or impaired relaxation due to myocardial ischaemia or severe sepsis. The resulting increase in end-diastolic pressure and associated pulmonary venous congestion can cause characteristic 'flash' pulmonary oedema. Patients with advanced diabetes or hypertension secondary to renal failure are at particular risk of diastolic dysfunction and flash pulmonary oedema. In diabetes, this is due to endomyocardial ischaemia caused by small vessel arteriopathy. In renal hypertension, blood flow from the epicardium to endomyocardium is impeded by ventricular wall hypertrophy and the resulting ischaemia impairs ventricular relaxation.

Bradycardia and tachycardia reduce CO. In tachycardia, this is due to either inadequate ventricular filling time or reduced contractility. Myocardial perfusion occurs during diastole, which is shortened during tachycardia causing myocardial ischaemia and impaired contractility.

2 Circuit factors

Although often overlooked, circuit factors are as important as myocardial contractility in determining CO because venous return determines EDV. Arterial 'conducting' vessels contain ~20% of the blood volume, where mean arterial pressure (MAP) is determined by force of myocardial ejection and downstream impedance. The venous 'capacitance' system contains ~70% of total blood volume and acts as a physiological reservoir ('unstressed volume'). When circulatory demand increases, sympathetic tone also increases causing reservoir contraction. The resultant 'autotransfusion' ('stressed volume') can increase venous return by up to 30%. Complex neurohormonal factors control the circulatory response including systemic adrenergic, renin-aldosterone, vasopressinergic and steroid systems, which are further modulated by local factors (e.g. endothelin, nitric oxide).

Disruption of peripheral vascular regulation, usually due to reduced responsiveness to sympathetic stimulation (e.g. spinal anaesthesia, anaphylaxis, sepsis), results in circulatory failure caused by venous pooling and inability to generate a 'stressed' volume. Management tends to focus inappropriately on arterial factors (i.e. SVR, afterload), whereas the problem is mainly due to impaired venous return. Fluid loading to restore effective intravascular volume (Chapters 9, 10, 11) should always precede the use of 'vasopressor' drugs (Chapter 12).

Clinical assessment (Chapters 1, 7)

• **Inspection:** look for features of poor perfusion and reduced CO including cool, pale limbs, peripheral cyanosis and prolonged capillary refill time (i.e. >2 secs for colour to return to an area of skin previously subjected to pressure). Confusion and reduced urine output also indicate poor CO.

• **Auscultation:** listen for leaking heart valves and check BP. Initially compensatory mechanisms (e.g. tachycardia, increased SVR) maintain BP, and CO has to fall by >20%, equivalent to 1 L of acute blood loss, before BP falls. Pulse pressure narrows during arterial vasoconstriction (e.g. hypovolaemia, cardiogenic shock). During vasodilation (e.g. sepsis), diastolic BP is low.

• **Palpation:** feel peripheral and central pulses for HR, rhythm and equality. Thready, fast pulses indicate a poor CO, whereas bounding pulses suggest sepsis.

In most patients, clinical assessment is reliable, adequate and ensures successful management. However, invasive measurement of physiological variables (e.g. CO, SVR, PCWP) may be required in critically ill patients to optimize circulatory performance (Chapter 3).

Management

Management includes fluid replacement, control of bleeding and restoration of HR, CO, BP and tissue perfusion. Good venous access must be established using wide-bore peripheral and central venous cannulae. Circulatory support utilizes a hierarchy of management:

• **Diagnosis** determines treatment (e.g. fluid restriction in left heart failure vs. fluid resuscitation in hypovolaemia). Life-threatening conditions such as haemorrhage, cardiac tamponade and massive pulmonary embolism must be detected and treated immediately.

• **Rate and rhythm:** both tachyarrhythmias (>180 beats/min) and bradycardia (e.g. vagal tone) can reduce CO. Restoring sinus rhythm and normal HR improve BP and CO. Electrolyte concentrations must be optimized (K^+ > 4.5 mmol/L, Mg^{2+} > 1.2 mmol/L) and arrhythmogenic drugs (e.g. salbutamol) withdrawn. Antiarrhythmic drugs, cardioversion or pacemakers may be required (Chapter 32).

• **Fluid therapy** aims to optimize preload (Figure 8b). In the absence of cardiac failure (i.e. raised central venous pressure (CVP) or coarse bilateral basal crepitations on lung auscultation), a '**fluid challenge**' (~0.5 L over <20 min) is given and the response assessed in terms of HR, BP and chest auscultation. The CVP response to a fluid challenge (Figure 8c) is a useful measure of the patient's fluid status (i.e. hypovolaemic, hypervolaemic). A transient increase in CVP, CO and BP suggests the need for further fluid. A sustained increase in CVP indicates that the heart is operating on the flat part of the Starling curve (Figure 8b) and further fluid administration risks pulmonary oedema.

If there is only a transient response to the initial fluid challenge, the challenge is repeated and the patient reassessed. Aim to restore systolic BP to >100 mmHg or normal (if known). Fluid management and the selection of the appropriate fluid for replacement (e.g. crystalloid vs. colloid) are discussed in Chapters 9, 10 and 11. In general, crystalloid solutions are used first or the fluid that is lost is replaced (e.g. blood during haemorrhage). Large volumes of maintenance fluid suggest ongoing loss and a cause should be sought. If haemorrhage is suspected, send blood for cross-matching.

• **Inotropic and vasopressor drugs:** if fluid resuscitation fails to achieve an adequate circulation or precipitates cardiac failure, alternative means of improving CO and tissue perfusion including inotropic or vasopressor drugs and mechanical ventricular support devices must be considered (Chapter 12).

9 Fluid management: pathophysiological factors

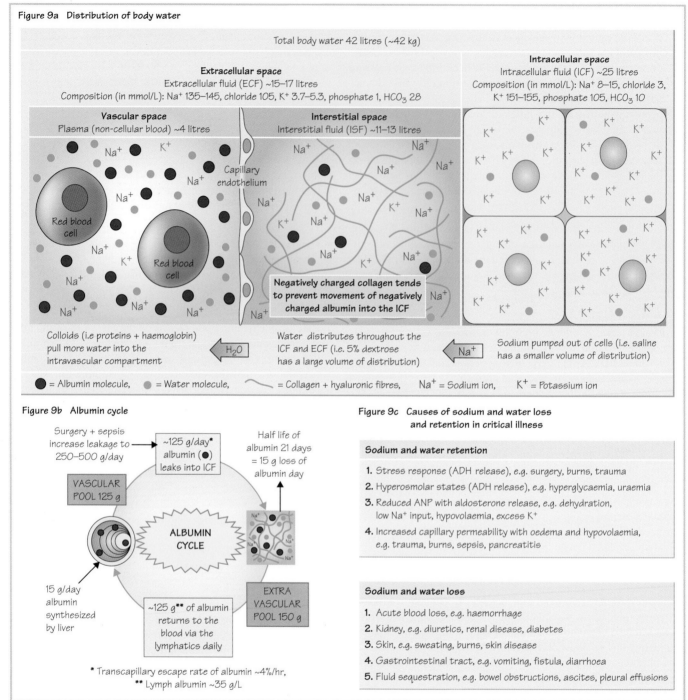

Figure 9a Distribution of body water

Total body water 42 litres (~42 kg)

Extracellular space
Extracellular fluid (ECF) ~15–17 litres
Composition (in mmol/L): Na^+ 135–145, chloride 105, K^+ 3.7–5.3, phosphate 1, HCO_3 28

Intracellular space
Intracellular fluid (ICF) ~25 litres
Composition (in mmol/L): Na^+ 8–15, chloride 3, K^+ 151–155, phosphate 105, HCO_3 10

Vascular space
Plasma (non-cellular blood) ~4 litres

Interstitial space
Interstitial fluid (ISF) ~11–13 litres

Red blood cell

Red blood cell

Capillary endothelium

Negatively charged collagen tends to prevent movement of negatively charged albumin into the ICF

Colloids (i.e proteins + haemoglobin) pull more water into the intravascular compartment

H_2O

Water distributes throughout the ICF and ECF (i.e. 5% dextrose has a large volume of distribution)

Na^+

Sodium pumped out of cells (i.e. saline has a smaller volume of distribution)

● = Albumin molecule, ● = Water molecule, 〰 = Collagen + hyaluronic fibres, Na^+ = Sodium ion, K^+ = Potassium ion

Figure 9b Albumin cycle

Surgery + sepsis increase leakage to 250–500 g/day

~125 g/day* albumin (●) leaks into ICF

Half life of albumin 21 days = 15 g loss of albumin day

VASCULAR POOL 125 g

ALBUMIN CYCLE

15 g/day albumin synthesized by liver

~125 g** of albumin returns to the blood via the lymphatics daily

EXTRA VASCULAR POOL 150 g

* Transcapillary escape rate of albumin ~4%/hr,
** Lymph albumin ~35 g/L

Figure 9c Causes of sodium and water loss and retention in critical illness

Sodium and water retention

1. Stress response (ADH release), e.g. surgery, burns, trauma
2. Hyperosmolar states (ADH release), e.g. hyperglycaemia, uraemia
3. Reduced ANP with aldosterone release, e.g. dehydration, low Na^+ input, hypovolaemia, excess K^+
4. Increased capillary permeability with oedema and hypovolaemia, e.g. trauma, burns, sepsis, pancreatitis

Sodium and water loss

1. Acute blood loss, e.g. haemorrhage
2. Kidney, e.g. diuretics, renal disease, diabetes
3. Skin, e.g. sweating, burns, skin disease
4. Gastrointestinal tract, e.g. vomiting, fistula, diarrhoea
5. Fluid sequestration, e.g. bowel obstructions, ascites, pleural effusions

When primitive sea organisms emerged onto land, they carried with them their own 'internal sea', the extracellular fluid (ECF). This allowed their cells to bathe in a constant chemical environment and to maintain water and salt balance in a new ecosystem low in both. The cells retained their primitive energy-consuming sodium (Na^+) pumps that ensured Na^+ was largely extracellular, while potassium (K^+) remained intracellular to neutralise negatively charged cellular proteins/ions (Figure 9a).

Water comprises 60% of body weight (slightly less in the obese) or ~42 L in a 70 kg man, of which ~25 L is intracellular and 15–17 L extracellular. The ECF comprises interstitial fluid (ISF; 11–13 L) and intravascular plasma (3–4 L), separated by the capillary endothelium, which is freely permeable to low molecular weight (MW) solutes (e.g. Na^+, K^+), increasingly impermeable to high MW solutes (e.g. albumin) and impervious to red blood cells.

Fluid administration

Daily fluid assessment and administration are essential daily tasks. Unfortunately under- and over-hydration (e.g. pulmonary oedema, peripheral oedema) are common, especially in older people and post-operatively. Fluid is best delivered by oral (or nasogastric) routes but intravenous (IV) fluids may be needed in patients who are acutely unwell and require resuscitation, have excessive fluid losses (e.g. diarrhoea, burns), or are unable to drink (e.g. coma, stroke, unsafe swallow) or absorb water (e.g. vomiting, paralytic ileus).

Aims of fluid administration

• Replace normal fluid and electrolyte losses and ensure a stable cellular and extracellular 'milieu'.
• Maintain blood pressure, cardiac output (CO) and tissue perfusion to satisfy metabolic needs, aid temperature regulation and facilitate waste removal.
• Replenish substantial deficits or ongoing losses.
• Adjust for renal function (see later).
• Avoid excessive tissue oedema.

Factors affecting fluid and electrolyte administration

1. **Compartmental distribution of water (±electrolytes)** is primarily dependent on the 'osmotic pressure' exerted by small diffusible ions (e.g. Na^+). *Osmotic pressure* reflects ion concentration gradients between compartments created by cellular ion pumps, such that Na^+ and chloride (Cl^-) ions are mainly extracellular, and K^+ and phosphate intracellular. For example, a saline infusion increases extracellular Na^+ and Cl^-, raises ECF osmotic pressure and attracts water out of intracellular compartments into the ECF.

2. **Intravascular volume** depends on:
   a. *Plasma oncotic (colloid) pressure (POP)*, which is the ability of large plasma proteins to 'bind' and retain water in the circulation. POP is normally ~3.4 kPa (26 mmHg) with 75% of the effect due to albumin, 20% haemoglobin and 5% globulins. Figure 9b illustrates the albumin cycle. The plasma albumin concentration is ~35–52 g/L and total body albumin is ~270 g (120 g intravascular, 150 g ISF). A gram of albumin 'binds' ~18 ml of water; thus, intravascular albumin binds ~2.25 L (18 × 120) of plasma water.
   b. *Vascular permeability*: normal albumin leakage across capillary membranes is limited to ~4–5%/hour (i.e. ~120 g/day) by its high MW and negative charge, which is repelled by similarly charged 'gel-like' interstitial space glycoproteins (e.g. collagen; Figure 9a). Thus, all the normal intravascular albumin content (~120 g) leaks into the ISF each day. It returns to the blood via the lymph and thoracic ducts at the same rate (Figure 9b). Inflammation (e.g. sepsis) increases vascular permeability and albumin leakage by up to 300%. Acute illness also impairs hepatic albumin synthesis reducing total albumin by ~15 g/day. Subsequent falls in plasma albumin reduce intravascular volume, while increases in ISF albumin cause oedema.
   c. *Circulatory hydrostatic pressure* (see later) increases leakage of intravascular water, while POP draws fluid into, and maintains, plasma volume as a proportion of the ECF (Starling effect).

3. *Normal daily water and electrolyte requirements* are 1.5–2.5 L water/day (25–35 ml/kg/day), ~70–100 mmol Na^+/day (~1–1.5 mmol/kg/day) and 40–70 mmol K^+/day (0.5–1 mmol/kg/day). These losses occur in ~1–1.5 L urine/day (~1 ml/kg/h) and 0.5–1 L 'insensible loss'/day as lung water vapor and sweat. Fever or high ambient temperatures can increase 'insensible losses' to >3 L/daily. Loss of skin or mucous membrane barriers (e.g. burns, ulcerative colitis), fluid-losing enteropathies (e.g. diarrhoea) and salt-losing polyuric renal failure are also associated with large fluid and electrolyte losses. Salt and/or water depletion stimulate antidiuretic hormone (ADH) release, which concentrates urine, retaining water (±salt), while the renin-angiotensin-aldosterone system (RAAS) reduces urinary sodium to <5 mmol/L. Excretion of a salt load is slower and depends on passive RAAS suppression, but the associated hyperchloraemic acidosis can reduce glomerular filtration and potentiate Na^+ retention. Figure 9c summarises causes of sodium and water imbalance.

4. *Renal function (clearance)* may alter fluid and electrolyte requirements. Daily urine solute load comprises normal urinary Na^+, K^+ and Cl^- losses (i.e. [NaClx2] = 70−100 × 2) + (KCl × 2 = 40−70 × 2]) plus 400 mosmol of normal urea waste equalling 620–740 mosmol/day. Normal kidneys achieve a maximum urine concentration of ~1000 mosmol/L. Therefore, the minimum urine volume to excrete the normal daily solute load is ~620–740 ml daily (or ~0.5 ml/kg/h; 35 ml/h). During acute illness (e.g. sepsis), renal solute excretion may be inadequate because urine production often falls, maximum urine concentrating capacity decreases to ~500 mosmol/L, catabolic metabolism increases the urea solute load (>1000 mosmol/day) and fluid resuscitation often includes large salt loads. These retained solutes (e.g. ions, acids) may be harmful (e.g. excess Cl^- ions cause hyperchloraemic acidosis).

5. *Response to stress:* acute illness/injury promotes salt and water retention (i.e. >10 L), which accumulates in interstitial spaces causing tissue or pulmonary oedema. Causes include impaired renal function with reduced free water excretion (±dilutional hyponatraemia), hormonal effects (e.g. ADH, RAAS, catecholamines) with K^+ depletion due to RAAS activity (i.e. renal K^+ excretion occurs in exchange for Na^+ reabsorption), increased urea waste production competing with Na^+ for excretion and, in severely ill patients, impaired energy production causing intracellular sequestration of Na^+ and water due to failure of the Na^+/K^+ ATPase pump, the 'sick cell syndrome'.

6. *Organ function* affects fluid management. Examples include gastrointestinal tract fluid flux in health or disease (e.g. gastroenteritis); chronic renal disease with polyuria or oliguria and variable ability to excrete metabolic waste and solutes (e.g. salt conserving or losing); and cardiac disease that alters contractility, preload and afterload, risking pulmonary oedema or low CO states (Chapters 7, 8, 34).

Fluid management: assessment and prescription

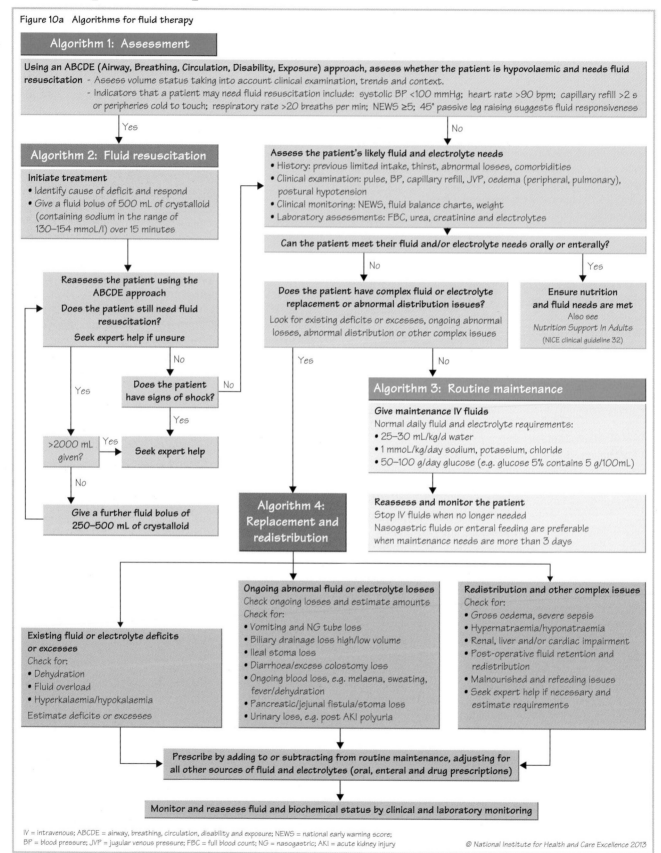

Figure 10a Algorithms for fluid therapy

Algorithm 1: Assessment

Using an ABCDE (Airway, Breathing, Circulation, Disability, Exposure) approach, assess whether the patient is hypovolaemic and needs fluid resuscitation - Assess volume status taking into account clinical examination, trends and context.
- Indicators that a patient may need fluid resuscitation include: systolic BP <100 mmHg; heart rate >90 bpm; capillary refill >2 s or peripheries cold to touch; respiratory rate >20 breaths per min; NEWS ≥5; 45° passive leg raising suggests fluid responsiveness

Yes → | No →

Algorithm 2: Fluid resuscitation

Initiate treatment
- Identify cause of deficit and respond
- Give a fluid bolus of 500 mL of crystalloid (containing sodium in the range of 130–154 mmoL/l) over 15 minutes

Assess the patient's likely fluid and electrolyte needs
- History: previous limited intake, thirst, abnormal losses, comorbidities
- Clinical examination: pulse, BP, capillary refill, JVP, oedema (peripheral, pulmonary), postural hypotension
- Clinical monitoring: NEWS, fluid balance charts, weight
- Laboratory assessments: FBC, urea, creatinine and electrolytes

Can the patient meet their fluid and/or electrolyte needs orally or enterally?

No | Yes

Reassess the patient using the ABCDE approach

Does the patient still need fluid resuscitation?

Seek expert help if unsure

Does the patient have complex fluid or electrolyte replacement or abnormal distribution issues?

Look for existing deficits or excesses, ongoing abnormal losses, abnormal distribution or other complex issues

Ensure nutrition and fluid needs are met

Also see
Nutrition Support In Adults
(NICE clinical guideline 32)

Yes | No

No

Yes →

Does the patient have signs of shock?

No →

Yes ↓

>2000 mL given? — Yes → **Seek expert help**

No ↓

Algorithm 3: Routine maintenance

Give maintenance IV fluids
Normal daily fluid and electrolyte requirements:
- 25–30 mL/kg/d water
- 1 mmoL/kg/day sodium, potassium, chloride
- 50–100 g/day glucose (e.g. glucose 5% contains 5 g/100mL)

Give a further fluid bolus of 250–500 mL of crystalloid

Algorithm 4: Replacement and redistribution

Reassess and monitor the patient
Stop IV fluids when no longer needed
Nasogastric fluids or enteral feeding are preferable when maintenance needs are more than 3 days

Ongoing abnormal fluid or electrolyte losses
Check ongoing losses and estimate amounts
Check for:
- Vomiting and NG tube loss
- Biliary drainage loss high/low volume
- Ileal stoma loss
- Diarrhoea/excess colostomy loss
- Ongoing blood loss, e.g. melaena, sweating, fever/dehydration
- Pancreatic/jejunal fistula/stoma loss
- Urinary loss, e.g. post AKI polyuria

Redistribution and other complex issues
Check for:
- Gross oedema, severe sepsis
- Hypernatraemia/hyponatraemia
- Renal, liver and/or cardiac impairment
- Post-operative fluid retention and redistribution
- Malnourished and refeeding issues
- Seek expert help if necessary and estimate requirements

Existing fluid or electrolyte deficits or excesses
Check for:
- Dehydration
- Fluid overload
- Hyperkalaemia/hypokalaemia
Estimate deficits or excesses

Prescribe by adding to or subtracting from routine maintenance, adjusting for all other sources of fluid and electrolytes (oral, enteral and drug prescriptions)

Monitor and reassess fluid and biochemical status by clinical and laboratory monitoring

IV = intravenous; ABCDE = airway, breathing, circulation, disability and exposure; NEWS = national early warning score;
BP = blood pressure; JVP = jugular venous pressure; FBC = full blood count; NG = nasogastric; AKI = acute kidney injury

© National Institute for Health and Care Excellence 2013

Critical Care Medicine at a Glance, Third Edition. Richard Leach. © 2014 John Wiley & Sons, Ltd. Published 2014 by John Wiley & Sons, Ltd.

Figure 10 illustrates the intravenous (i.v.) fluid management protocol. This directs the initial assessment of water and electrolyte requirements (algorithm 1). It identifies and manages patients who require resuscitation due to haemodynamic instability (algorithm 2); routine maintenance for normal daily losses in patients unable to take oral/enteral fluids (algorithm 3); and replacement of established deficits or excesses, ongoing losses or stress-induced compartmental redistributions (algorithm 4).

Assessment (algorithm 1)

Determine i.v. fluid requirements from:
- Clinical assessment of fluid balance including volume status (see later), jugular venous pressure (JVP)/central venous pressure (CVP), peripheral perfusion and the presence of fluid-related complications (e.g. peripheral oedema, lung crackles).
- Monitored variables including fluid charts of input (e.g. resuscitation fluids, feed) and output (e.g. urine output, gastrointestinal loss, drainage) and serial body weights.
- Daily measurements of serum (occasionally urinary) electrolytes, urea and creatinine. Arterial pH, base excess and serial lactate measurements may indicate poor tissue perfusion.

Day-to-day trends in these parameters often guide i.v. fluid prescription. The response to a 'fluid challenge' (~250 mls) may determine the need for volume replacement (Chapter 8).

Resuscitation (algorithm 2)

In acute illness, the need for immediate intervention limits initial assessment, which is based on the ABCDE approach (i.e. A-Airway, B-Breathing, C-Circulation, D-Disability and E-Exposure (Chapters 1, 5), clinical context, volume status (i.e. systolic pressure <100–110 mmHg, heart rate >90 beats/min, respiratory rate >20/min, cold peripheries with capillary refill >2 secs and response to a 45° passive leg raising) and national early warning scores (NEWS). Full clinical evaluation occurs in subsequent reviews.

Treatment should address the underlying cause (e.g. sepsis) and may include high-flow oxygen. After insertion of a wide-bore cannula, assess the response to a 500 ml bolus of crystalloid (containing sodium in the range of 130–154 mmol/L) given over ~15 min. Further boluses of 250–500 mls are given until haemodynamic improvement is achieved. Then continue fluid management using algorithms 3 and 4 (see later). If no improvement has occurred after 2 L fluid administration, seek further advice and consider other options (e.g. more fluid, inotropes).

Routine maintenance (algorithm 3)

After initial assessment of fluid status and exclusion of complex replacement issues (e.g. ongoing losses), clinically stable patients who are unable to take oral or enteral fluid (e.g. unsafe swallow) require replacement of normal daily water losses (~25–30 ml/kg/day; ~1.5 L urine and ~0.5 L insensible lung water/sweat), electrolytes (~1 mmol/kg/day of potassium, sodium and chloride in urine and sweat) and 50–100 g/day of glucose to prevent ketosis. Consider lower volumes (25 mls/kg/day) in older or obese patients, and those with renal or cardiac impairment. Many fluid combinations can be used (e.g. sodium chloride 0.18% in dextrose 4%) but, to avoid the risk of hyponatraemia, routine i.v. maintenance regimens should not exceed 25–35 ml/kg/day especially in older people. Initially fluid status should be re-assessed daily.

Replacement and/or redistribution (algorithm 4)

Critically ill patients cannot maintain water and electrolyte balance as hormonal responses alter compartmental distributions and inflammation increases leakage of plasma proteins and water into interstitial fluid (ISF). This causes 'intravascular' hypovolaemia, peripheral oedema and impaired gas exchange due to pulmonary oedema. In addition, initial fluid resuscitation with sodium-containing fluids, and catabolic urea production, increase solute loads that are difficult to excrete due to impaired renal function (Chapter 9). Water and electrolyte homeostasis is further complicated by losses from fistula, vomiting, burns or trauma.

Fluid prescription in complex cases with established deficits, fluid excesses/oedema (e.g. previous resuscitation), ongoing losses (e.g. high output ileal stomas and fluid/electrolyte redistributions requires careful adjustments of the normal daily fluid/electrolyte regimen in algorithm 3 (i.e. addition to, or subtraction from, normal daily maintenance requirements).

General fluid management

I.v. fluid prescriptions should include the type, rate and volume of fluid to be administered and frequency of re-assessment (i.e. at least daily, frequently in unstable patients). Correct for other fluid and electrolyte sources (e.g. drug regimens, blood transfusions). Fluid choice (Chapter 11) is determined by fluid and electrolyte requirements, electrolyte concentrations in available i.v. fluids and the clinical scenario. Stop i.v. fluids when patients are clinically stable and able to tolerate oral or enteral fluids.

Types of fluid

- **Crystalloid solutions** are water to which solutes (e.g. NaCl, glucose) have been added. They are inexpensive, isotonic and redistribute rapidly after i.v. infusion (~1–4 h) from intravascular to other fluid compartments (e.g. extracellular fluid [ECF], intracellular fluid [ICF]; Chapter 9). Consequently, large volumes are needed to maintain intravascular volumes, which may cause interstitial (peripheral) oedema. Low-sodium fluids (e.g. 5% dextrose) disperse throughout the ICF and ECF. In contrast sodium-containing fluids (e.g. normal saline) are restricted to ECF (i.e. cellular pumps remove ICF sodium) and therefore have a smaller volume of distribution (i.e. slightly more is intravascular), an advantage in resuscitation. The use of hypertonic crystalloids (e.g. 7.5% saline) for resuscitation (i.e. to osmotically 'pull' ICF water into the ECF) has not improved outcome in general trauma patients. However, the osmotic effects and small fluid resuscitation volumes may beneficially reduce cerebral oedema after head trauma.
- **Colloid solutions** are expensive and meta-analysis has shown no benefit, and potential harm, compared to crystalloids. Synthetic colloids include gelatin, dextran and hydroxyethel starch (HES). Theoretically, these large molecules remain intravascular longer, exerting an oncotic pressure that pulls water into, and expands, the intravascular compartment. It is often erroneously quoted that 4–5 times as much crystalloid is required for equivalent resuscitation as colloid but recent data showed that the volume ratio of 4% albumin to saline was 1:1.4. Albumin may be beneficial in hypoalbuminaemic (<15 g/dL) patients with severe sepsis and in acute respiratory distress syndrome to aid lung water clearance. Disadvantages of colloids include allergic reactions, clotting abnormalities and AKI. HES has recently been withdrawn from use following evidence of increased mortality and AKI.
- **Blood** is given to maintain haemoglobin concentration >70–80 g/L but young patients with renal disease, haemoglobinopathies or chronic anaemia may tolerate lower levels. A haemoglobin ≥100 g/L improves outcome in cardiac patients.
- **Bicarbonate** use is controversial but may be used in metabolic acidosis (pH < 7.2) due to renal or gastrointestinal losses.

11 Fluid management: fluid choice

Figure 11a Composition of crystalloids and colloids

Fluid	Na (mmol/L)	K (mmol/L)	Cl (mmol/L)	Osmolarity (mosmol/L)	Additions (mmol/L)	
Crystalloids						
Dextrose 5%	0	0	0	278	Glucose: 278	
0.9% saline	154	0	154	308	Nil	
Hartmann's	131	5.4	112	275	HCO_3 29; Ca 1.8	
Ringer's	130	4.2	109	273	Ca 2.2	
Colloids					T½ (hrs)	PVE
Gelofusin	154	0	154	279	~2	80%
Isoplex	145	4	105	284	~2	80%
5% Albumin	130–160	0	?	300	2–4h	100%
Voluven	154	0	154	308	~5	120%
10% HES	154	0	154	308	6–12	145%

T½ = Approximate effective plasma half life

PVE = Plasma volume expansion (% of volume given)

HES = Hydroxyethyl starch

MW = molecular weight

PVD = peripheral vascular disease

RES = reticuloendothelial system

Figure 11b Properties of colloid solutions

Colloid (MW in Da)	Properties	Disadvantages
Gelatins ~30,000	Cheap and rapidly degraded to water. Maximum volume 1.5–2.0 L daily	Allergic reactions
Dextrans ~40-70,000	~30% intravascular at 24hrs. ↓ serum viscosity, so used in PVD and as DVT prophylaxis. Renal and RES clearance	Bleeding risk. Interferes with blood tests. Allergy 5%. Osmotic diuresis and renal impairment
Hydroxyethyl starch ~50-500,000	Good plasma volume expansion and long intravascular times. Renal and RES clearance. Drug licence recently suspended due to possible ↑ in mortality	Accumulates in macrophages. Bleeding risk. ↑renal impairment. Possible↑in mortality. Pruritis
Albumin ~68,000	Few advantages over synthetic colloids. May improve outcome in severe sepsis. Expensive	Infection risks Allergic reactions

Large volume infusions of electrolyte containing crystalloid or colloid solutions engender substantial solute (i.e. Na^+/Cl^- ions) loads (Figures 11a and 11b), which may be difficult to excrete in critically ill patients with renal impairment. The retained solutes may have a significant physiological impact and can cause harm. For example, high chloride (Cl^-) levels following infusion of large volumes of NaCl-containing solutions (e.g. 0.9% saline, most colloids) may precipitate hyperchloraemic acidosis (HCA) with associated nausea, vomiting, confusion, oliguria and further renal impairment. In these circumstances, a physiologically balanced solution (PBS) with a lower Cl^- content (e.g. Hartmann's solution; Figure 11a) is preferred because HCA is less common.

Fluid choice

Selection of an appropriate intravenous fluid can be difficult and must balance the immediate clinical requirement with the consequences resulting from, or inability to subsequently excrete, the infused solution. For example, fluid resuscitation may be essential to maintain life in acute sepsis but the associated renal impairment may result in subsequent life-threatening fluid overload. Although fluid guidelines have been produced for some conditions (e.g. sepsis; Chapter 25), in general there are no specific/simple algorithms for fluid choice and benefits must be balanced against individual risks. However, there are a few basic principles:

• **For resuscitation**: Na^+-containing fluids (130–154 mmol/L) tend to have a smaller volume of distribution and best improve vascular expansion. Large volumes risk HCA (see earlier) and PBS (e.g. Hartmann's) with lower Cl^- contents may reduce this risk and should be considered. Crystalloid solutions are generally preferred because there is no conclusive evidence that colloids are more effective and some may be harmful (Figure 11b). In Europe, drug licences for hydroxyethyl starches have been withdrawn in

response to concerns about increased mortality and renal impairment risks.

• **In physiologically stable patients** requiring maintenance fluids, limited volumes (25–35 ml/kg/day) of low Na^+/electrolyte fluids (e.g. 0.18% or 0.45% saline) may be used to replace normal daily fluid and electrolyte losses. Larger volumes of these fluids risk hyponatraemia especially in older people.

• **Complex patients** may have significant fluid and electrolyte accumulation and redistribution due to acute illness (±fluid resuscitation) or physiological, stress-induced, homeostatic mechanisms that promote salt and water retention. These patients require careful adjustment of their routine fluid maintenance regimen to correct for established deficits, ongoing losses, previous excessive resuscitation and distribution abnormalities (Chapters 9, 10). Fluid choice must be individually tailored from available fluids (Figure 11a) to deliver the calculated daily fluid and electrolytes requirements.

For example, a post-operative patient will need their routine maintenance regimen corrected to address stress-induced physiological changes that increase ADH (vasopressin) secretion, causing significant water (±Na^+) retention that tends to promote hyponatraemia. In these circumstances, slightly less fluid (±higher Na^+ content) would reduce the risk of hyponatraemia. If the patient also had 2 L of nasogastric tube fluid loss, the associated water, Na^+, Cl^- and hydrogen ion (H^+) loss would need to be corrected by giving 2 L of 0.9% saline with large K^+ supplements. The K^+ is required to correct the associated metabolic (hypochloraemic) alkalosis by facilitating H^+/K^+ exchange in the kidney (i.e. renal K^+ loss to retain H^+). The haemoglobin should be maintained at ≥7–9 g/dL in the stable patient and ≥10 g/dL in unstable cardiac patients (e.g. ischaemic heart disease). Remember that large fluid requirements may indicate internal bleeding.

Critical Care Medicine at a Glance, Third Edition. Richard Leach. © 2014 John Wiley & Sons, Ltd. Published 2014 by John Wiley & Sons, Ltd.

12 Inotropes and vasopressors

Figure 12a   Properties of inotropic drugs

Vasoactive Agent	Receptors (▮ = main effect) or action	Midrange dose effects		
		Inotropic contractility	Chronotrope (heart rate)	Vaso-constrictor
Inoconstrictors				
Epinephrine	α, β₁, β₂	++++	+++	++
Dopamine	α, β₁, β₂	+++	++	– to ++
Inodilators				
Dobutamine	α, β₁, β₂	+++	+	– to ±
Milrinone	PDI (↑cAMP)	+++	0	– –
Enoximone	PDI (↑cAMP)	+++	0	–
Vasoconstrictor				
Norepinephrine	α, β₁	+/++	0	++++
Phenylephrine	α, β₁	+	0	++++

PDI=phosphodiesterase inhibitor;
cAMP=cyclic adenosine monophosphate;
– = vasodilation

Inotropes and vasopressors provide additional haemodynamic support if optimal fluid resuscitation (Chapters 8, 9) and heart rate control do not correct circulatory failure. The aim is to achieve effective tissue perfusion rather than a specific blood pressure (BP) that may differ between subjects (e.g. hypertensives require higher BP). Vasoactive drugs are relatively ineffective in volume-depleted patients and an adequate circulating volume is essential. Similarly, acidosis (pH < 7.1) and electrolyte derangements (e.g. hypokalaemia, hypomagnesaemia) impair inotropic drug actions and should be corrected to ensure maximal pressor effects. These agents must be administered through central lines to avoid tissue necrosis from extravasation.

Monitoring The effects of these agents in an individual case are unpredictable. The response must be closely monitored and therapy titrated to specific end points (e.g. mean arterial pressure [MAP] 65–70 mmHg, urine output). In general, all haemodynamically unstable patients receiving vasoactive drugs require continuous intra-arterial BP monitoring, preferably from a large artery (e.g. femoral), because smaller arteries (e.g. radial) often underestimate systemic pressures in shocked patients. Volume status is most conveniently assessed with a central venous catheter but in complex cases haemodynamic monitoring of cardiac output (CO), systemic vascular resistance (SVR), left-sided filling pressures and lung water may be necessary to maintain optimal tissue perfusion (Chapter 3).

Selection of appropriate vasopressor therapy requires an understanding of an agent's cardiovascular properties, knowledge of adrenergic receptor distribution and actions, and an accurate assessment of the underlying haemodynamic disturbance. The pharmacological properties and receptor activation of individual agents is presented in Figure 12a. Activation of α receptors causes peripheral vasoconstriction, β₁ **receptors** are chronotropic (i.e.

increase heart rate) and inotropic (i.e. increase the force and velocity of myocardial contractility and consequently BP and CO), whereas β₂ **receptors** cause vasodilation and bronchodilation. An individual drug may activate several receptors (e.g. epinephrine [adrenaline] has α, β₁, β₂ properties) but the balance varies (i.e. dobutamine also has α, β₁, β₂ properties but β₁, β₂ effects are greater than α properties). Ideally a single drug should be used but occasionally the correct balance of receptor stimulation may require drug combinations. Both vasopressin and low dose steroids (e.g. hydrocortisone 8 mg/h) may have a 'catecholamine sparing' effect, particularly in septic shock.

Opinions differ between institutions and countries as to optimal therapy in specific situations. In the absence of conclusive evidence, the controversy is likely to continue.

• **In septic shock**, profound vasodilation causes hypotension despite a high CO. Current evidence supports the initial use of norepinephrine (±epinephrine), which is primarily an α-vasoconstrictor, to maintain CO, BP and organ perfusion. However, prolonged sepsis may impair cardiac contractility requiring later addition of a β₁-inotropic agent to maintain CO (e.g. dobutamine).

• **In myocardial ischaemia**, dobutamine's β₁ properties increase cardiac contractility without raising myocardial oxygen consumption, while β₂-vasodilator properties reduce 'afterload' and increase CO. However, norepinephrine-mediated α-vasoconstriction may be required to offset hypotension induced by high-dose dobutamine β₂-vasodilation.

• **In systolic heart failure**, most catecholamines (e.g. dopamine, dobutamine, epinephrine) effectively support the circulation. Milrinone, a phosphodiesterase inhibitor increases cardiac contractility while reducing both systemic afterload and pulmonary hypertension due to vasodilation. It is often favoured in low output cardiac failure, diastolic dysfunction and catecholamine resistance (Chapter 34) but may be associated with an increased risk of atrial arrhythmias and hypotension.

• **'Renal protection'**: Augmentation of MAP to prevent or ameliorate renal failure can be achieved with many catecholamines (e.g. dopamine, norepinephrine). The concept that drug concentration influences receptor stimulation is controversial. In particular, there is no evidence that low-concentration 'renal dose' dopamine increases renal blood flow by stimulating dopaminergic receptors. It is no longer recommended.

Other methods of circulatory support are occasionally required. Cardiac pacemakers increase CO (Chapter 34) and ventilatory support reduces cardiorespiratory work, systemic afterload and pulmonary oedema (Chapter 18). Intra-aortic balloon pumps are valuable in ischaemic heart disease (IHD), ventricular septal defect (VSD) and while awaiting heart transplantation. They are sited in the descending aorta above the renal arteries. Diastolic balloon inflation enhances coronary and systemic perfusion pressures while systolic deflation increases CO by reducing afterload. Complications include renal and mesenteric ischaemia, infection and aortic dissection. Left ventricular assist devices are currently being developed.

Critical Care Medicine at a Glance, Third Edition. Richard Leach. © 2014 John Wiley & Sons, Ltd. Published 2014 by John Wiley & Sons, Ltd.

13 Failure of oxygenation and respiratory failure

Figure 13a Relationship between oxygen tension (P_O_2) and haemoglobin saturation (S_O_2)

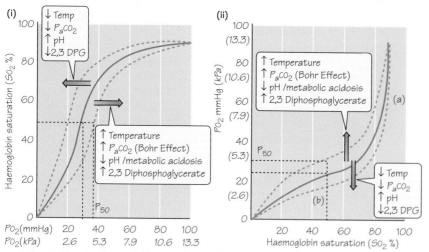

(i)
↓ Temp
↓ P_aCO_2
↑ pH
↓ 2,3 DPG

↑ Temperature
↑ P_aCO_2 (Bohr Effect)
↓ pH /metabolic acidosis
↑ 2,3 Diphosphoglycerate

(ii)
↑ Temperature
↑ P_aCO_2 (Bohr Effect)
↓ pH /metabolic acidosis
↑ 2,3 Diphosphoglycerate

↓ Temp
↓ P_aCO_2
↑ pH
↓ 2,3 DPG

Left: traditional oxyhaemoglobin curve showing effect of temperature, pH and 2,3 diphosphoglycerate.
Right: realigned to show its two key features (a) haemoglobin maintains high levels of saturation despite falling oxygen tension (i.e. pick up of oxygen in the lung is maintained despite reduced oxygen tension) (b) oxygen tension remains fairly stable as oxyhaemoglobin saturation falls (i.e. oxygen delivery to tissues maintained despite falling oxyhaemoglobin saturation)

Figure 13b Pathophysiological mechanisms of tissue hypoxia

Arterial Hypoxaemia
1. Low inspired partial pressure of oxygen (e.g. high altitude)
2. Alveolar hypoventilation (e.g. drugs, sleep apnoea)
3. Ventilation/perfusion mismatch (e.g. patchy consolidation)
4. Right to left shunts (e.g. atrial septal defect, PAVM)

Failure of oxygen-haemoglobin transport
1. Inadequate tissue perfusion
2. Low haemoglobin concentration (e.g. anaemia)
3. Reduced oxygen dissociation (e.g. haemoglobinopathies)
4. Failure of oxygen utilisation (e.g. sepsis, cyanide poisoning)

Figure 13d Effect of true shunt (Q_S/Q_T) and ventilation/perfusion mismatch on the arterial oxygen tension (P_aO_2) and inspired oxygen fraction (F_iO_2) relationship

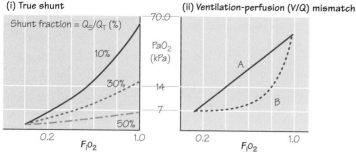

(i) True shunt
Shunt fraction = Q_S/Q_T (%)
10%
30%
50%

(ii) Ventilation-perfusion (V/Q) mismatch
A
B

Hypoxaemia caused by true right to left shunt is refractory to supplemental O_2 when 'shunt fraction' exceeds 30%

Reductions in P_aO_2 caused by V/Q mismatch respond to O_2 but the response depends on whether there are many units with mild V/Q mismatch (A) or a few units with very low V/Q ratios (B)

Figure 13c Alveolar oxygen tension and alveolar-arterial oxygen tension difference

Alveolar oxygen tension: as derived from the simplified alveolar gas equation

$$P_AO_2 = P_iO_2 - (1.25 \times P_aCO_2)$$

where

$P_iO_2 = F_iO_2 \times (\text{barometric} - \text{water vapour pressure})$
Breathing air; $P_iO_2 = 0.21 \times (101 - 6.2) = 19.9\,kPa$

$$P_AO_2 \text{ (breathing air)} = 19.9 - (1.25 \times 5.3)$$
$$= \sim13.5 \text{ kPa}$$

Alveolar-arterial oxygen tension difference

$$P_{(A-a)}O_2 = P_AO_2 - P_aO_2$$
$$= \sim13.5 - \sim13 = <1.0 \text{ kPa (breathing air)}$$

P_AO_2 = alveolar oxygen tension, P_iO_2 = Inspired oxygen tension, F_iO_2 = fractional concentration of oxygen in inspired air, $P_{(A-a)}O_2$ = alveolar-arterial oxygen tension difference, P_aO_2 = arterial oxygen tension, P_aCO_2 = arterial CO_2 tension

Figure 13e Calculation of shunt fraction or venous admixture (Q_S/Q_T)

$$Q_S/Q_T = (C_cO_2 - C_aO_2) / (C_cO_2 - C_vO_2)$$
Where C denotes oxygen content and c, a and v denote end capillary, arterial or venous
(end capillary and calculated alveolar oxygen tensions are assumed to be equivalent)

$$C_{c,a,v}O_2 = [(Hb \times S_aO_2 \times k) + (P_aO_2 \times 0.023)]$$
Where: Hb = haemoglobin (g/l); k= coefficient of Hb oxygen binding capacity (1.36 ml O_2/g Hb); $P_aO_2 \times 0.023$ = oxygen dissolved in plasma*

Venous admixture in a man breathing air with a Hb 100 g/L, S_aO_2 85% and S_vO_2 50% is:
$$Q_S/Q_T = ([100 \times 0.98 \times 1.36] - [100 \times 0.85 \times 1.36]) / ([100 \times 0.98 \times 1.36] - [100 \times 0.5 \times 1.36]) = (135-115) / (135-68) = 0.3 = 30\% \text{ venous admixture}$$

The 'true shunt' (i.e. corrected for partial V/Q mismatch) is calculated using 100% O_2.
In this case on 100% O_2 the S_aO_2 was 95% and S_vO_2 = 60%
$$Q_S/Q_T = ([100 \times 1 \times 1.36] - [100 \times 0.95 \times 1.36]) / ([100 \times 1 \times 1.36] - [100 \times 0.6 \times 1.36]) = (136-129) / (136-82) = 0.13 = 13\% \text{ shunt}$$

Q_S/Q_T = shunt fraction; $C_{c,a,v}O_2$ = Oxygen content (ml/L); P_aO_2 = arterial O_2 tension; S_aO_2 = arterial oxygen saturation; S_vO_2 = mixed venous oxygen saturation; Hb = haemoglobin; V/Q = ventilation/perfusion ratio; P_aCO_2 = arterial CO_2 tension; *Oxygen dissolved in plasma is insignificant (i.e. not included in calculations)

Critical Care Medicine at a Glance, Third Edition. Richard Leach. © 2014 John Wiley & Sons, Ltd. Published 2014 by John Wiley & Sons, Ltd.

Tissues require oxygen for survival. Oxygen delivery (Do_2) depends on adequate ventilation, gas exchange and circulatory distribution. **Tissue hypoxia** occurs within 4 minutes of cardiorespiratory arrest because tissue, blood and lung oxygen reserves are small. **Causes** of tissue hypoxia (Figure 13b) can be classified into those resulting in: (a) arterial hypoxaemia, and (b) failure of the oxygen–haemoglobin transport system without arterial hypoxaemia.

Six pathophysiological mechanisms cause arterial hypoxaemia:
1 Low inspired oxygen partial pressure (Po_2) occurs at high altitude due to reduced barometric pressure, during fires due to O_2 combustion and after toxic fume inhalation.
2 Hypoventilation: failure to replenish alveolar O_2 as quickly as it is removed by haemoglobin uptake.
3 Shunt refers to venous blood that bypasses lung gas-exchange and passes directly into the systemic arterial system. Increasing inspired O_2 concentration (F_iO_2) has little effect on P_aO_2 when the 'true' shunt fraction is $\geq 30\%$ (Figure 13d[i]).
4 Ventilation/perfusion (V/Q) mismatch is the most frequent cause of hypoxaemia even in diseases like pulmonary fibrosis where diffusion limitation might be expected to predominate. Figure 13d(ii) illustrates that hypoxaemia due to venous admixture from many lung units with mild V/Q mismatch (Figure 13d[ii]: A) readily corrects with low-dose oxygen, whereas hypoxaemia due to a few lung units with severe V/Q mismatch (Figure 13d[ii]: B) (i.e. very poorly ventilated units) requires high-dose oxygen. Unventilated lung units produce true shunt (i.e. resulting hypoxaemia cannot be corrected with oxygen). Figure 13e illustrates the calculation of venous admixture due to V/Q mismatch and true shunt fraction. High V/Q units contribute to deadspace but not hypoxaemia.
5 Impaired diffusion is rarely clinically significant but may prevent equilibration of alveolar gas with capillary blood if capillary transit time is reduced (e.g. high cardiac output [CO], exercise).
6 Venous saturation: venous blood with a very low S_aO_2 returning to the right heart usually has little effect on arterial P_aO_2, but in patients with impaired gas exchange or low CO it may reduce P_aO_2.

Clinical features of tissue hypoxia are non-specific (e.g. altered mental state, dyspnoea, hyperventilation, arrhythmias, hypotension). Nevertheless, early recognition is required for successful therapy. **Central cyanosis** is detected when deoxygenated haemoglobin is >1.5–5 g/dl. It is an unreliable sign of hypoxia because it can be absent in hypoxic, anaemic patients but apparent in normoxic, polycythaemic subjects.

The oxygen-haemoglobin relationship is usually illustrated as in Figure 13a(i) but realignment as in Figure 13a(ii) demonstrates its key characteristics: (a) haemoglobin saturation remains high despite marked reductions in P_aO_2, and (b) P_aO_2 remains relatively stable as saturation declines. Temperature, pH and 2,3 diphosphoglycerate modulate this relationship. Compensatory mechanisms (e.g. rightward shift of the dissociation curve) ensure adequate tissue Do_2 in chronic hypoxia.

Monitoring oxygenation (Chapter 3)

• **Arterial Po_2** (P_aO_2) is the tension driving oxygen into tissues. **Arterial So_2** (S_aO_2) reflects how much oxygen is being carried by haemoglobin molecules. **Pulse oximetry** and **blood gas analysis** measure S_aO_2 and P_aO_2 respectively, and are the principal measures used to initiate, monitor and adjust oxygen therapy. However, they can be normal when tissue hypoxia is caused by low CO, anaemia or impaired oxygen utilization. In these circumstances, **mixed venous oxygen saturation** (S_vO_2) <55–60% (normal $>70\%$) reflects inadequate Do_2 better (Chapter 3).
• **P_aO_2/F_iO_2 ratio** is a convenient index of oxygen exchange that adjusts for F_iO_2.
• **Alveolar-arterial oxygen gradient** ($P_{(A-a)}O_2$) determines efficiency of gas exchange. The P_AO_2 is calculated from the simplified alveolar gas equation (Figure 13c), which by incorporating P_aCO_2 eliminates hypoventilation and hypercapnia as causes of hypoxaemia (i.e. high P_aCO_2 lowers P_AO_2). The A – a gradient – is increased by shunts, V/Q mismatch and diffusion impairment. It is normally ~ 0.2–0.4 kPa but increases with age and F_iO_2.
• **Individual organ ischaemia** is difficult to detect. Most techniques have significant limitations (e.g. gastric tonometry).

Respiratory failure (RF) may be acute, chronic or acute-on-chronic. It is due to inadequate gas exchange and is defined as an arterial oxygen (P_aO_2) <8 kPa or arterial carbon dioxide (P_aCO_2) >6 kPa. These patients must be monitored (e.g. S_aO_2) in an appropriate facility (e.g. high dependency unit [HDU]) and treatment directed at the underlying cause:
• **Type I RF is due to failure of oxygenation**: it occurs when blood bypasses or is not fully oxygenated in the lungs causing **hypoxaemia** (i.e. low P_aO_2). P_aCO_2 is normal or low because ventilation is unchanged or increased due to breathlessness. **Causes** include V/Q mismatch (e.g. pneumonia), right to left shunts (e.g. heart defects), low F_iO_2 (e.g. altitude) and impaired diffusion (e.g. during exercise in pulmonary fibrosis). P_aO_2 usually improves with oxygen therapy (Chapter 13) but re-expansion/recruitment of collapsed alveoli and reduction of V/Q mismatch may be equally effective (Chapters 13, 17). For example, continuous positive airways pressure may improve oxygenation by recruiting collapsed lung.
• **Type II RF is due to failure of ventilation**: hypoventilation reduces CO_2 clearance causing **hypercapnia** (high P_aCO_2) with, or occasionally without, hypoxaemia. Hypoventilation is either due to inadequate respiratory drive or ineffective ventilation. **Causes** include neuromuscular weakness (e.g. motor neurone disease), chest wall deformity (e.g. kyphoscoliosis), impaired respiratory drive (e.g. opioid overdose) and increased work of breathing (WoB) due to primary lung disease (e.g. chronic obstructive pulmonary disease [COPD]). In critical illness, the WoB required to ventilate abnormal lungs may be $>30\%$ of total O_2 consumption (normally $<5\%$). Ventilation is improved and WoB reduced by treating the precipitating cause, decreasing airways resistance (e.g. bronchodilation) and improving compliance (e.g. alveolar recruitment). If hypercapnia and acidosis persist, non-invasive ventilation (NIV) is often effective and widely available (Chapter 16).

Indications for mechanical ventilation in RF include a respiratory rate (RR) >35/min, $P_aO_2 < 8$ kPa on $>50\% F_iO_2$; $P_aCO_2 > 7.5$ kPa, pH < 7.25, decreased conscious level (Glasgow Coma Score [GCS] <8), poor secretion clearance, exhaustion and failure to improve after 1–4 hours on NIV.

Pearl of wisdom
Hypoxaemia due to a shunt fraction (Qs/Qt) > 30% can rarely be corrected with oxygen alone; consider alveolar recruitment techniques

14 Oxygenation and oxygen therapy

Figure 14a Indications for acute oxygen therapy

1. Cardiac and respiratory arrest
2. Hypoxaemia (P_aO_2 <8kPa, S_aO_2 <90%)
3. Hypotension (systolic BP <100mmHg)
4. Low cardiac output
5. Metabolic acidosis (bicarbonate <18mmol/l)
6. Respiratory distress (respiratory rate >24/min)

Figure 14b Oxygen prescription chart

Drug: Oxygen	Time (h)	Date/time administered Initials and S_aO_2						
Circle target oxygen saturation								
88–92% 92–98% (94–98%) Other		4/8	5/8					
Starting device/flow rate *NC 2l/min*	06	*Rl* 94%	*Rl* 92%					
PRN/Continuous (see O_2 guidelines)	09	*Rl* 90%						
Tick here if saturation not indicated* __	14	*Rl* 94%						
Signature and date *PPolly 4/8/09*	18	*Rl* 95%						
PRINT NAME Dr Pretty Polly	22	*Rl* 94%						

*Saturation is indicated in most cases except palliative terminal care
NC = nasal cannulae

Figure 14d Indications for acute oxygen therapy

1. Variable performance devices

Air is entrained during breathing whilst oxygen is delivered from a reservoir (i.e. mask, reservoir bag, nasopharynx)

The F_iO_2 delivered to the lungs depends on the oxygen flow rate, the patient's inspiratory flow, respiratory rate and the amount of air entrained

e.g. Figure (i) 'Low-flow face masks', O_2 flows at ~2–10 L/min into the mask and is supplemented by air drawn into the mask. The F_iO_2 achieved depends on ventilation

Ventilation = 5 L/min
O_2 flow = 2 L/min; Air (21% O_2) flow = 3 L/min
F_iO_2 = (2+0.21 x 3)/5 x 100 = **53%**

Ventilation = 25 L/min
O_2 flow = 2 L/min; Air (21% O_2) flow = 23 L/min
F_iO_2 = (2+0.21 x 23)/25 x 100 = **27%**

These devices cannot be used if accurate control of F_iO_2 is desirable, e.g. COPD with hypercapnia

Examples of variable performance devices are 'low-flow' facemasks (see i), nasal cannulae (see ii) and non-rebreathing facemasks with reservoir bags (see iii)

2. Fixed performance devices

Are independent of the patient's pattern of breathing and inspiratory volume

Figure (iv) illustrates that a fixed O_2 flow through a Venturi valve entrains the correct proportion of air to achieve the required O_2 concentration

This system delivers more gas than is inspired (i.e. >30 L/min). Consequently, F_iO_2 is less affected by the breathing pattern. The resulting masks are high flow, low concentration and fixed performance

Used in patients with COPD and respiratory failure to avoid CO_2 retention

Figure 14c Risks associated with high dose oxygen therapy

1. **Carbon dioxide retention:**
   ~10% of breathless patients, mainly COPD, have type II respiratory failure (RF). ~40–50% of COPD patients are at risk of type II RF
2. **Rebound hypoxaemia:**
   occurs if oxygen is suddenly withdrawn in type II RF
3. **Absorption collapse**
   O_2 in poorly ventilated alveoli is rapidly absorbed causing collapse; whereas N_2 absorption is slow
4. **Pulmonary oxygen toxicity**
   F_iO_2>60% may damage alveolar membranes causing ARDS if inhaled for >24–48 hrs (chapter 42). Hyperoxia can cause coronary and cerebral vasospasm
5. **Fire**
   Deaths and burns occur in smokers during O_2 therapy
6. **Paul-Bert effect**
   Hyperbaric O_2 can cause cerebral vasoconstriction and epileptic fits

(i) 'Low-flow' facemask

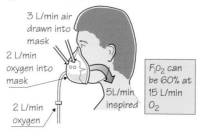

3 L/min air drawn into mask

2 L/min oxygen into mask

2 L/min oxygen

5L/min inspired O_2

F_iO_2 can be 60% at 15 L/min

O_2 flows at ~2–15 L/min into the mask and is supplemented by air drawn into the mask. Flow rate must be > 5 L/min to prevent CO_2 rebreathing

(ii) Nasal cannulae

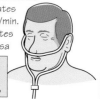

O_2 flow rates up to 4 L/min. Higher rates dry mucosa

F_iO_2 is between 24–35%

The O_2 flow is constant so F_iO_2 varies with ventilatory volume. More comfortable and not removed during eating or coughing. O_2 inhaled even when mouth breathing

(iii) Non-rebreathing and anaesthetic masks

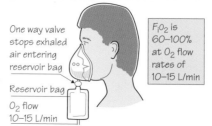

One way valve stops exhaled air entering reservoir bag

Reservoir bag

O_2 flow 10–15 L/min

F_iO_2 is 60–100% at O_2 flow rates of 10–15 L/min

High (10–15 L/min) flow rates of O_2 provide high F_iO_2 >60% and up to 100%

Non-rebreathing masks have a reservoir bag which should be filled before use. They increase F_iO_2 by preventing O_2 loss during expiration

(iv) 'High-flow' (Venturi), low concentration facemask

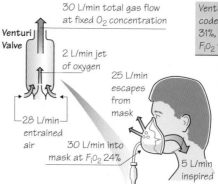

30 L/min total gas flow at fixed O_2 concentration

Venturi Valve

2 L/min jet of oxygen

25 L/min escapes from mask

28 L/min entrained air

30 L/min into mask at F_iO_2 24%

5 L/min inspired

Venturi valves are colour coded and deliver 24%, 28%, 31%, 35%, 40% or 60% F_iO_2 for a fixed flow rate

Continuous positive airways pressure (CPAP) masks
Use a tight fitting mask and a flow generator to deliver a fixed F_iO_2 with a positive pressure (5–10 cm/H_2O) throughout the respiratory cycle

Critical Care Medicine at a Glance, Third Edition. Richard Leach. © 2014 John Wiley & Sons, Ltd. Published 2014 by John Wiley & Sons, Ltd.

Management of arterial hypoxaemia requires: (a) treatment of the cause (e.g. pneumonia), (b) supplemental oxygen to increase inspired oxygen concentration (F_iO_2), and (c) reduction of ventilation/perfusion (V/Q) mismatch (Chapter 13) by ensuring optimal ventilation, sputum clearance, bronchodilation and alveolar recruitment.

Oxygen therapy

Oxygen is widely available and commonly prescribed. When given correctly, it is a life-saving drug, but it is often used without evaluation of potential benefits and side effects. Figure 14a lists indications for initiating oxygen therapy. It should be prescribed on the drug chart (i.e. dose, delivery method, duration, target saturation), signed for by the doctor and documented by nursing staff at each drug round (Figure 14b). Initial oxygen saturation (S_aO_2) and associated F_iO_2 should be recorded. In emergency situations, oxygen is often started without prescription but therapy should be documented retrospectively. Immediate 'ABC' assessment (i.e. airway, breathing, circulation) is essential and confirms airway patency and good circulation.

The therapeutic aims of oxygen therapy depend on the risk of developing hypercapnic respiratory failure (HCRF).
- **In normal patients** (i.e. low risk of HCRF), aim to achieve a S_aO_2 of 94–98% if <70 years old and 92–98% if >70 years old (i.e. wider normal range in older people). These ranges ensure haemoglobin (Hb) is fully saturated (i.e. on the plateau of the oxygen–Hb dissociation curve). Consequently, increasing P_aO_2 further has no impact on oxygen delivery because little oxygen is dissolved in plasma (Chapter 13).
- **In patients at risk of HCRF** (e.g. neuromuscular disease, chronic obstructive pulmonary disease [COPD]), the target SaO_2 should be 88–92% pending arterial blood gas (ABG) analysis. A higher S_aO_2 has few advantages but results in hypoventilation, hypercapnia and respiratory acidosis in patients dependent on hypoxaemic respiratory drive.

Figure 14d illustrates the important features of oxygen delivery systems. Initial oxygen dose and delivery method depend on cause:
- **High-dose supplemental oxygen (≥60%)** is delivered through a non-rebreathing, reservoir mask at 10–15 L/min. It is given during cardiac or respiratory arrests, shock, major trauma, sepsis, carbon monoxide (CO) poisoning and other critical illness. Once clinical stability has been restored, the oxygen dose is reduced, while maintaining a S_aO_2 of 92–98%. Seriously ill patients at risk of HCRF are initially treated with high-dose oxygen pending ABG analysis.
- **Moderate-dose supplemental oxygen (40–60%)** is given in serious illnesses (e.g. pneumonia), through nasal cannulae (2–6 L/min) or simple facemasks (5–10 L/min), aiming for a S_aO_2 of 92–98%. A reservoir mask is substituted if the target S_aO_2 is not achieved.
- **Low-dose (controlled) supplemental oxygen (24–28%)** is delivered through a fixed performance Venturi mask. It is indicated in patients at risk of HCRF including COPD, neuromuscular disease, chest wall disorders, morbid obesity and cystic fibrosis. Long-term smokers >50 years old, with exertional dyspnoea and without another cause for breathlessness, are treated as COPD. The target S_aO_2 is 88–92% while awaiting ABG results. If P_aCO_2 is normal, S_aO_2 is adjusted to 92–98% (except in patients with previous HCRF) and ABG rechecked at 1 hour. If an air compressor is not available, nebulizers are driven with oxygen but for ≤6 min to

limit the risk of HCRF. A raised P_aCO_2 and bicarbonate with normal pH suggests longstanding hypercapnia and the target S_aO_2 should be 88–92% with repeat ABG at 1 hour. If the patient is hypercapnic ($P_aCO_2 > 6$ kPa) and acidotic (pH < 7.35), consider non-invasive ventilation (NIV), especially if the acidosis has persisted for >30 min despite appropriate therapy. Venturi masks are replaced with nasal cannulae (1–2 L/min) when the patient is stable. An oxygen alert card and Venturi mask are issued to patients with previous HCRF to warn future emergency staff of the potential risk.

Oxygen therapy is of little benefit in 'normoxic' patients because haemoglobin is fully saturated and oxygen solubility is low even at high P_aO_2. Early restoration of tissue blood flow is often more important in these cases. Oxygen therapy is of little value in myocardial infarction, drug overdoses, metabolic disorders, hyperventilation or non-hypoxic pregnant women in labour. It may be harmful in normoxic patients with strokes, paraquat poisoning, bleomycin lung injury or acid inhalation, and to the foetus in normoxic obstetric emergencies. However, in **CO poisoning**, high-dose oxygen is essential, despite a normal P_aO_2, to reduce carboxyhaemoglobin half-life (Chapter 76). Figure 14c reports the dangers of oxygen therapy.

Monitoring S_aO_2 should be measured regularly in all breathless patients and recorded on the observation chart with the oxygen dosage. In unstable patients, S_aO_2 is monitored continuously in high dependency areas. S_aO_2 is observed for 5 minutes after starting or changing oxygen dose and adjusted to achieve the target SaO_2. If possible, an ABG is measured before and within 1 hour of starting oxygen therapy, especially in those at risk of HCRF, and then at intervals to assess the response.

Stop oxygen therapy when the patient is clinically stable on low-dose oxygen (e.g. 1–2 L/min) and S_aO_2 is within the desired range on two consecutive occasions. Monitor S_aO_2 for 5 minutes after stopping oxygen and recheck at 1 hour. If S_aO_2 remains within the desired range, oxygen has been safely discontinued.

Other techniques to improve oxygenation

1 Anaemia: failure of tissue oxygen delivery is best corrected by blood transfusion (Chapter 5).
2 Secretion retention requires physiotherapy, mucolytic agents (e.g. N-acetylcysteine) and occasionally bronchoscopy to remove impacted sputum plugs and improve alveolar ventilation.
3 Fluid restriction reduces alveolar oedema in settings of increased alveolar permeability (e.g. acute respiratory distress syndrome [ARDS]).
4 Alveolar recruitment improves oxygenation by reducing V/Q mismatch and shunt (Chapter 13). Simple postural changes, regular turning and prone positioning improve secretion drainage and oxygenation in supine patients. Sitting upright optimizes V/Q matching in the alert patient. Techniques that increase mean alveolar pressures (e.g. positive end-expiratory pressure [PEEP], continuous positive airways pressure [CPAP], increased I : E ratio) also improve alveolar recruitment and oxygenation (Chapters 18, 42).
5 Ventilatory support (e.g. NIV) improves oxygenation by correcting hypoventilation and associated hypercapnia (Chapter 16).

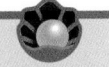

Pearl of wisdom

Oxygen is like any other medication; it should be prescribed, monitored and stopped when appropriate

15 Airways obstruction and management

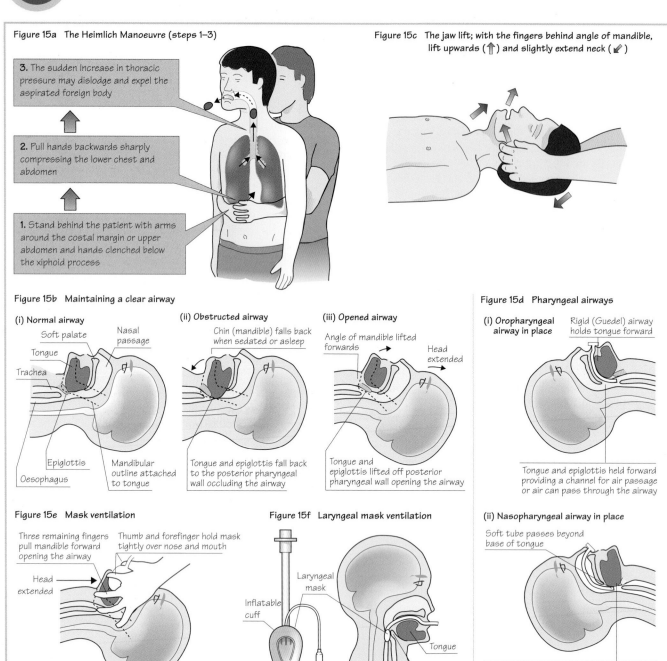

Figure 15a The Heimlich Manoeuvre (steps 1–3)

3. The sudden increase in thoracic pressure may dislodge and expel the aspirated foreign body

2. Pull hands backwards sharply compressing the lower chest and abdomen

1. Stand behind the patient with arms around the costal margin or upper abdomen and hands clenched below the xiphoid process

Figure 15c The jaw lift; with the fingers behind angle of mandible, lift upwards (⬆) and slightly extend neck (✎)

Figure 15b Maintaining a clear airway

(i) Normal airway
Soft palate
Nasal passage
Tongue
Trachea
Epiglottis
Oesophagus
Mandibular outline attached to tongue

(ii) Obstructed airway
Chin (mandible) falls back when sedated or asleep
Tongue and epiglottis fall back to the posterior pharyngeal wall occluding the airway

(iii) Opened airway
Angle of mandible lifted forwards
Head extended
Tongue and epiglottis lifted off posterior pharyngeal wall opening the airway

Figure 15d Pharyngeal airways

(i) Oropharyngeal airway in place
Rigid (Guedel) airway holds tongue forward
Tongue and epiglottis held forward providing a channel for air passage or air can pass through the airway

Figure 15e Mask ventilation
Three remaining fingers pull mandible forward opening the airway
Thumb and forefinger hold mask tightly over nose and mouth
Head extended

Figure 15f Laryngeal mask ventilation
Laryngeal mask
Inflatable cuff
Tongue
Epiglottis

(ii) Nasopharyngeal airway in place
Soft tube passes beyond base of tongue
Tongue held forward providing a channel for air passage or air can pass through the airway

Critical Care Medicine at a Glance, Third Edition. Richard Leach. © 2014 John Wiley & Sons, Ltd. Published 2014 by John Wiley & Sons, Ltd.

Airways obstruction is a life-threatening emergency and is particularly perilous when cardiorespiratory function is compromised. Within minutes it causes arterial hypoxaemia, hypoxic brain injury, coma and death. Consequently, all emergency personnel must be able to establish and maintain a patent airway and ventilation.

Upper airways obstruction

Complete or partial upper airways obstruction (UAO) may occur at any level in the respiratory tract from the mouth to the trachea.

- **Complete obstruction** is characterized by absent air flow and breath sounds, chest wall intercostal recession, accessory muscle use and paradoxical abdominal movement (i.e. the abdomen is pulled in as the chest inflates, rather than the normal outward movement as the diaphragm descends).

- **Partial obstruction** reduces air flow despite increased respiratory effort and is usually noisy. Inspiratory stridor suggests laryngeal obstruction, snoring follows partial nasopharyngeal occlusion by the tongue (±palate), a distressing 'crowing' occurs during laryngeal spasm and expiratory wheeze indicates airways obstruction.

Recognition of airways obstruction utilizes the 'look, listen and feel' approach:

- **Look** for respiratory effort, paradoxical chest and abdominal wall movement, accessory muscle use (e.g. neck, shoulder) and tracheal tug. Examine the mouth for the cause of the obstruction (e.g. foreign bodies, secretions). Central cyanosis is a late sign.

- **Listen and feel** for airflow and reduced, absent, noisy or characteristic (e.g. stridor) breath sounds. Movement of air at the patient's mouth is detected by placing your cheek or hand immediately in front of the patient's mouth.

Oropharyngeal obstruction is often caused by the tongue, which falls backwards when normal muscle tone is reduced in drowsy, sedated or unconscious patients, obstructing normal airflow. Solid particulate matter (e.g. food, coins, teeth or vomit), laryngeal oedema (e.g. allergy, burns, inflammation), tumours and laryngeal spasm (e.g. due to foreign bodies, blood, secretions, inhaled toxic gas) may also cause oropharyngeal obstruction.

Tracheobronchial obstruction is caused by aspiration of particulate matter, bronchospasm, tumours or pulmonary oedema.

Airways management

In many cases of UAO, simple measures open the airway and aid ventilation. These include:

- **The Heimlich Manoeuvre** (Figure 15a): following aspiration of an object (e.g. food) that completely occludes the larynx or trachea, the subject is unable to speak or breathe and becomes rapidly cyanosed; a scenario that is often termed the 'café coronary' when partially masticated food is aspirated during swallowing. If a sharp blow to the back of the chest fails to dislodge the object, the Heimlich manoeuvre is attempted. The attendant stands behind the patient with his arms around the upper abdomen, just adjacent to the costal margin, and the hands clenched below the xiphoid process. The hands are pulled backwards sharply, compressing the upper abdomen and lower costal margin. The sudden increase in thoracic pressure may dislodge the object, which is then exhaled.

- **Airway clearance**: foreign bodies (e.g. dentures) and secretions are detected and removed by sweeping the index finger around the oral cavity. Head tilt, chin lift and jaw thrust (Figure 15b), whilst slightly extending the neck and lifting the mandible forward, relieves nasopharyngeal obstruction due to the tongue and upper airway structures. This restores the airway and airflow. Jaw thrust is the technique of choice in patients with potential cervical spine injury (Figure 15c).

- **Mechanical oropharyngeal airways** are firm plastic tubes, inserted through the nose or mouth, to bypass the relaxed tongue and establish an airway when manipulation of the mandible and neck is unsuccessful. They are useful during mask ventilation (see later), especially in edentulous patients.
  - **Rigid oropharyngeal (Guedel) airways (OPAs)** lift the tongue and epiglottis away from the posterior pharyngeal wall (Figure 15d[i]) and act as a 'bite-block' to reduce damage during jaw clenching. The airways are inserted upside down and rotated 180° into the functional position. Care is required to avoid damaging the teeth or increasing obstruction by pushing the tongue backwards. OPAs should only be used in obtunded patients because they provoke gag reflexes, vomiting and laryngospasm, and they should be removed when consciousness returns.
  - **Soft nasopharyngeal airways (SNPA)**: are firm (but compressible) tubes available in different sizes and diameters. After insertion, they extend beyond the base of the tongue creating an airway (Figure 15d[ii]). As they provoke less gag reflex, SNPAs are useful in alert patients and facilitate nasopharyngeal secretion removal. Topical nasal anaesthesia and lubrication (e.g. lidocaine [lignocaine] gel) reduce insertion discomfort although traumatic epistaxis is not uncommon. Continuous use risks infective (e.g. sinusitis) and erosive complications. Contraindications to SNPA include coagulopathy, nasal obstruction and basilar skull fractures.

- **Mask ventilation** enables ventilatory support and oxygen therapy in non-intubated patients. In conjunction with jaw lift, the increased oropharyngeal pressure delivered during ventilation alleviates UAO. **Anaesthetic facemasks** are available in many shapes and sizes to ensure a tight fit. OPAs alleviate difficulty associated with edentulous patients. Firm downward pressure on the mask with the thumb and forefinger maintains a seal while the mandible is simultaneously lifted with the three remaining fingers and the head extended to optimize the airway during ventilation (Figure 15e). A two-handed technique with an assistant to squeeze the bag may be required. Unfortunately, mask ventilation is occasionally impossible.

- **Laryngeal mask airways** are useful if intubation fails or is difficult. They sit over the laryngeal inlet allowing temporary positive pressure ventilation in sedated or obtunded patients (Figure 15f). Potential problems (e.g. aspiration, laryngospasm, gastric inflation, poor ventilation) limit intensive care unit (ICU) use.

- **Combitube** is an oesophageal-tracheal double lumen airway for use in pre-hospital emergencies by those without specialist airways skills. It is blindly inserted into the oropharynx up to the indicated markings and after inflation of the appropriate cuffs may aid ventilation.

If a patent airway and adequate ventilation cannot be achieved, consider **endotracheal intubation** by an appropriately trained clinician (Chapter 17). Occasionally, an **emergency cricothyroidotomy** or **surgical tracheostomy** is required to establish an airway (Chapter 19).

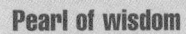

Pearl of wisdom

'Silent' respiratory distress in a 'choking, cyanosed' patient indicates complete upper airways obstruction; partial obstruction is usually noisy

16 Non-invasive ventilation

Figure 16a Benefits and limitations of positive pressure NIV

Benefits	Limitations

• Avoids complications associated with MV
  – pulmonary infection
  – pressure induced damage
• Avoids ETT complications
  – mini-aspiration
  – upper airway trauma
• Allows rest periods
• Preserves cough
• Allows oral nutrition
• Speech (+ decision making)
• Allows earlier mobilization
• Allows time to decide if MV is appropriate
	• Lack of airways protection
	• No endotracheal suction
	• Less complete correction of blood gases than with MV
	• Mask discomfort; eye damage
	  – prolonged use difficult
	• Ulceration over nasal bridge
	• Gastric dilation + vomiting
	  – may need NG tube
	• Limits ventilatory capacity
	• Increases nursing time
	• Needs patient reassurance
	• Intolerance + distress
	• Impedes sputum clearance

ETI = endotracheal intubation, MV= mechanical ventilation,
ETT = endotracheal tube; NIV= non-invasive ventilation;
CPAP = continuous positive airways pressure; NG = nasogastric

Figure 16b NIV/CPAP mask

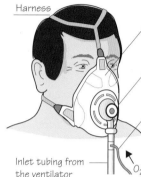

Harness

NIV/ CPAP masks may cover the nose and mouth or just the nose. Mouth leaks limit the value of nasal masks

Outlet valves may determine the expiratory positive airways pressure

Oxygen is entrained into the circuit. Therefore the F_iO_2 cannot be set only the O_2 flow rate (L/min)

Inlet tubing from the ventilator

O_2

Figure 16d Gastric dilation with CPAP

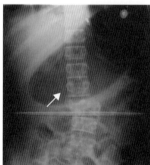

Gastro-oesophageal sphincter pressure is ≤12 cm H_2O. NIV masks may push air into the stomach causing dilation (→), risking vomiting/aspiration and bradycardia. A NG tube avoids this, but mask leaks can occur

Figure 16c Setting up non-invasive ventilation, problem solving and contraindications to NIV

Setting up a non-invasive ventilator

1. Set Mode
Pressure support ⌐ (assists inspiration e.g. in
Pressure control ⌐ acute hypercapnic COPD
CPAP (improves oxygenation e.g. in pneumonia, pulmonary oedema)

2. Set inspiratory positive airway pressure (IPAP)
Improves ventilation
Increases P_aO_2
Decreases P_aCO_2

9. Insert a filter
– bacterial or
– bacterial/viral

10. Ensure correct mask size to reduce leaks

4. Set timed inspiratory phase (Ti)
Only in pressure control
Set at 0.8–1.2 secs in acute hypercapnic COPD exacerbation

3. Set expiratory positive airway pressure (EPAP)
Improves oxygenation
Increases P_aO_2
May cause CO_2 retention

5. Set trigger sensitivity
Only in pressure control

11. Check an ABG before and within 1 hr of starting NIV

6. Set low flow alarm
Indicates circuit occlusion
(e.g. sputum plug)

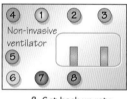

Non-invasive ventilator

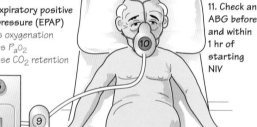

7. Set high flow alarm
Indicates excess leak
(e.g. circuit disconnection)

8. Set back up rate for apnoea

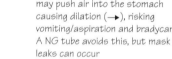

Problem solving in NIV

1. If P_aCO_2 remains elevated
Increase IPAP or decrease EPAP

2. If P_aO_2 remains low
Increase EPAP or IPAP or both
Increase F_iO_2

3. If patient-ventilator synchronization is poor
Adjust trigger sensitivity or adjust EPAP
Check mask size and fit

4. If the machine is cycling at the back up rate
The patient has either stopped breathing or is not triggering breaths

5. Factors that indicate NIV has failed
Failure of P_aCO_2 to decrease by 4–6 hrs
Failure of P_aO_2 to increase by 4–6 hrs
Reducing conscious level

Contraindications to NIV (but may be used if ceiling of therapy)
Facial trauma/burns/surgery
Oesophageal surgery
Severe hypoxaemia
Haemodynamic instability
Coma/confusion/claustrophobia
Active TB/epistaxis
Vomiting/bowel obstruction
Copious respiratory secretions
Fixed upper airway obstruction
Focal consolidation on CXR
Undrained pneumothorax

Figure 16e Factors associated with success and failure in NIV

Success
• High P_aCO_2
• Low A-a O_2 gradient
• pH 7.3–7.35
• Improvement in pH, P_aCO_2 and respiratory rate within 1 hr of NIV
• Good conscious level

Failure
• Pneumonia on CXR
• pH <7.25–7.3
• Copious respiratory secretions
• Edentulous/mask leak
• Poor patient–ventilator synchrony
• Poor nutritional status
• Impaired consciousness/confusion
• High APACHE score

Critical Care Medicine at a Glance, Third Edition. Richard Leach. © 2014 John Wiley & Sons, Ltd. Published 2014 by John Wiley & Sons, Ltd.

Non-invasive ventilation provides respiratory support, aids alveolar recruitment and reduces work of breathing (WoB) without the need for endotracheal intubation (ETI) and mechanical ventilation (MV). Negative and positive pressure techniques are available.

Negative pressure ventilation

Negative pressure ventilation (NPV) developed to support victims of poliomyelitis-induced respiratory paralysis. Affected patients were placed in **tank ventilators** ('iron lungs') sealed at the neck. Lowering tank pressure expanded the chest causing inspiration; expiration was passive. However, inadequate nursing access, poor carbon dioxide (CO_2) clearance and secretion retention limited use. Current techniques include **jacket (cuirass) ventilators** that localize external negative pressure to the chest region and **rocking beds** that utilize gravity to enhance diaphragmatic movement. NPV has been superseded by positive pressure techniques and use is now limited to specialist rehabilitation (e.g. spinal injury) or hypoventilation (e.g. kyphoscoliosis) centres.

Positive pressure ventilation

Positive pressure ventilation (PPV) is particularly effective in acute respiratory failure. It is delivered through full facemasks or helmets (Figure 16b). Nasal masks are more comfortable in stable patients. Figure 16a lists the benefits and disadvantages. PPV is most successful in alert, co-operative, haemodynamically stable patients who can protect and clear their airways (Figure 16e).

1 **Non-invasive ventilation (NIV)** refers to PPV that assists inspiration. Pressure-controlled (PC) modes compensate for mask leaks and have largely replaced volume-controlled modes (Chapter 18). Tidal volume is determined by lung ($\pm$chest wall) compliance and circuit resistance.

- **Pressure support (PS)**: the patient determines breath timing and frequency as respiratory effort 'triggers' the ventilator (i.e. assisted spontaneous breathing). Only pressure ($\sim$10–30 cmH$_2$O) is adjusted to support inspiration. Most PS ventilators have a 'back-up' breath rate of 6–8/min for patients who make no respiratory effort.
- **Bi-level pressure support** combines inspiratory positive airways pressure (IPAP; $\sim$30 cmH$_2$O) to aid inspiration and expiratory positive airways pressure (EPAP; $\sim$5 cmH$_2$O) to recruit underventilated lung and 'stent' open upper airways. EPAP also offsets intrinsic positive end-expiratory pressure (PEEP), which aids ventilator triggering (Chapter 18). These ventilators are cheap and easy to use.
- **Pressure-controlled ventilation (PCV)**: the decelerating flow of a PC breath improves distribution of ventilation. Inflation pressure, frequency and inspiratory time (T_i) are selected as required (e.g. T_i is set at $\sim$0.8–1.2 secs in acute hypercapnic chronic obstructive pulmonary disease [COPD]). A preset number of mandatory breaths are delivered in the absence of patient effort. Although patient triggering can occur, the breaths are identical to mandatory breaths. Triggered breaths delay (i.e. synchronize) the next machine-delivered breath (i.e. the spontaneous/timed [S/T] mode on NIV machines).

2 **Continuous positive airways pressure (CPAP)** is maintained throughout inspiration and expiration (e.g. 5–10 cm/H$_2$O) by a flow generator; it does not assist inspiration. Resulting alveolar recruitment (i.e. inflation of collapsed lung) reduces ventilation/perfusion (V/Q) mismatch and improves oxygenation. Consequently, CPAP is most effective in heart failure or acute lung injury (ALI). In obstructive sleep apnoea (OSA), it prevents upper airways collapse during sleep. Although CPAP is not usually considered respiratory support, the increase in functional residual capacity reduces WoB by making the lungs easier to inflate (i.e. the steep upstroke of the lung pressure–volume relationship). In patients with hyperinflation due to airways obstruction, further increases in lung volume may be detrimental, but, by offsetting intrinsic PEEP (e.g. in COPD), CPAP can reduce WoB, increase ventilation and reduce P_aCO_2 (Chapters 40, 41).

Indication for NIV and CPAP

NIV is most beneficial in patients with respiratory acidosis (pH < 7.35). Arterial blood gas (ABG) measurement is usually required in patients with acute breathlessness, neuromuscular disease, chest wall deformity, obesity or acute confusional states. Before starting, decide whether NIV will be the ceiling of treatment (e.g. end-stage COPD) or a therapeutic trial leading to ETI in the event of failure. Figure 16c illustrates how to optimize NIV and lists contraindications. Try NIV/CPAP if ABG do not rapidly improve with oxygen and medical therapy in patients with:

1 **Acute hypercapnic respiratory failure:**
- **COPD exacerbations**: mortality, MV rates and complications (e.g. pneumonia) are reduced with early NIV. In addition, pH, P_aCO_2 and respiratory rate usually improve within 1 hour.
- **Neuromuscular disease/chest wall deformity** (e.g. kyphoscoliosis): NIV is the treatment of choice in acute decompensation. In chronic respiratory failure, home NIV achieves 80% 5-year survival depending on bulbar involvement and severity.

2 **Cardiogenic pulmonary oedema**: CPAP reduces mortality and MV rates in patients who are hypoxaemic despite maximal medical treatment. NIV is less effective.

3 **OSA**: CPAP and NIV are equally effective in decompensated OSA. Bi-level pressure support is required in patients with respiratory acidosis.

4 **Weaning**: NIV may aid weaning of COPD patients from MV.

5 **Other conditions**: NIV is used with varying success in chest wall trauma, ALI and post-operative respiratory failure.

6 **When MV is inappropriate** (e.g. end-stage respiratory disease).

Monitoring includes clinical evaluation (e.g. comfort, conscious level, respiratory rate, chest wall motion), continuous S_aO_2 monitoring and ABG measurements 1 hour after starting NIV and at 4–6 hours if the earlier sample showed little improvement.

Treatment success and failure (Figures 16c, 16e) Patients who benefit from NIV are ventilated as much as possible during the first 24 hours, with breaks for meals, drugs and physiotherapy. A nasogastric tube prevents gastric distension and reduces aspiration risk (Figure 16d). Benefit is usually evident at 1 hour and certainly after 4–6 hours of NIV. The point at which treatment is considered to have failed and should be withdrawn, or MV considered, depends on respiratory failure severity, patient wishes and whether other factors (e.g. secretions) could be better managed following ETI. **Follow-up**: measure spirometry and ABG before discharge in those who benefit. Patients with chronic hypercapnic hypoventilation (e.g. obesity) should be referred for home NIV assessment.

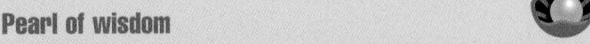

Pearl of wisdom

Non-invasive ventilation (NIV) is less likely to be successful in pneumonia and delayed mechanical ventilation (MV) risks a poor outcome

17 Endotracheal intubation

Rapid sequence anaesthetic induction (RSI)

Figure 17a   Be prepared

1. Equipment
Tight-fitting facemask
Oxygen + spare oxygen source
Breathing circuit with bag-valve mask
Suction (on max)
– switched on, easily to hand
– rigid Yankauer and flexible suction catheters
Ventilator
Endotracheal tubes (ETT)
– 2 sizes
– check cuff
– lubricating gel
– syringes (for cuff inflation)
Laryngoscopes
– long + short blades
– check bulbs
Magill forceps
Bougie
Flexible stylet
Scissors
Tape to secure ETT

2. Patient
• **Check intubation conditions**
– History of difficult intubation
– Neck movement
– Teeth (remove dentures)
– Mouth opening (Mallampati test)

• **Position patient correctly**
– Neck flexed (one pillow)
– Head extended 'sniffing the morning air'

Observe facial muscles for fasciculations during paralysis

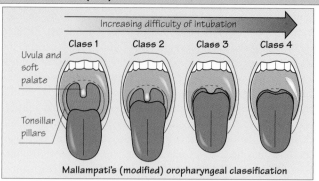

Increasing difficulty of intubation

Class 1   Class 2   Class 3   Class 4

Uvula and soft palate

Tonsillar pillars

Mallampati's (modified) oropharyngeal classification

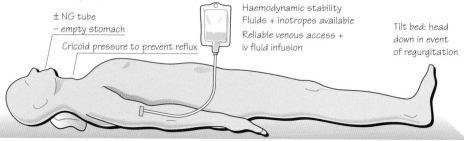

± NG tube
– empty stomach

Cricoid pressure to prevent reflux

Haemodynamic stability
Fluids + inotropes available
Reliable venous access + iv fluid infusion

Tilt bed: head down in event of regurgitation

3. Monitoring
Blood pressure, ECG, saturation, end tidal CO_2

4. Drugs
Draw up all drugs and label (including infusions)
– Anaesthetic (e.g. propofol, midazolam)
– Muscle relaxant e.g. Suxamethonium, rocuronium are used for modified RSI
– Analgesic e.g. fentanyl
– CVS stabilisers (e.g. atropine/ephedrine in bradycardic patients
   metaraminol (α-agonist vasoconstrictor) in tachycardic patients)

5. Appropriate personnel
Trained assistant nurse

Figure 17b   Procedure

4. Cricoid pressure
Assistant applies cricoid pressure to prevent aspiration

3. Anaesthetic induction
Anaesthesia induced with predetermined dose of induction agent (e.g. midazolam, propofol)

2. Check: patient position and equipment again

1. Preoxygenate
100% O_2 for >3 mins or >4 deep vital capacity breaths

Differences from a normal intubation
In a normal intubation
– Patient starved to empty stomach
– No cricoid pressure
– Use long acting muscle relaxant
– Ensure able to ventilate before giving paralysis

5. Muscle relaxant given with anaesthetic induction
– to paralyse cords, prevent cough, etc.
   e.g. suxamethonium, rocuronium

6. Intubation
– Allow 45-90 secs for paralysis
– Position patient 'neck flexed + head extended'
– laryngoscopy (see fig)
– intubation (i.e. pass the ETT between the vocal cords and into the trachea)
– inflate cuff + 'bag' patient
– auscultate both sides of chest to confirm ventilation
– only release cricoid pressure when the ETT position is confirmed

7. Follow-up
– end-tidal CO_2 measurement is the gold standard for tube placement
– check tube position on CXR
– tie ETT in place
– start continuous sedative infusions

Laryngoscopy: Assesses difficulty of intubation

Tongue
Laryngoscope blade
Epiglottis
Vocal cords
Arytenoids

Grade 1

Grade 2

Grade 3

Increasing difficulty of intubation

Grade 4

Critical Care Medicine at a Glance, Third Edition. Richard Leach. © 2014 John Wiley & Sons, Ltd. Published 2014 by John Wiley & Sons, Ltd.

Most intubations in critically ill patients are emergency procedures rendered particularly hazardous by haemodynamic instability, hypoxaemia, co-existing disease and potential aspiration of stomach contents. Whenever possible, appropriately trained clinicians, skilled in airways management, should perform endotracheal intubation (ETI). However, in order to assist during emergencies, all critical care team members should be familiar with basic airways management (Chapter 15), ETI techniques and failed intubation drills.

Indications for ETI

• **Clinical indications** include respiratory failure (Chapter 14), airways protection from aspiration of oral secretions or gastric contents, decreased conscious level (Glasgow Coma Score [GCS] ≤8), sputum clearance, upper airways obstruction and surgical procedures.
• **Objective measures** suggesting the need for ventilatory support and ETI (if non-invasive ventilation is not possible), include a respiratory rate >35/min; vital capacity <15 ml/kg; $P_aO_2 < 8$ kPa on >50% O_2 and $P_aCO_2 > 7.5$ kPa (except in chronic retainers).

Preparation for ETI (Figure 17a)

• **Airways assessment** predicts ~50% of difficult ETI (incidence ≤1:65). **History**: when feasible, review anaesthetic notes and ask about previous difficult ETI. **General examination**: assess cardiorespiratory status including oxygen requirements. Obesity, short necks, distorted neck anatomy (e.g. goitres), beards or pregnancy often present problems. **Airway examination**: evaluate features associated with difficult ETI including: (a) absence of key anatomical landmarks during oropharyngeal inspection with tongue protrusion (e.g. faucial pillars, soft palate, uvula) as described in Mallampati's modified classification (Figure 17a); (b) short thyromental distance (i.e. <3 fingerbreadths or 6 cm from thyroid cartilage to chin); (c) restricted mouth opening (i.e. <4 cm); (d) reduced neck extension; (e) oral factors (e.g. large tongue, buck teeth).
• **Intubation routes**: oral endotracheal tubes are preferred. They are relatively wide, which reduces airways resistance and improves secretion clearance. Nasotracheal tubes are rarely used (e.g. oral trauma).
• **Preparation for ETI**: ensure equipment and drugs are immediately available (Figure 17a). Establish intravenous access and start fluid (±electrolyte) resuscitation. In emergencies, clinical circumstances rarely permit full resuscitation. **Preoxygenation** using tight-fitting facemasks to deliver 100% oxygen (O_2) increases the time available before desaturation fivefold (Chapters 14, 15). **Suction apparatus** is required to clear oropharyngeal secretions. **Laryngoscopes** enable laryngeal visualization (Figure 17b). In adults, curved Macintosh blades are most popular. **Endotracheal tubes (ETTs)** should be available in a number of sizes. The usual tube size is 8–9 mm (internal diameter in mm) in adult males and 7–8 mm in adult females. Most ETT have low-pressure, high-volume cuffs to limit mucosal damage. **Drugs** include anaesthetic, analgesic, muscle relaxant and vasoactive agents (e.g. atropine, ephedrine, metaraminol) because most anaesthetic agents are vasodilators. **Monitoring** should include end-tidal carbon dioxide (CO_2) measurement.

Intubation

Critically ill patients are assumed to be at high risk of aspiration because fasting status is unknown or <6 hours and gastric emptying may be impaired (e.g. obstruction, diabetes, opiates). These patients require rapid sequence rather than normal induction.

• **Rapid sequence induction (RSI**; Figure 17b) rapidly secures the airway reducing the risk of aspiration. Following preoxygenation, an induction agent (e.g. propofol) is administered, quickly followed by a rapidly acting muscle relaxant (e.g. suxamethonium). Simultaneously, an assistant applies anterior pressure to the cricoid cartilage, which closes the oesophagus preventing gastric regurgitation (Sellick manoeuvre). The patient is positioned with the **neck flexed** (i.e. one pillow beneath the occiput) and **head extended** ('sniffing the morning air') to align the glottis, pharynx and oral cavity and achieve the best view on laryngoscopy. Intubation rapidly follows *without mask ventilation*. Cricoid pressure is released only after confirmation of correct ETT placement and cuff inflation. **Modified RSI** using a non-depolarizing muscle relaxant (e.g. rocuronium) is recommended in situations where suxamethonium is contraindicated (i.e. hyperkalaemia in renal failure, neuromuscular disorders, trauma).
• **Normal intubation** differs from RSI in that the patient is usually stable, has fasted for >6 hours to ensure an empty stomach and does not require cricoid pressure; mask ventilation is established before giving the muscle relaxant, then continued for 2–3 minutes to ensure complete paralysis before intubation.

Difficult intubation

• **Difficult intubation aids** include **gum elastic bougies/flexible stylets** to aid ETI when the tracheal opening is anterior to the visual axis. **Fibreoptic endoscopy** and **video laryngoscopes** allow direct visualization of ETI. **Specialist laryngoscope blades** (e.g. McCoy blade) lift the epiglottis improving the laryngoscopic view.
• **Failed intubation drill (FID)**: initial intubation fails in ≤1:300 intubations. The FID is as follows:
  1 Summon experienced help. Consider waking the patient, but this may not be an option in emergencies.
  2 Mask-ventilate the patient, or, if this is not possible, consider laryngeal mask ventilation (Chapter 15), until senior help arrives.
  3 If ventilation is inadequate with these methods, consider an emergency cricothyroidotomy (Chapter 19).
Experienced personnel may consider alternative approaches to intubation (e.g. fibreoptic endoscopy).

Complications

ETI complications include failure, oesophageal intubation, hypoxaemia, gastric aspiration, bronchospasm and trauma (e.g. lips, teeth, mucosa, vocal cords, cervical spine).

Endotracheal tube care

Check the ETT position on chest radiograph (CXR). The tip should be level with the lower border of the clavicles. The right main bronchus is intubated if the ETT is inserted too far, impairing ventilation of the left lung. The distance from the lips to the tube tip should be ~22–24 cm. The tip will move ~4 cm from full neck flexion to extension. Avoid high-cuff inflation pressures (>20 cmH$_2$O), head movement and prolonged intubation (>7–14 days) because these cause pressure-induced ischaemic ulcers, granulation tissue and, eventually, tracheal stenosis. Long ETT tubes increase airways resistance and impair ventilation.

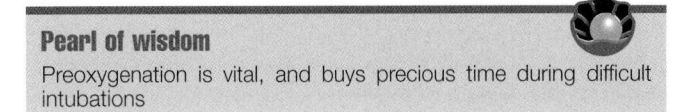

Pearl of wisdom
Preoxygenation is vital, and buys precious time during difficult intubations

18 Mechanical ventilation

Figure 18a Invasive and non-invasive ventilatory support

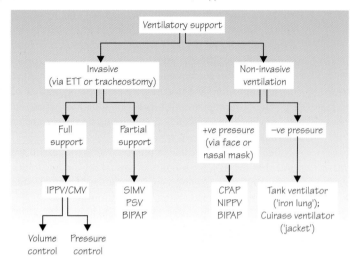

Figure 18b Indications for mechanical ventilation

Surgical
- General anaesthesia; post-operative

Respiratory centre depression
- Head injury and raised intracranial pressure
- Hypercapnia; P_aCO_2 >7–8 kPa
- Drug overdose, e.g. opiates, barbiturates
- Status epilepticus, encephalitis, meningitis, tumours

Lung disease
- ARDS, pneumonia, acute asthma, COPD
- Aspiration, smoke inhalation

Circulatory
- Cardiac arrest, pulmonary oedema, shock

Trauma
- Cervical cord trauma above C4; neck fractures

Neuromuscular disorders
- Guillain–Barré, myasthenia gravis, poliomyelitis

Chest wall disorders
- Kyphoscoliosis; traumatic flail segment

Other factors
- Poor nutrition → respiratory muscle weakness
- Abdominal distension/pain = splints diaphragm

Figure 18c Setting up the ventilator

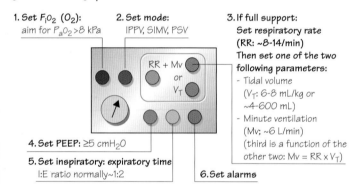

1. Set F_iO_2 (O_2): aim for P_aO_2 >8 kPa
2. Set mode: IPPV, SIMV, PSV
3. If full support:
   Set respiratory rate (RR: ~8-14/min)
   Then set one of the two following parameters:
   - Tidal volume (V_T: 6-8 mL/kg or ~4-600 mL)
   - Minute ventilation (Mv; ~6 L/min) (third is a function of the other two: Mv = RR x V_T)

RR + Mv or V_T

4. Set PEEP: ≥5 cmH$_2$O
5. Set inspiratory: expiratory time
   I:E ratio normally ~1:2
6. Set alarms

Figure 18d Pressure-time, flow-time curves in spontaneous and mechanical ventilation

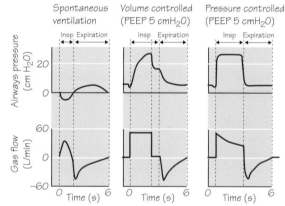

Figure 18e Pressure profiles in different types of ventilation

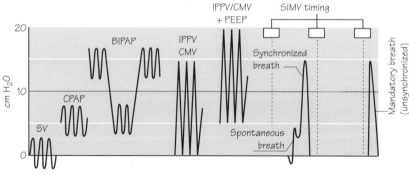

With SIMV, if a spontaneous breath occurs within the set time period it triggers a synchronized ventilator breath. If not, a mandatory breath is given immediately after the time period

Figure 18f Complications of mechanical ventilation

- Risks associated with ETT or tracheostomy (see Chapters 17, 19)
- Oxygen toxicity (see Chapter 14)
- Impaired cardiac output (see text)
- Fluid retention
- Ventilator-associated pneumonia
  - microaspiration
- Stress ulceration
- Barotrauma
  - pneumothorax, subcutaneous emphysema
- Volutrauma
- Bronchopulmonary dysplasia
- Ventilator failure/disconnection

BIPAP = bilevel positive pressure ventilation, CMV = controlled mechanical ventilation, CPAP = continuous positive airways pressure, ETT = endotracheal tube, IPPV = intermittent positive pressure ventilation, NIPPV = nasal-intermittent positive pressure ventilation, PEEP = positive end-expiratory pressure, PSV = pressure support ventilation, SIMV = synchronized intermittent mandatory ventilation, SV = spontaneous ventilation

During critical illness, ventilatory support (Figure 18a) may be required to maintain gas exchange and reduce work of breathing (WoB). Mechanical ventilation (MV) is usually delivered through an endotracheal tube or tracheostomy and provides complete or partial respiratory support. Non-invasive ventilation (NIV) aids spontaneous ventilation (SV) and avoids the need for endotracheal intubation (Chapter 16).

Indications for mechanical ventilation

The main indication for MV, after surgical procedures, is respiratory failure (Figure 18b). However, its value in the support of other organs, especially during shock, is increasingly recognized. Apart from in emergencies (e.g. cardiac arrest), the difficult decision is when and whether to ventilate a deteriorating patient. There are no simple guidelines but hypoxaemia ($P_a o_2 < 8$ kPa on $F_i o_2 > 0.5$), hypercapnia ($P_a co_2 > 7.5$ kPa), respiratory/metabolic acidosis (pH < 7.2) and physical factors (e.g. exhaustion, poor cough) may indicate the need for MV. Trends in these variables are often more helpful than absolute values. In general, MV is only appropriate when there is a reasonable chance of survival. In terminal illness, support is often limited to NIV, after discussion with the patient and family.

Ventilator set-up

Typical initial adult intermittent positive pressure ventilation (IPPV) settings are tidal volume (V_T) ~6–8 ml/kg, respiratory frequency (f) ~8–14 breaths/min and minute ventilation ($M_V = V_T \times f$) ~6 L/min (Figure 18c). $F_i o_2$ and M_V are adjusted to maintain $P_a o_2 > 8$ kPa and $P_a co_2 < 6$ kPa respectively, but acceptable values depend on individual diseases. Initially, positive end-expiratory pressure (PEEP) is set at ≥ 5 cmH$_2$O and the inspiratory : expiratory time (I : E ratio) at ~1 : 2. Disease-specific ventilatory strategies are discussed in individual chapters.

Ventilatory mode

Mode of ventilation describes whether a breath is: (a) fully or partially supported; (b) volume or pressure controlled; (c) mandatory (delivered by the ventilator regardless of patient respiratory effort) or spontaneously triggered (Figures 18a, 18e). Duration of a breath may be fixed (i.e. timed) or variable (i.e. dependent on T_v delivery). Modern ventilators with microprocessor controls provide considerable flexibility allowing a change from mandatory, full support modes to partial support modes that minimize sedation requirements and allow patients to be conscious but comfortable.

• **Full (mandatory) support modes** (e.g. IPPV, controlled mechanical ventilation [CMV]) are uncomfortable and require sedation because no allowance is made for SV. They are used in respiratory disease, circulatory instability or if respiratory drive is absent. Volume- or pressure-controlled (VC, PC) modes are available but the PC pattern of gas flow achieves better gas exchange.

  • **Volume-controlled IPPV/CMV** (Figure 18d) is often used post-operatively. Each breath is delivered at a preset volume over a fixed time. Airway pressure varies with lung compliance.

  • **Pressure-controlled IPPV/CMV** (Figure 18d) delivers preset pressures but there is no control of T_v, which depends on inspiratory time, lung compliance and airways resistance. PC ventilation protects lungs by limiting peak inspiratory pressure (PIP) and encourages alveolar recruitment.

• **Partial support modes** 'support' SV and beneficially reduce sedation requirements. Breaths are patient initiated and detected by sensitive flow/pressure triggers in the ventilator, which then provides inspiratory support.

• **Assist control** – the ventilator delivers a breath when triggered by inspiratory effort or independently if the patient does not breathe within a certain time.

• **Synchronized intermittent mandatory ventilation (SIMV)** delivers a set number of mechanically imposed breaths to achieve a minimum M_V but also allows pressure-supported SV. Imposed breaths are reduced as the patient becomes ventilator independent during weaning.

• **Pressure support**: a preset pressure supports each spontaneous breath. The patient determines breath rate. Gradual pressure reductions make it a comfortable and effective mode of weaning (Chapter 19).

• **PEEP** describes a positive pressure, maintained throughout expiration, that increases functional residual capacity (i.e. alveolar recruitment), prevents alveolar collapse, reduces ventilation/perfusion (V/Q) mismatch and decreases alveolar oedema by increasing lymphatic drainage. PEEP improves oxygenation for any given mode of ventilation, provided that cardiac output (CO) is not reduced by the associated increase in intrathoracic pressure.

Physiological responses to mechanical ventilation

1 **Cardiovascular responses to MV** are due to alveolar overdistension and increased intrathoracic pressure (IPr):

  • **Right ventricular (RV) preload reduction** is due to increased right atrial pressure that reduces venous return and RV CO. However, fluid infusion rapidly restores venous return and CO.

  • **Left ventricular (LV) afterload reduction** is due to reduced LV transmural pressure, which decreases LV work. In the normal heart, any beneficial effect of LV afterload reduction is offset by reduced venous return. However, in the failing heart, CO is relatively unaffected by preload changes but very sensitive to afterload reduction (Chapter 8, 34). Consequently, MV may increase CO in heart failure, a useful therapeutic effect.

The overall response to raised IPr depends on the state of the heart, vasomotor tone and fluid status (e.g. hypovolaemia). MV also increases lung volumes but overinflated alveoli compress alveolar blood vessels causing pulmonary hypertension. Subsequent RV distension displaces the septum into the LV cavity, reducing LV filling and CO, an effect known as 'interventricular dependence'.

2 **Respiratory effects**: MV reduces WoB, and increases blood flow to other potentially ischaemic organs. Re-expansion of collapsed alveoli also improves oxygenation. Unfortunately, supine position, reduced surfactant and ventilation of poorly perfused lung may increase V/Q mismatch.

3 **Fluid retention** is due to antidiuretic hormone secretion.

Complications of mechanical ventilation

Figure 18f lists complications of MV. 'Barotrauma' refers to pressure-induced lung damage (e.g. pneumothorax, airway disruption) caused by high PIP (>35 cmH$_2$O) due to reduced lung compliance (e.g. acute respiratory distress syndrome [ARDS]). 'Volutrauma' describes damage to healthy alveoli due to overdistension. 'Protective' ventilation strategies use low T_v (~6 ml/kg) to avoid volutrauma, PIP <35 cmH$_2$O and maintain alveolar recruitment with PEEP (Chapter 16, 42). Disease-specific complications are discussed in relevant chapters.

Pearl of wisdom
Low tidal volumes limit lung damage while PEEP improves oxygenation

Respiratory management, weaning and tracheostomy

Figure 19a Factors involved in failure to wean

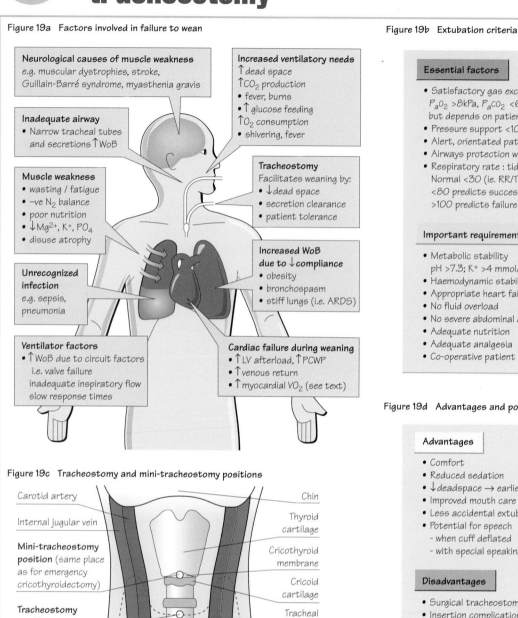

Neurological causes of muscle weakness
e.g. muscular dystrophies, stroke, Guillain-Barré syndrome, myasthenia gravis

Increased ventilatory needs
↑dead space
↑CO_2 production
• fever, burns
• ↑ glucose feeding
↑O_2 consumption
• shivering, fever

Inadequate airway
• Narrow tracheal tubes and secretions ↑WoB

Tracheostomy
Facilitates weaning by:
• ↓dead space
• secretion clearance
• patient tolerance

Muscle weakness
• wasting / fatigue
• –ve N_2 balance
• poor nutrition
• ↓Mg^{2+}, K^+, PO_4
• disuse atrophy

Increased WoB due to ↓compliance
• obesity
• bronchospasm
• stiff lungs (i.e. ARDS)

Unrecognized infection
e.g. sepsis, pneumonia

Ventilator factors
• ↑WoB due to circuit factors i.e. valve failure inadequate inspiratory flow slow response times

Cardiac failure during weaning
• ↑LV afterload, ↑PCWP
• ↑venous return
• ↑myocardial VO_2 (see text)

Figure 19c Tracheostomy and mini-tracheostomy positions

Carotid artery

Internal jugular vein

Mini-tracheostomy position (same place as for emergency cricothyroidectomy)

Tracheostomy positions

Manubrium sterni and clavicles

Chin

Thyroid cartilage

Cricothyroid membrane

Cricoid cartilage

Tracheal cartilages

Thyroid and isthmus

Figure 19b Extubation criteria

Essential factors

• Satisfactory gas exchange
P_aO_2 >8kPa, P_aCO_2 <6kPa on F_iO_2 <0.3
but depends on patient (i.e. CO_2 retainers)
• Pressure support <10 cmH₂O; PEEP ≤5 cmH₂O
• Alert, orientated patient
• Airways protection with adequate cough
• Respiratory rate : tidal volume (L/min) ratio
Normal <30 (ie. RR/T_V = 12/0.7 = 17.1)
<80 predicts success in 95% of cases
>100 predicts failure in 95% of cases

Important requirements

• Metabolic stability
pH >7.3; K^+ >4 mmol/L, PO_4 >0.8 mmol/L
• Haemodynamic stability
• Appropriate heart failure therapy
• No fluid overload
• No severe abdominal distension
• Adequate nutrition
• Adequate analgesia
• Co-operative patient

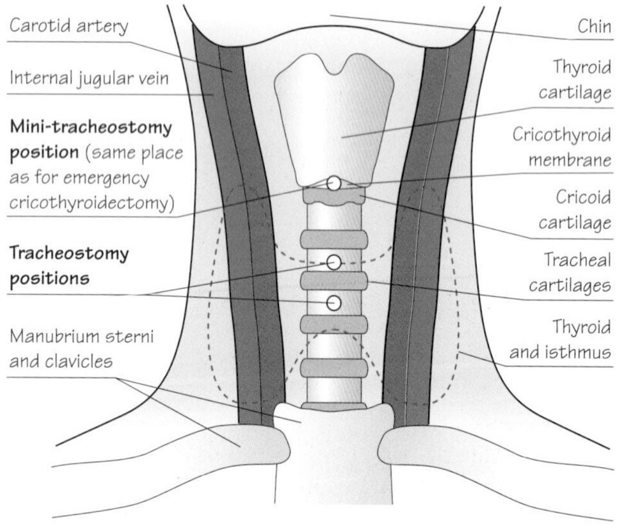

Figure 19d Advantages and potential risks of tracheostomy

Advantages

• Comfort
• Reduced sedation
• ↓deadspace → earlier and easier weaning
• Improved mouth care
• Less accidental extubations
• Potential for speech
  - when cuff deflated
  - with special speaking tube

Disadvantages

• Surgical tracheostomy requires theatre time
• Insertion complications
  - haemorrhage (~6% with PCT and ST)
  - false tract formation
  - tracheal wall damage
• Secondary skin infection (~10% with ST)
• Long-term complications
  - Tracheal stenosis (~1:200 with PCT)
  - Erosion into oesophagus

PCT = Percutaneous tracheostomy
ST = Surgical tracheostomy

Critical Care Medicine at a Glance, Third Edition. Richard Leach. © 2014 John Wiley & Sons, Ltd. Published 2014 by John Wiley & Sons, Ltd.

General respiratory management includes: (a) oxygen therapy (Chapter 14); (b) secretion clearance; (c) treatment of infection; (d) reducing work of breathing (WoB) by lowering airways resistance (e.g. bronchodilators) and improving compliance (e.g. treating oedema); and (e) optimizing functional residual capacity (FRC) by recruiting alveoli (e.g. continuous positive airways pressure [CPAP]) when FRC is low (e.g. pneumonia) and avoiding hyperinflation and raised intrathoracic pressure (Chapters 40, 41) when FRC is high (e.g. asthma).

Management of ventilated patients

Important considerations are:

• **Sedation (±paralysis)** improves synchronization and prevents patients 'fighting the ventilator' during uncomfortable ventilatory strategies. In agitated subjects, other problems (e.g. pneumothorax, pain) should be excluded before administering sedation.

• **Ventilator dependence**: control of breathing is abolished in sedated (±paralysed) patients. Ventilator alarms must be set for:

  • *Minimum ventilation*: to identify disconnection/failure.

  • *Maximum airways pressures*: to avoid barotrauma.

Ventilated patients cannot compensate for metabolic derangements (e.g. hyperventilation in acidosis). Therefore, ventilator settings must be adjusted and treatment given (e.g. bicarbonate infusion) to correct for monitored blood gas abnormalities.

• **Airways management**: regular suctioning, physiotherapy and 'positioning' facilitate secretion clearance and prevent airways obstruction or distal alveolar collapse. Inspired gas is humidified and warmed to reduce viscid secretions. Endotracheal tube (ETT) care is essential (Chapter 17). Chest radiograph (CXR) confirms ETT position and monitors respiratory disease. Bronchoscopy facilitates secretions removal, sampling (e.g. microbiology) and investigation.

• **Ventilator management** (Chapters 18, 38–44) includes:

  • **'Protective' strategies** to reduce ventilator-induced damage (e.g. barotrauma) when high pressures are required to achieve normal tidal volumes (T_V) in diseased lungs (e.g. fibrosis, atelectasis, acute respiratory distress syndrome [ARDS]). Low T_V (~6 ml/kg) ventilation and low peak inspiratory pressures (i.e. <30 cmH$_2$O) decrease volutrauma and barotrauma respectively. Increased mean airways pressures (e.g. positive end-expiratory pressure [PEEP]) and reversed I:E ratios (e.g. 2:1) promote alveolar recruitment and improve oxygenation.

  • **'Asthma' strategies** increase alveolar ventilation and carbon dioxide (CO$_2$) clearance by reducing gas trapping when airways resistance or FRC are high (e.g. asthma, chronic obstructive pulmonary disease [COPD]). Reduced breathing frequency and low I:E ratios (<1:2) increase expiratory time and hence expiratory volume. Likewise, modest PEEP levels hold open potentially collapsible airways during expiration increasing expiratory volumes. The resulting fall in FRC increases inspiratory volumes and improves minute ventilation.

  • **'Oxygenation' strategies** aim to reduce shunt fraction (Chapters 13, 14). For example, prone positioning (i.e. face down) improves oxygenation in >50% of severely hypoxaemic patients with dependent consolidation by improving ventilation/perfusion (V/Q) matching and recruiting poorly ventilated basal lung segments They do not improve survival.

Extubation and weaning

Weaning is the process of reducing and then removing respiratory support. It is usually required in patients who have undergone prolonged ventilation with associated muscle weakness. It is rarely necessary following short periods of ventilation (i.e. postoperative). A simple trial of breathing through the ETT and comparing the ratio of respiratory rate (RR) to T_V (L/min) often determines the likelihood of successful extubation. The normal RR/T_V ratio is <30 (i.e. 12/0.7 = 17.1); <80 or >100 strongly predicts success or failure, respectively. **Extubation criteria**: Figure 19b lists essential requirements prior to extubation.

Weaning techniques improve respiratory muscle strength by slowly reducing respiratory support.

1 **Partial support modes** (Chapters 16, 18) include the following:

  • **Synchronized intermittent mandatory ventilation (SIMV)** allows supported spontaneous breaths between gradually decreasing mandatory (i.e. imposed) breaths.

  • **Pressure support (PS) ventilation** is slowly decreased for patient triggered breaths until the patient is doing all the work. PS compensates for the work imposed by the ETT and breathing circuit.

  • **Bi-level positive pressure ventilation (BIPAP)** delivers two levels of pressure in phase with respiration. The higher pressure provides inspiratory support and augments T_V; the lower pressure is applied during expiration and increases FRC. It can be delivered via an ETT or facemask.

2 **Continuous positive airways pressure (CPAP)** increases FRC, in the same way as PEEP, in a spontaneously breathing patient (Chapter 16). It can be delivered through an ETT or facemask.

3 **Non-invasive ventilation** allows weaning after extubation.

Potential weaning difficulties are illustrated in Figure 19a. After extubation, cardiac dysfunction and pulmonary oedema may occur due to: (a) increases in left ventricular (LV) afterload, pulmonary capillary 'wedge' pressure and venous return (Chapter 8), or (b) inability to sustain the increased cardiac output, myocardial oxygen consumption and work required for spontaneous breathing. Cardiac support with diuretics, afterload reduction (e.g. angiotensin-converting enzyme [ACE] inhibitors) and inotropes may be necessary.

Tracheostomy (Figure 19c)

Despite the low-pressure, high-volume cuffs used in modern ETTs, prolonged intubation risks damage to the vocal cords and/or tracheal stenosis. Tracheostomy is usually considered after 7–14 days, or earlier, if it is evident that prolonged intubation will be required.

• **Advantages and potential risks** are reported in Figure 19d. Bedside **percutaneous tracheostomy** has the advantages of simplicity, reduced cost, saved theatre time and fewer complications (e.g. infection, tracheal stenosis) compared with surgical tracheostomy.

• **Tracheostomy tubes (±cuffs)** are available in a variety of sizes and types. Some have inner tubes that facilitate cleaning, prevent obstruction and reduce the frequency of tube changes (i.e. ~30 days). Others have long flanges for obese necks.

• **Removal** follows a period of cuff deflation and tube capping to ensure respiratory independence. The remaining stoma is covered with an airtight dressing and heals within a few days.

• **Mini-tracheostomy**: a small tube (~5 mm) is inserted through the cricothyroid membrane (Figure 19c), through which a suction catheter can be passed. These are useful for secretion clearance when cough or conscious level is temporarily impaired.

20 Arterial blood gases and acid-base balance

Figure 20a Calculating arterial oxygen partial pressure (PaO_2) from the alveolar gas equation

The simplified alveolar gas equation

$$P_AO_2 = F_iO_2 \, (P_b - P_{H_2O}) - (1.25 \times P_aCO_2)$$

Breathing air at sea-level where P_b ~101 kPa

$$P_AO_2 = 0.21 \, (101 - 6.2) - (1.25 \times 5.3)$$
$$= 19.9 - 6.63 = \sim 13\text{-}14 \text{ kPa}$$

P_aO_2 slightly lower than P_AO_2 because of normal shunt fraction (~3%) ~12.5-13 kPa

Thus, P_AO_2 (and P_bO_2) breathing air at 4500 m altitude where Pb ~53 kPa will be ~7-8 kPa

P_AO_2 = alveolar oxygen tension,
F_iO_2 = fractional concentration of oxygen in inspired air,
P_b = barometric pressure,
P_{H_2O} = water vapour pressure (6.2 kPa),
P_aO_2 = arterial oxygen tension,
P_aCO_2 = arterial CO_2 tension,

Figure 20b The bicarbonate buffer system and the Henderson-Hassalbach equation

The bicarbonate buffer system

Carbonic anhydrase
$$CO_2 + H_2O \leftrightarrow H_2CO_3 \leftrightarrow HCO_3^- + H^+$$

The Henderson-Hasselbach equation

→ $K = [HCO_3^-] \times [H^+] / [H_2CO_3]$
From the law of mass action
K = dissociation constant

→ $K_A = [HCO_3^-] \times [H^+] / [H_2CO_3]$
At equilibrium $[CO_2] \, \alpha \, [H_2CO_3]$
K_A = corrected dissociation constant

→ $\log K_A = \log [H^+] + \log ([HCO_3^-] / [CO_2])$

→ $-\log [H^+] = -\log K_A + \log ([HCO_3^-] / [CO_2])$

→ $pH = pK_A + \log ([HCO_3^-] / [CO_2])$
(Henderson-Hasselbach equation)

Figure 20c The relationship between pH, HCO_3^- and PCO_2

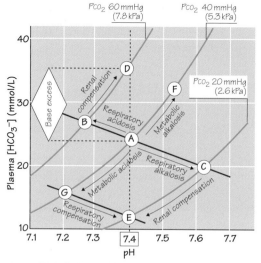

The line BAC is the buffer line for whole blood; changes in PCO_2 alter HCO_3^- and pH along this line. Point A represents normal conditions (pH 7.4, HCO_3^- 24 mmol/L, PCO_2 5.3 kPa). An acute rise in PCO_2 (e.g. hypoventilation) decreases the HCO_3^- : PCO_2 ratio and hence pH. This respiratory acidosis is represented by a move from A to B. A to C represents a respiratory alkalosis (e.g. hyperventilation). Sustained respiratory acidosis (e.g. chronic respiratory failure) is compensated for by renal HCO_3^- reabsorption and H^+ excretion. The HCO_3^- : PCO_2 ratio is restored and pH returns to normal. This renal compensation is described by the arrow B to D. Conversely a respiratory alkalosis may be compensated for by increased renal excretion of HCO_3^- (C to E). Metabolic acidosis (G) may be partially compensated by increased ventilation and a reduction in PCO_2 (G to E). There is little respiratory compensation of metabolic alkalosis (F).

Figure 20d Fenley acid-base nomogram

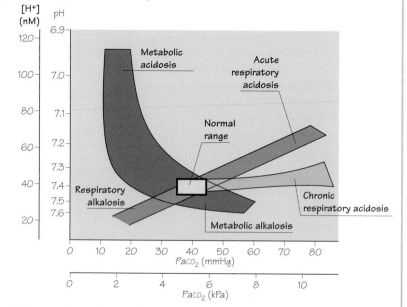

Figure 20e Disorders of acid-base balance

1. Metabolic acidosis
Normal anion gap (= hyperchloraemic acidosis)
• Renal HCO_3^- loss: proximal RTA, tubular damage (e.g. heavy metals)
• Loss of HCO_3^- from the gut: diarrhoea, ileostomy, hyperparathyroidism
• Decreased renal H^+ secretion: distal RTA, hypoaldosteronism
Increased anion gap; organic acid accumulation
• Lactic acidosis: Type A (sepsis, cardiac arrest, hypotension, methanol), Type B (insulin deficiency, metformin, decreased hepatic metabolism)
• Ketoacidosis: insulin deficiency (e.g. diabetic ketoacidosis), starvation
• Exogenous acids: salicylates

2. Metabolic alkalosis
• H^+ loss: vomiting, renal loss (with hypokalaemia, hyperaldosteronism), diuretics, low Cl^- states
• HCO_3^- gain: sodium HCO_3^- (excess antacid), lactate, citrate administration

3. Respiratory acidosis
• Airways obstruction, pneumonia, ARDS, pulmonary oedema
• Respiratory muscle weakness: myasthenia, Guillain-Barré, polio
• Trauma: flail segment, lung contusion
• Respiratory depression: head trauma, opiates

4. Respiratory alkalosis
• High levels of anxiety or pain
• Altitude
• Excessive mechanical ventilation
• Respiratory stimulants: salicylate overdose
• Pulmonary embolism, asthma, oedema

HCO_3^- = bicarbonate, H^+ = hydrogen ion, RTA = renal tubular acidosis, Cl^- = chloride ion, ARDS = acute respiratory distress syndrome

Critical Care Medicine at a Glance, Third Edition. Richard Leach. © 2014 John Wiley & Sons, Ltd. Published 2014 by John Wiley & Sons, Ltd.

Arterial blood gases (ABGs)

Understanding ABGs is essential to the management of acutely ill patients. Full interpretation requires knowledge of the clinical context, serum electrolyte concentrations and, occasionally, serum albumin and lactate levels.

Blood gas analysers typically display the following:

1 Arterial partial pressure of oxygen ($P_a o_2$), which is measured directly. Its relationship with the fractional inspired oxygen concentration ($F_i o_2$) is described by the alveolar gas equation (Figure 20a). When breathing air at sea level (i.e. barometric pressure ~101 kPa) the partial pressure of inspired oxygen ($P_i o_2$) is ~21 kPa. This falls to ~19.9 kPa when fully saturated with water in the upper airways. In the alveolus, oxygen is taken up and replaced with CO_2, which reduces the alveolar oxygen partial pressure ($P_A o_2$) to ~13–14 kPa. $P_a o_2$ is slightly lower than $P_A o_2$ because of the normal pulmonary shunt fraction (~3%). Normal $P_a o_2$ is ~13 kPa (~100 mmHg) at the age of 20 years and ~11 kPa at 65 years.

2 Arterial partial pressure of carbon dioxide ($P_a co_2$), which is measured directly and is normally ~5.3 kPa (40 mmHg).

3 pH, the negative logarithm$_{10}$ of the hydrogen ion concentration ($[H^+] = 40$ nmol/L (i.e. 40 nM) = pH 7.4).

4 Standard bicarbonate, which is calculated from the CO_2 and pH using the Henderson–Hasselbach equation (Figure 20b). It is the concentration of bicarbonate $[HCO_3^-]$ in a sample equilibrated to 37°C and $P_a co_2$ 5.3 kPa. It allows assessment of the metabolic component of acid–base balance. Normal values are ~21–27 mmol/L.

5 Actual bicarbonate, which reflects the contribution of both respiratory and metabolic components. In venous blood it is normally 21–28 mmol/l.

6 Base excess (BE), which is a measure of the amount of acid or alkali (in mmol/L) that must be added to a sample, under standard conditions (37°C, $P_a co_2$ 5.3 kPa), to return the pH to 7.4. It quantifies metabolic acid–base status by comparing the 'corrected' $[HCO_3^-]$ with the 'normal' $[HCO_3^-]$ (i.e. ~24 mmol/L at pH 7.4). It is calculated automatically from pH and $P_a co_2$ and adjusted for haemoglobin. The normal range is +2 mmol/L to −2 mmol/L.

A simple method to analyse arterial blood gases

1 Note the $P_a o_2$ and $F_i o_2$.
2 Assess pH: a pH < 7.35 defines acidaemia and >7.45 alkalaemia.
3 Assess the respiratory component: $P_a co_2$ > 6 kPa (45 mmHg) defines respiratory acidosis, $P_a co_2$ < 4.5 kPa (35 mmHg) defines respiratory alkalosis.
4 Assess the metabolic component: $[HCO_3^-]$ > 33 mmol/L defines metabolic alkalosis, $[HCO_3^-]$ < 23mmol/L defines metabolic acidosis.
5 Determine if there is metabolic or respiratory compensation: see 'Acid–base balance' later.
6 Consider the anion gap (AG): this is the difference between the sum of serum sodium and potassium ion concentrations (cations) and the sum of serum chloride and bicarbonate ions concentration (anions): $([Na^+] + [K^+]) − ([Cl^-] + [HCO_3^-])$. The normal AG (~12 ± 2 mmol/L) is a reflection of the kidney-excreted mineral acids (e.g. phosphates). An increased AG indicates an accumulation of anions including keto, lactic and exogenous (e.g. salicylates) acids. A normal or reduced AG (i.e. hyperchloraemic acidosis) suggests HCO_3^- loss or renal tubular acidosis.

Acid-base balance

Maintenance of a stable hydrogen ion concentration ($[H^+]$; 45–35 nM) or pH 7.35–7.45 is essential for intracellular enzyme function. Normally acids are generated by the hydration of CO_2 ('respiratory acids') or metabolic processes ('metabolic' acids; typically phosphoric, sulphuric and lactic). In disease states, $[H^+]$ rises due to lactate production (e.g. ischaemia), ketoacid generation (e.g. diabetes), alcohol ingestion (e.g. methanol) or failure of excretion (e.g. renal, respiratory or liver failure). Loss of H^+ (e.g. vomiting) or HCO_3^- (e.g. diarrhoea) also effects acid–base balance. **Causes** are listed in Figure 20e.

Control of acid-base balance

The body prevents pH change by regulating two pathways for eliminating acid: respiratory and renal. However, ~100 times more acid equivalents are expired each day in the form of CO_2/carbonic acid than are excreted as fixed acids by the kidneys. **Buffers** bind or release H^+ according to the pH; this limits the change in pH that occurs when acid is added. The relationship between the amount of acid added to a buffer-containing solution and the change in pH is known as the **buffer line** (Figure 20c). Buffers are most effective when pH is close to their pK_A (log of the dissociation constant K_A; Figure 20b).

The most important blood buffer systems are:

1 Bicarbonate (HCO_3^-; Figure 20b): CO_2 combines with water to form carbonic acid (H_2CO_3), which dissociates to HCO_3^- and H^+. The relationship between pH, Pco_2 and $[HCO_3^-]$ is described by the Henderson–Hasselbach equation. In normal blood, $[HCO_3^-]$ is 24 mmol/L, Pco_2 5.3 kPa and pH calculates to 7.4. If the ratio $[HCO_3^-]:Pco_2$ remains at 20, pH will remain at 7.4. Although the pK_A of the bicarbonate system (6.1) is further away from the blood pH (7.4) than would seem ideal for a buffer, the fact that Pco_2 and HCO_3^- are independently controlled by ventilation and the kidneys means that in practice it makes an effective buffer system.

2 Haemoglobin (Hb), especially when deoxygenated. Buffering capacity improves significantly in whole blood compared with plasma. All other blood proteins have <20% of the buffering capacity of Hb.

The relationship between pH, HCO_3^- and Pco_2

This is illustrated using Davenport diagrams (Figure 20c). Acute CO_2 changes cause **respiratory acidosis or alkalosis**. When CO_2 changes persist (e.g. type 2 respiratory failure), pH is slowly corrected by renal compensation (i.e. increase/decrease $[HCO_3^-]$). The terms **metabolic acidosis and alkalosis** are used to describe alterations in acid–base status due to changes in HCO_3^- rather than CO_2 – as a result, for example, of renal disease or increased H^+ production (e.g. diabetic ketoacidosis). A metabolic acidosis may be partially compensated by increased ventilation. However, there is little respiratory compensation for a metabolic alkalosis as this may require unsustainable falls in ventilation. **Mixed metabolic and respiratory** acid–base disorders may occur. For example, respiratory acidosis due to respiratory failure (i.e. increased Pco_2) may be combined with a metabolic acidosis due to associated hypoxia. The **Flenley nomogram** is a useful diagnostic aid because only one type of disturbance is likely if pH and Pco_2 fall within a specific band (Figure 20d).

Pearl of wisdom

A pH of 7.4 is 40nM $[H^+]$ (i.e. 40nmol/L $[H^+]$), pH 7.1 = 79nM $[H^+]$, pH 6.9 = 126nM $[H^+]$ and pH 7.6 = 25nM $[H^+]$ (Small physiological changes in hydrogen ion concentration $[H^+]$ are easier to understand as absolute values (as for other ions like Na^+) rather than as pH (which was originally developed to measure the major $[H^+]$ changes associated with chemical reactions.)

Analgesia, sedation and paralysis

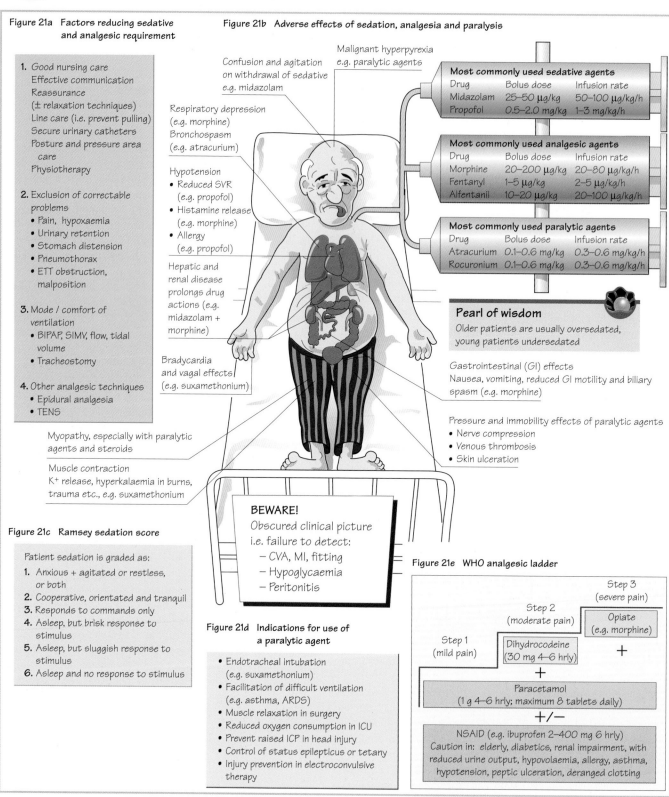

Figure 21a Factors reducing sedative and analgesic requirement

1. Good nursing care
   Effective communication
   Reassurance
   (± relaxation techniques)
   Line care (i.e. prevent pulling)
   Secure urinary catheters
   Posture and pressure area
   care
   Physiotherapy

2. Exclusion of correctable
   problems
   • Pain, hypoxaemia
   • Urinary retention
   • Stomach distension
   • Pneumothorax
   • ETT obstruction,
     malposition

3. Mode / comfort of
   ventilation
   • BIPAP, SIMV, flow, tidal
     volume
   • Tracheostomy

4. Other analgesic techniques
   • Epidural analgesia
   • TENS

Figure 21b Adverse effects of sedation, analgesia and paralysis

Confusion and agitation
on withdrawal of sedative
e.g. midazolam

Malignant hyperpyrexia
e.g. paralytic agents

Respiratory depression
(e.g. morphine)
Bronchospasm
(e.g. atracurium)

Hypotension
• Reduced SVR
  (e.g. propofol)
• Histamine release
  (e.g. morphine)
• Allergy
  (e.g. propofol)

Hepatic and
renal disease
prolongs drug
actions (e.g.
midazolam +
morphine)

Bradycardia
and vagal effects
(e.g. suxamethonium)

Myopathy, especially with paralytic
agents and steroids

Muscle contraction
K⁺ release, hyperkalaemia in burns,
trauma etc., e.g. suxamethonium

Most commonly used sedative agents		
Drug	Bolus dose	Infusion rate
Midazolam	25–50 µg/kg	50–100 µg/kg/h
Propofol	0.5–2.0 mg/kg	1–3 mg/kg/h

Most commonly used analgesic agents		
Drug	Bolus dose	Infusion rate
Morphine	20–200 µg/kg	20–80 µg/kg/h
Fentanyl	1–5 µg/kg	2–5 µg/kg/h
Alfentanil	10–20 µg/kg	20–100 µg/kg/h

Most commonly used paralytic agents		
Drug	Bolus dose	Infusion rate
Atracurium	0.1–0.6 mg/kg	0.3–0.6 mg/kg/h
Rocuronium	0.1–0.6 mg/kg	0.3–0.6 mg/kg/h

Pearl of wisdom
Older patients are usually oversedated,
young patients undersedated

Gastrointestinal (GI) effects
Nausea, vomiting, reduced GI motility and biliary
spasm (e.g. morphine)

Pressure and immobility effects of paralytic agents
• Nerve compression
• Venous thrombosis
• Skin ulceration

BEWARE!
Obscured clinical picture
i.e. failure to detect:
– CVA, MI, fitting
– Hypoglycaemia
– Peritonitis

Figure 21c Ramsey sedation score

Patient sedation is graded as:

1. Anxious + agitated or restless,
   or both
2. Cooperative, orientated and tranquil
3. Responds to commands only
4. Asleep, but brisk response to
   stimulus
5. Asleep, but sluggish response to
   stimulus
6. Asleep and no response to stimulus

**Figure 21d Indications for use of
a paralytic agent**

• Endotracheal intubation
  (e.g. suxamethonium)
• Facilitation of difficult ventilation
  (e.g. asthma, ARDS)
• Muscle relaxation in surgery
• Reduced oxygen consumption in ICU
• Prevent raised ICP in head injury
• Control of status epilepticus or tetany
• Injury prevention in electroconvulsive
  therapy

Figure 21e WHO analgesic ladder

Step 1
(mild pain)

Step 2
(moderate pain)
Dihydrocodeine
(30 mg 4–6 hrly)
+

Step 3
(severe pain)
Opiate
(e.g. morphine)
+

Paracetamol
(1 g 4–6 hrly; maximum 8 tablets daily)

+/–

NSAID (e.g. ibuprofen 2–400 mg 6 hrly)
Caution in: elderly, diabetics, renal impairment, with
reduced urine output, hypovolaemia, allergy, asthma,
hypotension, peptic ulceration, deranged clotting

Critical Care Medicine at a Glance, Third Edition. Richard Leach. © 2014 John Wiley & Sons, Ltd. Published 2014 by John Wiley & Sons, Ltd.

Effective relief of pain and anxiety is essential. Analgesic and sedative requirements vary according to patient psychology, pathology, surgical procedure and need for mechanical ventilation. Good nursing care, comfortable modes of ventilation and epidural analgesia reduce drug doses and side-effects (Figure 21a). The aims, type and route of therapy depend on the clinical scenario:

1 **Self-ventilating patients** usually communicate their needs, which aids choice of therapy (i.e. drug type, route), guides dosage and permits early recognition of side-effects. Oral therapy and regional anaesthesia (e.g. epidural) may be possible.

2 **Ventilated patients** should be comfortable but able to communicate and co-operate. Heavy sedation may be required for intracranial pressure reduction, uncomfortable ventilatory modes (i.e. inverse I:E ratio) or epilepsy. Assess sedation levels regularly and stop sedative infusions briefly each day to allow a degree of 'awakening'. The Ramsay Scale (Figure 21c) is the most frequently used sedation-scoring system. Levels 2–5 are appropriate for most patients. Adverse effects of over-sedation are illustrated in Figure 21b. Under-sedation with unrelieved pain and/or anxiety causes hypertension, tachycardia, atelectasis, immobility and reduced immunity.

3 **Paralysed, ventilated patients** are sedated to unconsciousness. Distress in 'awake' patients is recognized as hypertension, tachycardia, sweating and lacrimation. Limited electroencephalography helps confirm sedation. A peripheral nerve stimulator is the best measure of level of paralysis. Paralytic agents are used infrequently (Figure 21d) and with caution because unrecognized extubation is fatal.

Analgesics

The World Health Organization (WHO) 'analgesic ladder' recommends a stepwise approach to pain relief (Figure 21e), using regularly prescribed, preferably oral, medication, tailored to the patient's needs.

• **Step 1 Non-opioid analgesia:** regular **paracetamol** (1 g 6 hourly) is an effective first-line antipyretic analgesic with few side-effects. Add **non-steroidal anti-inflammatory drugs** (NSAIDs) at any stage for their intrinsic analgesic effect and to potentiate paracetamol and opioid efficacy. Renal toxicity, peptic ulceration, drug interactions and deranged clotting limit NSAID use.

• **Step 2 Add mild opioid analgesics** (e.g. **dihydrocodeine or codeine** [15 mg 6 hourly]) to regular paracetamol (±NSAID) if pain remains uncontrolled. Inadequate paracetamol doses may result with use of combination paracetamol/weak opioid tablets (e.g. coproxamol).

• **Step 3 Use strong opioid analgesics** instead of mild opioids, in combination with regular paracetamol (±NSAID), if pain persists. Analgesic and sedative responses to opioid receptor (μ, κ, σ) stimulation are variable and gradual titration is essential in older or debilitated patients. **Side-effects** include hypotension, respiratory depression, constipation, euphoria, biliary spasm, meiosis, histamine release, tolerance and withdrawal symptoms. Nausea, vomiting and gastroparesis hamper enteral nutrition.

• **Tramadol** is a medium-strength opioid analgesic, useful in post-operative or protracted pain. It has fewer side-effects, notably constipation, respiratory depression and addiction.

• **Morphine** is a potent, rapid-onset analgesic/anxiolytic with little cardiovascular instability. Renal or hepatic failure impairs clearance and prolongs action. Ventilated patients need high doses, with benzodiazepines, to cause unconsciousness. Reduced respiratory drive may aid patient-ventilator synchronization but can cause apnoea.

• **Fentanyl**, a synthetic opioid, has a short duration of action after single doses. Protracted use allows accumulation in, and subsequent slow release from, fat stores, which prolongs action.

• **Alfentanil and remifentanil** are short-acting agents.

• **Naloxone** is an effective but short-acting opioid antagonist.

Sedative-anxiolytics

No drug has all the properties of an ideal sedative (i.e. anxiolysis, analgesia, amnesia, predictability, titratability, no side-effects and rapid elimination) in the ventilated patient. A multi-drug approach using analgesics, anxiolytic-sedatives and occasional paralyzing agents is required. Choice depends on patient needs, drug properties and side-effects. Most drugs are administered as continuous intravenous infusions and titrated to the required effect.

• **Benzodiazepines** provide excellent sedation, anxiolysis, amnesia, muscle relaxation and anticonvulsant effects with few cardiorespiratory consequences. They do not relieve pain but reduce analgesic requirements by relieving anxiety. Hepatic metabolism and excretion prolong action in liver disease, whereas liver enzyme induction (e.g. alcoholics, epileptics) engenders large doses to achieve therapeutic effects. **Midazolam** is lipid soluble, allowing rapid onset of action (i.e. blood–brain barrier penetration), but accumulation in fat prolongs drug withdrawal. **Lorazepam** differs in that it has no hepatic metabolism or active metabolites. **Flumazenil** is a short-acting benzodiazepine antagonist but may precipitate withdrawal.

• **Propofol** is an easily titrated, short-acting and rapidly reversible sedative, with no analgesic properties. Hypotension occurs in 30% of patients and limits use in haemodynamic instability. The drug vehicle (i.e. egg and soyabean emulsion) can cause allergic reactions or become infected causing bacteraemia. Infusions must be prepared under sterile conditions and changed at short intervals. Metabolism is neither hepatic nor renal.

• **Haloperidol** and benzodiazepine combinations are better than either agent alone, if carefully titrated, in agitated patients. Barbiturates and phenothiazines have few advantages over other sedatives and cause significant side-effects (e.g. dystonic reactions).

Neuromuscular paralytic agents

• **Depolarizing neuromuscular agents** resemble acetylcholine (ACh) and depolarize neuromuscular junctions (NMJ) but are not metabolized by acetylcholinesterases. Depolarization lasts until the drug diffuses out of the NMJ and is degraded by plasma cholinesterases. **Suxamethonium/succinylcholine** is short acting (<10 min) with a rapid onset of action that is ideal for intubation. Depolarization causes muscle contraction and associated K^+ release limits use in renal failure, rhabdomyolysis, burns and trauma. Vagal stimulation prevents use of continuous infusions.

• **Non-depolarizing neuromuscular agents** passively occupy ACh-binding sites, prevent ACh action and block depolarization. Onset takes 2–3 minutes and duration of action is 20–60 min. **Atracurium** and **rocuronium** infusions are non-cumulative and often used in intensive care units. Prolonged paralysis, particularly with steroid therapy, results in severe myopathy. Side-effects include vagal blockade (e.g. pancuronium) and histamine release with bronchospasm (e.g. atracurium).

Many factors potentiate (e.g. acidosis, hyponatraemia, gentamicin) and inhibit (e.g. oedema, phenytoin) neuromuscular blockade. **Complications** (Figure 21b) include malignant hyperthermia (Chapter 23). **Pseudocholinesterase deficiency** affects 1 in 2500 people and prolongs paralysis (i.e. >6 hours).

Enteral and parenteral nutrition

Figure 22a Nutritional requirements

1. Energy (calorie) requirement

a. Determine basal metabolic rate (BMR) from Schofield equation

b. Adjust BMR for stress, activity and thermogenesis

BMR in kcal/day by age and gender		
Age (yrs)	Female	Male
15–18	13.3W + 690	17.6W + 656
18–30	14.8W + 485	15.0W + 690
30–60	8.1W + 842	11.4W + 870
>60	9.0W + 656	11.7W + 585

W = weight in kg, #=fractures
IBD = inflammatory bowel disease

Starvation (>10% weight loss)	– 0–15%
Mild infection, IBD, post-operative	+ 0–13%
Moderate infection, long bone #	+ 10–30%
Severe sepsis, multiple trauma	+25–50%
Burns 10-90%	+10–70%
Bed-bound, immobile	+10%
Bed-bound, mobile/sitting	+20%
Mobile around the ward	+25%

Or determine energy expenditure from:
  (a) Direct bedside calorimetry: measures O_2 consumption + CO_2 production
  (b) The Fick principle in patients with pulmonary artery catheters

Or calculate from lean body weight:
  Normally ~30 kcal/kg/day, increasing to >60 kcal/kg/day in severe stress (e.g. burns). Non-protein sources supply ~80% of calories (e.g. carbohydrate 30-70%, fat 15–30%)

2. Protein requirement:
Can be determined from 24 hour urinary nitrogen loss; but not necessary Nitrogen intake should be ~0.2 g/kg/day, given as protein ~1.25 g/kg/day.

3. Vitamin and trace elements
Especially Vitamin K, thiamine, folic acid and zinc. Other trace elements serve key physiological and metabolic roles

4. Basal water and electrolyte requirements/kg/day
Water 30 ml, sodium ~1 mmoL, potassium 0.7–1 mmoL, magnesium 0.1 mmoL, calcium 0.1 mmoL, phosphorus 0.4 mmoL

Figure 22c Starter feeding regime

Initially feed at 30 mls/hr
Check gastric aspirates 4 hrly

↓

If GRV <200 mls increase feed to 60 mls/hr
Check gastric aspirates 4 hrly

If GRV <200 mls increase feed to 75 mls/hr or target volume
Check gastric aspirates 4 hrly

Feed with target volume for 20 hrs
Daily rest period 4 hrs
Check gastric aspirates 4 hrly until feeding established

GRV=gastric residual volume

Figure 22b Disease-specific nutritional requirements

Starvation
Electrolyte depletion (PO_4^-, K^+, Mg^{2+}) and glucose intolerance result in impaired cardiac contractility and respiratory muscle function. Electrolyte and glucose imbalance must be corrected. Refeeding syndrome occurs after prolonged starvation

Renal failure (RF)
High energy feed is used (i.e. 2 kcal/mL) to reduce volume. In TPN essential amino acids (AA) may stimulate protein synthesis and reduce urea by recycling nitrogen into non-essential AA. Low Na^+ and K^+ feeds with supplemental vitamins may be required

Nutritional requirements in disease states

COPD
Malnutrition is common. Ventilation in respiratory failure has a high energy expenditure. Overfeeding with carbohydrate causes high CO_2 production. Feeds should contain less carbohydrate and more fat. Fat oxidation produces 30% less CO_2

Hepatic failure
Impaired fat metabolism and carbohydrate intolerance are common. Use of branched chain (instead of aromatic) amino acids may improve mental status in hepatic encephalopathy. TPN must contain less sodium and volume due to aldosterone-induced water retention

Figure 22d Complicatons of enteral and parenteral nutrition

Enteral nutrition (EN)

Parenteral nutrition (TPN)

NG tube problems:
sinusitis, tube obstruction, perforation + ulceration

Aspiration pneumonia:
Prevented by avoiding gastric distention + 30° elevation of the head of the bed

Impaired gastric emptying

Feeding 'Intolerance'
(i.e.>200 mL/h residual volume) causes gastric + abdominal distention, vomiting and ileus

Bacterial overgrowth:
Due to pH-neutralizing effects of EN in stomach. Predisposes to chest and GIT infections

Diarrhoea (35%):
not always due to EN (e.g. Clostridium difficile, antibiotic colitis, drugs)

Faecal impaction:
rare; due to fibre in feed

Metabolic problems:
mainly with TPN (~5–10%) over the first 24–48 hrs
• Hyperglycaemia
• Hypoglycaemia (i.e. if feeding stops abruptly. Replace with 10% glucose infusion)
• Hypokalaemia
• Hypomagnesaemia
• Hypophosphataemia
• Metabolic Acidosis

Catheter-related:
• line infection, sepsis
• thrombosis, phlebitis
• air embolism, occlusion

Fluid overload

↓K^+, ↓Mg, ↓PO_4 especially in the first 24 hrs

Hepatobiliary:
• abnormal liver function tests (~90% ± jaundice)
• liver fatty infiltration
• intrahepatic cholestatsis
• cholecystitis

Intestinal:
Mucosal + villous atrophy
Bacterial translocation

Trace element deficiency
e.g. zinc, iron

Vitamin deficiency:
e.g. K, B_{12}, folate

Other TPN problems:
Hyperchloraemic metabolic acidosis due to amino-acid solutions with high Cl^- content. Replace some Cl^- with acetate in TPN solution Refeeding syndrome (see text) Bone pain (prolonged TPN)

Critical Care Medicine at a Glance, Third Edition. Richard Leach. © 2014 John Wiley & Sons, Ltd. Published 2014 by John Wiley & Sons, Ltd.

Nutritional assessment is essential in the critically ill patient. Clinical evaluation (e.g. weight loss, subcutaneous fat loss, muscle wasting, oedema, ascites, gastro-intestinal symptoms) is more effective than objective measurements (e.g. skin-fold thickness), which may be obscured by oedema, or laboratory features (e.g. transferrin, albumin, lymphocyte count) that fall independently in acute illness.

Effects of malnutrition include impaired immune function, reduced plasma protein and oncotic pressure, delayed wound healing and impaired respiratory muscle strength. **Refeeding syndrome** occurs when food intake is resumed after a period of starvation. As glucose is reintroduced, increased insulin promotes cellular ion uptake, resulting in hypophosphataemia, hypokalaemia, hypomagnesaemia and metabolic acidosis. Adenosine triphosphate (ATP) and 2,3 diphosphoglycerate (DPG; ±thiamine) depletion causes tissue hypoxia and inhibits metabolism, leading to cardiorespiratory failure, paraesthesia and seizures.

Timing and benefits of nutritional support (NSt) are controversial. Although NSt reduces protein catabolism and improves markers of nutritional status (e.g. lymphocyte counts, plasma proteins), evidence that specific regimes improve outcome is limited. Generally, early NSt is recommended for pre-existing malnutrition, hypermetabolic states and protracted illness but is unnecessary in well-nourished, short-stay patients. Current guidelines recommend starting NSt in any patient unlikely to recommence oral intake within 5–10 days.

Nutritional route: enteral nutrition (EN) is usually preferred to total parenteral nutrition (TPN) because it is cheaper and may reduce infective complications. However, complications also occur in EN (e.g. tube misplacement, aspiration).

Assessment of nutritional requirements

• **Energy expenditure (calories)** is usually calculated from equations that determine basal metabolic rate (BMR) from weight, age and sex, corrected for stress, activity and fever. The Schofield equation is currently used (Figure 22a). Indirect calorimetry (i.e. measures of oxygen [O_2] consumption and carbon dioxide [CO_2] production) or calculations from the Fick principle (i.e. pulmonary artery catheter measurements) offer little additional benefit. Adjustments are required in chronic obstructive pulmonary disease (COPD) and renal and hepatic failure (Figure 22b). Many clinicians have discarded energy expenditure measurements and simply deliver ~30 kcal/kg/day.
• **Protein:** daily nitrogen provision of 0.2 g/kg/day (1.25 g protein/kg/day) is usually adequate but 0.3 g/kg/day (2 g protein/kg/day) may be required in severely catabolic patients (e.g. burns). Urinary urea nitrogen measurements are generally unhelpful.
• **Vitamins and micronutrients:** the need for vitamins A, K, thiamine (B_1), B_3, B_6, C and folic acid increase in severe illness. Vitamin K, folic acid and thiamine are prone to deficiency during TPN and zinc, iron and selenium deficits have been reported. Renal replacement therapy risks loss of water- soluble vitamins.
• **Water and electrolytes:** requirements vary considerably. Basal intakes are shown in Figure 22a.

Enteral nutrition

EN improves splanchnic perfusion; prevents stress ulceration; protects mucosal integrity, which stops bacterial translocation (±sepsis); increases gut-associated lymphoid tissue, which enhances immunity; supplies complex nutrients (e.g. medium-chain fatty acids); stimulates gallbladder emptying; and promotes insulin gastrin (±gut hormones) and pancreatic secretions. **Feeding formulas:** standard commercial feeds provide 1–1.5 kcal/ml (~45% carbohydrate, ~25% lipid) and most electrolytes and micronutrients. They are isotonic, polymeric (i.e. complex protein, fat and carbohydrate molecules) and gluten/lactose free. Elemental diets (i.e. amino acids, oligosaccharides) require minimal digestion (e.g. in chronic pancreatitis). **Administration** is continuous, initially through a wide bore (12–14 F) nasogastric tube that allows gastric residual volumes to be aspirated at 4-hourly intervals. Once feeding is established, this is replaced by a more comfortable fine bore tube. A daily 4-hour feeding rest period inhibits stomach bacterial overgrowth by restoring normal gastric pH (<7.1) and reduces the risk of aspiration pneumonia. EN can usually be achieved despite abdominal distension, absence of bowel sounds or diarrhoea. Figure 22c illustrates a typical starter feeding regime. **Complications** are illustrated in Figure 22d. **Contraindications** include intestinal obstruction, ischaemia and anatomical disruption. **Difficulty establishing EN:** initially measure gastric aspirates every 4 hours. Gastric residual volumes (GRV) >400 ml risk pulmonary aspiration and feeding should be stopped and reintroduced at a lower infusion rate. Treat GRV consistently >200 ml with prokinetic agents, initially metoclopramide (10 mg 8 hourly), a dopamine antagonist, and then erythromycin (250 mg 12 hourly), a motilin-receptor agonist that stimulates gastric emptying. Endoscopically placed nasojejunal or surgical jejunostomy tubes bypass the stomach and feed directly into the bowel.

Total parenteral nutrition

TPN is required if EN is contraindicated or cannot be established (e.g. ileus). The main energy source is fat emulsion (i.e. ~35%) because excess glucose causes metabolic derangement (i.e. hyperglycaemia, CO_2 production, lipogenesis). Unfortunately, lipid infusions impair neutrophil function and TPN may be immunosuppressive. Nitrogen is supplied as amino acids but glutamine and tyrosine are unstable and absent. Insulin is often added to ensure normoglycaemia. Consequently, TPN is nutritionally incomplete, irritant and often hyperosmolar. **Administration:** most TPN is prepared aseptically in hospital pharmacies as a single bag that is infused continuously over 24 hours through a dedicated central venous catheter lumen. If TPN is given into a peripheral vein, large volumes with low glucose concentrations are used to reduce osmolality-induced phlebitis. Nevertheless, new line sites may still be required at 2- to 3-day intervals. **Complications** are illustrated in Figure 22d. Catheter-related sepsis is reduced by using antimicrobial-coated lines, dedicated lumens and strict aseptic handling (Chapter 26). Subcutaneous tunnelling is not beneficial. Liver dysfunction is reduced by lowering TPN glucose content.

Immunonutrition

Immunonutrition uses compounds that, although unproven, may improve metabolic and immune responses in critical illness. Glutamine, an amino acid and primary energy source for enterocytes, preserves intestinal integrity. Arginine stimulates immune (e.g. T-cell) function and nitrogen balance. Omega-3-polyunsaturated fatty acids, from fish oils, are anti-inflammatory agents and immune modulators.

23 Hypothermia and hyperthermia

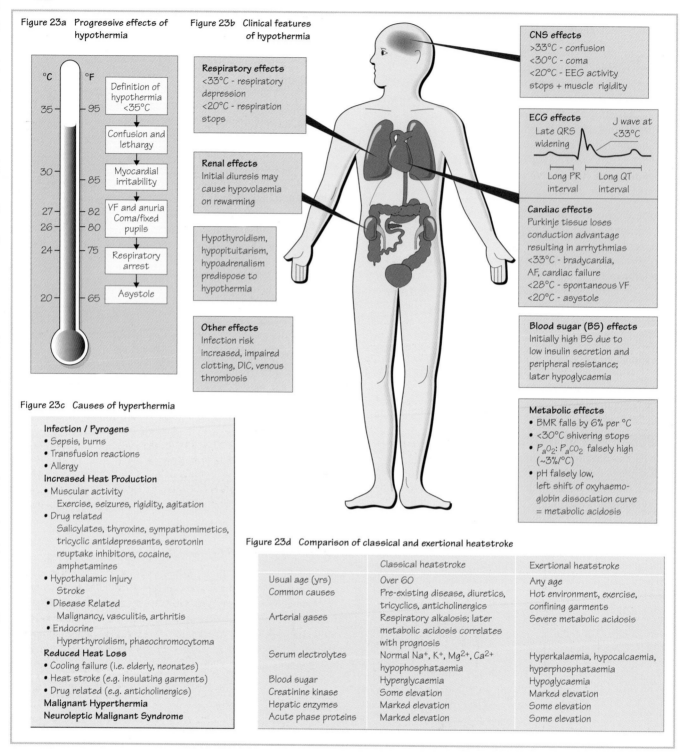

Figure 23a Progressive effects of hypothermia

°C   °F

35 — 95   Definition of hypothermia <35°C

↓

Confusion and lethargy

30 — 85   Myocardial irritability

27 — 82   VF and anuria
26 — 80   Coma/fixed pupils
24 — 75   Respiratory arrest

20 — 65   Asystole

Figure 23b Clinical features of hypothermia

Respiratory effects
<33°C - respiratory depression
<20°C - respiration stops

Renal effects
Initial diuresis may cause hypovolaemia on rewarming

Hypothyroidism, hypopituitarism, hypoadrenalism predispose to hypothermia

Other effects
Infection risk increased, impaired clotting, DIC, venous thrombosis

CNS effects
>33°C - confusion
<30°C - coma
<20°C - EEG activity stops + muscle rigidity

ECG effects
Late QRS widening   J wave at <33°C
Long PR interval   Long QT interval

Cardiac effects
Purkinje tissue loses conduction advantage resulting in arrhythmias
<33°C - bradycardia, AF, cardiac failure
<28°C - spontaneous VF
<20°C - asystole

Blood sugar (BS) effects
Initially high BS due to low insulin secretion and peripheral resistance; later hypoglycaemia

Metabolic effects
• BMR falls by 6% per °C
• <30°C shivering stops
• P_aO_2: P_aCO_2 falsely high (~3%/°C)
• pH falsely low, left shift of oxyhaemoglobin dissociation curve = metabolic acidosis

Figure 23c Causes of hyperthermia

Infection / Pyrogens
• Sepsis, burns
• Transfusion reactions
• Allergy
Increased Heat Production
• Muscular activity
  Exercise, seizures, rigidity, agitation
• Drug related
  Salicylates, thyroxine, sympathomimetics, tricyclic antidepressants, serotonin reuptake inhibitors, cocaine, amphetamines
• Hypothalamic Injury
  Stroke
• Disease Related
  Malignancy, vasculitis, arthritis
• Endocrine
  Hyperthyroidism, phaeochromocytoma
Reduced Heat Loss
• Cooling failure (i.e. elderly, neonates)
• Heat stroke (e.g. insulating garments)
• Drug related (e.g. anticholinergics)
Malignant Hyperthermia
Neuroleptic Malignant Syndrome

Figure 23d Comparison of classical and exertional heatstroke

	Classical heatstroke	Exertional heatstroke
Usual age (yrs)	Over 60	Any age
Common causes	Pre-existing disease, diuretics, tricyclics, anticholinergics	Hot environment, exercise, confining garments
Arterial gases	Respiratory alkalosis; later metabolic acidosis correlates with prognosis	Severe metabolic acidosis
Serum electrolytes	Normal Na^+, K^+, Mg^{2+}, Ca^{2+} hypophosphataemia	Hyperkalaemia, hypocalcaemia, hyperphosphataemia
Blood sugar	Hyperglycaemia	Hypoglycaemia
Creatinine kinase	Some elevation	Marked elevation
Hepatic enzymes	Marked elevation	Some elevation
Acute phase proteins	Marked elevation	Some elevation

Hypothermia

Hypothermia is defined as a core temperature <35°C; mild hypothermia is 32–35°C, moderate 28–32°C and severe <28°C. Severity and cause determine mortality (e.g. hypothermia [28–32°C] alone ~20%; with an underlying cause >60%).

Causes

Accidental hypothermia is usually multifactorial, involving exposure to low environmental or water immersion temperatures (e.g. drowning), alcohol intoxication, a primary neurological insult (e.g. cerebrovascular accident [CVA]), thermoregulatory compromise

Critical Care Medicine at a Glance, Third Edition. Richard Leach. © 2014 John Wiley & Sons, Ltd. Published 2014 by John Wiley & Sons, Ltd.

(e.g. spinal cord injury), predisposing factors (e.g. hypopituitarism), surgery (i.e. exposure, anaesthetic drugs, impaired shivering) and drugs that alter cold perception, cause vasodilation or inhibit heat generation (e.g. alcohol, barbiturates). Hypothyroidism is a factor in 10% of cases and impairs heat production, temperature perception and shivering. Induced hypothermia during cardiac or neurosurgery provides cerebral protection.

Clinical features

Initially, hypothermia stimulates protective peripheral vasoconstriction, shivering and increased metabolism. As core body temperature falls, physiological and organ dysfunction develop (Figure 23a), including cardiorespiratory and neurological depression, renal diuresis, tissue hypoperfusion and metabolic derangement (Figure 23b). Below 33 °C, cardiac conduction and pacemaker activity are progressively impaired and myocardial irritability increases, with atrial fibrillation and heart block common. Ventricular fibrillation, resistant to cardioversion, is precipitated by rough handling or cardiopulmonary resuscitation (CPR) below 28 °C. Cardiac output falls by 50% at 28 °C due to bradycardia and impaired contractility. Initial neurological effects include reduced respiratory drive, lethargy and confusion. Coma and fixed pupils occur below 30 °C. Cerebral oxygen consumption halves during a 10 °C temperature fall, which partially protects against the reductions in cerebral perfusion.

Management

1 **General management** includes gentle handling, close monitoring, oxygen therapy and treatment of underlying causes. Fluid resuscitation may require central access due to intense peripheral vasoconstriction. Arrhythmias and heart block usually respond to rewarming alone. Prolonged CPR is often successful in hypothermic patients but cardioversion is often ineffective below 30 °C. Consequently, rewarming to >35 °C is essential before death is declared.

2 **Rewarming strategies** depend on hypothermia severity:
- **Passive, external rewarming** (i.e. warm environment (>30 °C), insulating covers) is adequate in mild hypothermia (i.e. >33 °C) without circulatory compromise.
- **Active, external rewarming** (i.e. warming blankets, immersion) is recommended in moderate to severe hypothermia with no circulatory collapse. However, caution is required because rapid peripheral vasodilation may increase organ hypoperfusion (±mortality). Convective (forced air) warming (e.g. Bair Hugger) at 43 °C increases body temperature by 2–3 °C/h.
- **Internal, core rewarming** is indicated in severe hypothermia with physiological instability, circulatory failure or cardiac arrest when rapid rewarming is necessary. Techniques include warm intravenous (i.v.) fluids or inhaled gas (1 °C/h), bladder, pleural or peritoneal lavage (2–3 °C/h) and haemodialysis (5 °C/h). Cardiopulmonary bypass (10 °C/h) is only necessary during cardiac arrest.

Hyperthermia

Hyperthermia is defined as a core temperature >37.5 °C (99 °F). Fever increases metabolic rate and carbon dioxide (CO_2) production. Sweating and vasodilation cause hypovolaemia. Metabolic acidosis, epilepsy, neurological impairment, renal failure, rhabdomyolysis and myocardial ischaemia may follow. Severe hyperthermia (>42 °C) is potentially lethal and even short periods may cause permanent cerebral damage.

Causes

Figure 23c lists the causes of hyperthermia; ~50% are due to infection. In addition to thyroid storm (Chapter 51), five non-infectious causes of hyperthermia require immediate recognition and treatment:
- **Exertional heatstroke** follows prolonged exercise in warm, humid environments. It often affects athletes, firefighters, military recruits and those wearing garments that restrict heat loss. It presents with hyperthermia, confusion, hypotension and tachypnoea followed by shock, rhabdomyolysis and renal failure. Figure 23d presents the metabolic consequences. Mortality is ~10% even with rapid cooling.
- **Classical (non-exertional) heatstroke** affects sedentary, older, city dwellers with co-existent illness during heatwaves. Patients with thermoregulatory disorders (e.g. hypothalamic stroke), inability to dissipate heat (e.g. skin disease) and those using drugs that impair heat loss (e.g. anticholinergics, diuretics) or generate heat (e.g. tricyclics) are at greater risk. It presents with hyperthermia, hot (dry) skin and confusion followed by shock and organ failure. Figure 23d reports metabolic effects. Hypovolaemia and rhabdomyolysis occasionally cause renal failure. Most deaths (~80%) occur in those >50 years old.
- **Drug-induced hyperthermia**: due to serotonin receptor stimulation by amphetamine derivatives (e.g. methylene dioxymethamphetamine [MDMA; 'ecstasy']), serotonin reuptake inhibitors (e.g. imipramine) or serotonin agonists (e.g. lithium).
- **Malignant hyperthermia (MH)**: a rare autosomal dominant trait, causes excessive muscle heat production due to altered calcium kinetics after anaesthetic drug exposure. Muscle rigidity, sudden hyperpyrexia (41–45 °C), tachycardia, metabolic acidosis and hypercarbia occur. Halothane and succinylcholine precipitate 80% of cases. Early recognition has reduced mortality to <10%.
- **Neuroleptic malignant syndrome (NMS)**: an idiosyncratic reaction to neuroleptic drugs (e.g. haloperidol, phenothiazines, metoclopramide) due to hypothalamic dopamine-receptor blockade. Muscle rigidity, encephalopathy, catatonia, extrapyramidal symptoms and autonomic effects (e.g. sweating, labile hypertension, tachycardia) are common. Organ failure (e.g. renal) and death (10–15%) may occur.

Management

1 **General management**: early recognition is lifesaving. Stop causative drugs, replace fluid and correct electrolyte imbalance. Renal replacement therapy and seizure prophylaxis may be required.

2 **Cooling**: spray unclothed skin with tepid water and use a fan to encourage evaporation. Ice packs (e.g. axilla, groin) are often useful. Cold water immersion may prevent heat loss due to cutaneous vasoconstriction. Additional measures include cold i.v. fluids, iced gastric or peritoneal lavage and haemofiltration.

3 **Drug therapy**: paracetamol (±NSAID) is ineffective. I.v. dantrolene, a muscle relaxant that uncouples excitation-contraction mechanisms by inhibiting intracellular calcium release is the only specific therapy for MH, NMS and MDMA toxicity. Anticholinergics and muscle relaxants may be helpful, and bromocriptine in NMS. Alkaline diuresis and mannitol may reduce myoglobin-induced renal damage.

> **Pearl of wisdom**
> In hypothermic cardiac arrests, ventricular fibrillation is resistant to cardioversion, so rewarming to >35 °C is essential before death is declared

24 Assessment of the patient with suspected infection

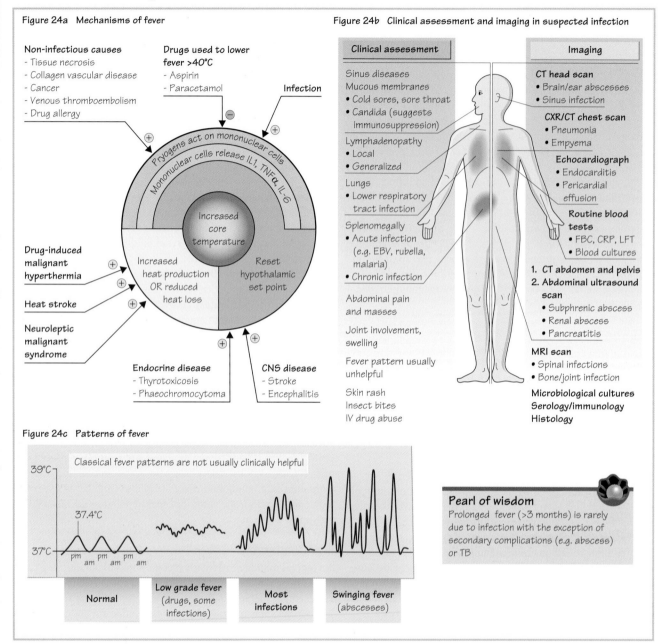

Figure 24a Mechanisms of fever

Non-infectious causes
- Tissue necrosis
- Collagen vascular disease
- Cancer
- Venous thromboembolism
- Drug allergy

Drugs used to lower fever >40°C
- Aspirin
- Paracetamol

Infection

Pryogens act on mononuclear cells
Mononuclear cells release IL1, TNFα, IL-6

Increased core temperature

Drug-induced malignant hyperthermia

Heat stroke

Neuroleptic malignant syndrome

Increased heat production OR reduced heat loss

Reset hypothalamic set point

Endocrine disease
- Thyrotoxicosis
- Phaeochromocytoma

CNS disease
- Stroke
- Encephalitis

Figure 24b Clinical assessment and imaging in suspected infection

Clinical assessment

Sinus diseases
Mucous membranes
• Cold sores, sore throat
• Candida (suggests immunosuppression)
Lymphadenopathy
• Local
• Generalized
Lungs
• Lower respiratory tract infection
Splenomegally
• Acute infection (e.g. EBV, rubella, malaria)
• Chronic infection

Abdominal pain and masses

Joint involvement, swelling

Fever pattern usually unhelpful

Skin rash
Insect bites
IV drug abuse

Imaging

CT head scan
• Brain/ear abscesses
• Sinus infection
CXR/CT chest scan
• Pneumonia
• Empyema
Echocardiograph
• Endocarditis
• Pericardial effusion
Routine blood tests
• FBC, CRP, LFT
• Blood cultures
1. CT abdomen and pelvis
2. Abdominal ultrasound scan
• Subphrenic abscess
• Renal abscess
• Pancreatitis
MRI scan
• Spinal infections
• Bone/joint infection
Microbiological cultures
Serology/immunology
Histology

Figure 24c Patterns of fever

39°C

Classical fever patterns are not usually clinically helpful

37.4°C

37°C

pm am pm am pm am

Normal

Low grade fever (drugs, some infections)

Most infections

Swinging fever (abscesses)

Pearl of wisdom
Prolonged fever (>3 months) is rarely due to infection with the exception of secondary complications (e.g. abscess) or TB

Although 'fever' is a cardinal feature of infection, there are many non-infective causes (Figure 24a). Normal hypothalamic set point for body temperature varies between individuals (oral range 36–37.7 °C), diurnally (e.g. evening peaks) and with hormonal cycles (e.g. menstrual). Hyperthermia (Chapter 23) can occur in the absence of infection due to excess heat production or reduced loss (e.g. heat stroke), hypothalamic damage (e.g. stroke) or rare drug-induced syndromes (e.g. neuroleptic malignant syndrome). Fever may also be due to exogenous pyrogens. During infection, these are breakdown products of infectious agents or their toxins. In malignancy, connective tissue disease (CTD) or drug reactions pyrogens include immune complexes and lymphocytes.

History

A comprehensive history is paramount in suspected infection. Although some patients take their own temperature, the presence of fever is often surmised from symptoms of hot or cold 'chills' or excessive perspiration. Drenching night sweats (e.g. requiring nightwear or bed-linen changes) may occur in tuberculosis (TB) or lymphoproliferative disorders. Rigors often accompany bacteraemia and weight loss accompanies chronic infection (e.g. TB).

History should include:
- **Duration and pattern of fever**, which aid diagnosis. Few infectious agents cause prolonged fever (>2–3 months) with the exception of secondary complications (e.g. abscess) or TB.
- **Symptom localization**: focal symptoms may indicate the cause (e.g. pleurisy). Non-specific features (e.g. myalgia) occur in generalized infections (e.g. septicaemia).
- **Infection source**: explore recent travel (Chapter 27), occupation (e.g. leptospirosis in sewage workers), animal contact, tick bites acquired in forest or heathland (e.g. Lyme disease), exposure to local diseases (e.g. malaria) or epidemic conditions (e.g. cholera). Consider viral infections related to blood transfusion.
- **Sexual history**: assess HIV risk.
- **Immune status**: infection is common in the immunocompromised.
- **Past medical history**: assess recurrent conditions (e.g. cholecystitis, urinary tract infection [UTI]), implanted prosthetic material (e.g. valves), instrumentation (e.g. post-catheter sepsis) and pre-existing disease (e.g. liver). Vaccination makes some infections unlikely (e.g. measles) but can be less reliable (e.g. TB can occur despite previous BCG vaccination).
- **Drug history**: immunosuppressive drugs predispose to opportunistic infections. Drug reactions or traditional remedies may also cause fever, while other drugs including corticosteroids, antibiotics and antipyretics may reduce fever or modify clinical presentation.
- **Social and family history**: close contact is important in meningiococcal infection (e.g. military camps, student halls) and norovirus transmission (e.g. cruise ships). Overcrowding, poverty and famine (e.g. refugee camps) are associated with louse-borne infections and epidemic typhus. Gastroenteritis affecting recipients of a shared meal suggests food poisoning (e.g. *Campylobacter*) but in general food histories are unhelpful. Rarely, family history may suggest inherited familial periodic fevers (Chapter 28).
- **Likely causative organism**: determined from age, environment (e.g. hospital), immune status, site of instrumentation, geography, travel history, symptom duration, organs affected and medical history.

Assessment

Comprehensive clinical examination is essential (Figure 24b) because symptoms may not be organ specific. Fever pattern is generally unhelpful (Figure 24c) although a high 'swinging' fever may indicate an abscess.

Investigation

Routine blood tests should include:
- **Full blood count**: normochromic/normocytic anaemia may indicate chronic infection. Neutrophil leucocytosis (toxic granulation) suggests bacterial infection, although leukopaenia can occur in overwhelming sepsis, especially in older people, due to failure to mount an immune response. The total white cell count (WCC) is usually normal or reduced in viral infections although a raised lymphocyte counts may occur, and if associated with atypical lymphocytes suggests Epstein–Barr virus (EBV) or cytomegalovirus (CMV) infection. In some bacterial infections (e.g. typhoid, brucellosis), lymphocyte counts may be elevated. A low lymphocyte count should raise the possibility of human immunodeficiency virus (HIV). Eosinophilia occurs in schistosomiasis and other parasitic infections. A low platelet counts suggest malaria, dengue fever, parovirus 19 infection or disseminated intravascular coagulation (DIC) in sepsis.
- **Inflammatory markers**: C-reactive protein (CRP) rises within 4–8 hours of infection and has a circulation half-life of 8 hours. It indicates the recent onset of infection. Erythrocyte sedimentation rate (ESR), the rate at which red cells settle through plasma, increases with age and depends on sex, red-cell characteristics, immunoglobulins and acute phase proteins like fibrinogen. During infection or inflammation, it rises slowly over 2–3 weeks.
- **Liver, renal and clotting function tests** assess the consequences of infection and rise with local infective processes (e.g. hepatitis, cholecystitis) or severe, disseminated infections (e.g. sepsis, leptospirosis, TB).
- **Microbiology and culture**: simple microscopy alone may detect some micro-organisms (e.g. stool parasites) but often requires specific stains (e.g. gram stains for bacteria; Ziehl–Neelson for mycobacteria, fluorescent linked antibodies for some viruses). Electron microscopy identifies rotavirus in stool and herpes viruses (e.g. varicella–zoster from chicken pox lesions). Culture is the definitive diagnostic technique for most bacteria and fungi and some viruses, and utilizes a variety of growth media. Antibiotic discs on culture plates allow determination of antibiotic sensitivities.
- **Serology** assesses the host's immune response to infection by measuring the rise in IgM and IgG antibodies (acute and convalescent titres) over 10–14 days. It is helpful in the diagnosis of hepatitis and EBV infection.
- **Histology**: specific pathological features may aid diagnosis (e.g. caseating granulomata in TB, fungal hyphae in aspergillosis, lymphoma).
- **Molecular techniques**, including nuclear acid hybridization (e.g. chlamydia) and polymerase chain reaction (PCR) amplification to detect small amounts of nucleic acid from 'difficult to culture' organisms (e.g. herpes simplex) or to quantify viral load (e.g. HIV), are increasingly important.
- **Imaging**: chest radiography, ultrasound examinations (e.g. cholecystitis), computed tomography, nuclear imaging and echocardiography (e.g. endocarditis) aid detection of the cause and site of infection.

If clinical assessment and early investigation do not reveal a cause, consider stopping all unnecessary drugs, re-culture all possible infected sites and consider non-infective causes of fever (e.g. vasculitis, CTD). Avoid empirical antibiotics unless the patient is very unwell, when broad spectrum antibiotics should be used.

Bacteraemia, SIRS and sepsis

Figure 25a Terminology for SIRS, sepsis, severe sepsis and septic shock

Infection	Invasion of sterile host tissue by microorganisms
Bacteraemia	Viable bacteria in the blood
Systemic Inflammatory Response Syndrome (SIRS)	An inflammatory response to infective and non-infective conditions (e.g. pancreatitis, trauma, burns) defined as ≥2 of 4 criteria: 1. Temperature >38 or <36°C 2. Heart rate >90 /min 3. Respiratory rate >20 /min, P_aCO_2 <32 mmHg (4.3kPa) 4. White cell count >12000 or <4000 cells /mm^3 or >10% immature (band) forms
Sepsis	SIRS due to infection
Severe sepsis	Sepsis plus sepsis-induced organ dysfunction or tissue hypoperfusion (i.e. hypotension, ↑ lactate, ↓ UO). Where sepsis-induced hypotension is defined as SBP <90 mmHg, or MAP <70 mmHg, or a SBP fall of >40 mmHg
Septic shock	Sepsis-induced hypotension persisting despite adequate fluid resuscitation (i.e. shock, inadequate organ perfusion)
Multiple organ dysfunction	Development of impaired organ function in SIRS. Multiple organ failure may follow

Pearl of wisdom

The characteristic inflammatory response of 'sepsis' is not always due to infection. An infective cause is only found in 65% of cases

Figure 25b Septic shock

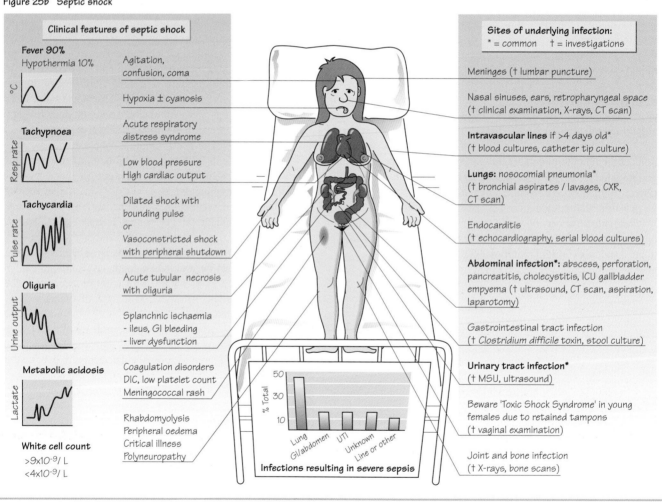

Definitions

The inflammatory response that characterizes 'sepsis' is not always due to infection. A potential infective cause is detected in ~65% of cases. Blood cultures are positive in <25%. Figure 25a presents the current terminology used to describe the systemic inflammatory response syndrome (SIRS) and sepsis. *Severe sepsis* implies sepsis-induced organ dysfunction or tissue hypoperfusion and *septic shock* persistent hypotension despite fluid resuscitation.

Critical Care Medicine at a Glance, Third Edition. Richard Leach. © 2014 John Wiley & Sons, Ltd. Published 2014 by John Wiley & Sons, Ltd.

Epidemiology

In the USA, ~500,000 patients (average age 55 years) develop sepsis annually. Half of intensive care unit patients are on antibiotics at any one time and in ~50% the infection was acquired after admission. Sepsis is the leading cause of multiple organ failure, acute respiratory distress syndrome (ARDS), acute renal injury and late death following trauma. The most common organisms are:

- Gram positive (e.g. *Staphylococcus* spp., pneumococci) ~60–65%.
- Gram negative (e.g. *E.coli*, *Pseudomonas* spp.) 35–40%.
- Fungi (e.g. *Candida* spp.) 2–5%.

Pathophysiology

Invasive micro-organisms or bacterial endotoxins stimulate the host's immune response. Initial cytokine release (e.g. TNFα) activates polymorphs, platelets, complement and coagulation pathways. The activated white cells adhere to and damage vascular endothelium allowing fluid and cell leakage into the interstitial space. Endothelial inflammatory mediators (e.g. nitric oxide) cause vasodilation, microcirculatory thrombosis and myocardial dysfunction. Tissue oxygen usage is impaired by sepsis-mediated cellular enzyme inhibition.

Clinical presentation

The clinical features of sepsis and potential sources of infection are illustrated in Figure 25b. Haemodynamic changes are variable (Chapter 7,) and circulatory assessment may reveal either a hyperdynamic (i.e. 'warm, dilated') patient with bounding pulses, or a hypotensive, vasoconstricted (i.e. cold, clammy') patient (i.e. mimics myocardial infarction [MI] or pulmonary embolism [PE]). *Examination* may reveal a focus of infection or diagnostic clues (e.g. meningococcal rash, splinter haemorrhages in endocarditis). Chest infection is the most common source of sepsis.

Management

The updated 'Surviving Sepsis Campaign' management guidelines (2013) apply to all acute wards. As in MI, the speed and appropriateness of initial therapy influences outcome.

a. *Diagnosis of sepsis*
- *Identify the cause* because this guides therapy (e.g. antibiotic choice, abscess drainage, tissue debridement, line removal).
- *Essential investigations*: include routine blood tests, C-reactive protein, plasma lactate, coagulation profile, arterial blood gases (ABGs), urinalysis, chest radiography, electrocardiogram and if possible central venous SO_2 ($S_{cv}O_2$).
- *Monitor* vital signs, urine output, biochemistry, ABGs and, if possible, central venous pressure (CVP).
- *Culture* blood, sputum, urine, cerebrospinal fluid or wound pus, as required, before antibiotic therapy, providing this does not delay treatment. At least two blood cultures (≥ 1 percutaneous sample and one through each vascular access device >48 hours old) are recommended.
- *Specific investigations* (Figure 25b) depend on the suspected cause (e.g. ultrasonography in abdominal sepsis) and patient mobility (e.g. CT scans).

b. *Initial resuscitation (first 6 hours) and antibiotic therapy*
- *Protocolized fluid* resuscitation must start immediately in hypoperfused (i.e. lactate >4 mmol/L, raised $S_{cv}O_2$) or hypotensive patients. Aim to achieve: (a) mean arterial pressure (MAP) ≥ 65 mmHg; (b) urine output ≥ 0.5 ml/kg/h; (c) CVP ≥ 8 mmHg (≥ 12 mmHg if ventilated); and (d) $S_{cv}O_2 \geq 70\%$ using crystalloid (1 L) or colloid (0.5 L) fluid challenges (Chapters 10, 11). If the $S_{cv}O_2$ target is not achieved, consider packed red cell transfusion to a haemocrit $\geq 30\%$ or a dobutamine infusion (max 20 μg/kg/min) to increase oxygen delivery and $S_{cv}O_2$. Reduce/stop fluid therapy if CVP increases without haemodynamic improvement.
- *Antibiotic therapy* should start as soon as possible and always within <1 hr. Initial empiric therapy uses broad spectrum agents with good tissue penetration. Antibiotic selection depends on the clinical features, whether community or hospital acquired (Chapters 26, 38, 39), the primary site of infection and local antibiotic resistance patterns. In the absence of an obvious cause, treatment options include:
- Community-acquired sepsis: penicillin with a β-lactamases inhibitor (e.g. co-amoxiclav) or a second- or third-generation cephalosporin (e.g. cefuroxime).
- Hospital-acquired sepsis: carbenopenem (e.g. meropenem), ceftazidime or antipsuedomonal penicillin with a β-lactamase inhibitor and an antistaphylococcal drug. Aminoglcosides may be added in critically ill patients or if resistant organisms are suspected. Vancomycin should be used if methicillin-resistant staphylococcus aureus (MRSA) infection is suspected (i.e. recent hospitalization).
- In neutropaenic patients or those with possible Pseudomonas infection (e.g. cystic fibrosis), use combination therapy.

Microbiology results guide subsequent therapy. Stop unnecessary antibiotics (i.e. aim for monotherapy after 3–5 days) and review daily. Stop all antibiotics after 5–14 days depending on response and organism isolated.

c. *Haemodynamic support and adjunctive therapy*
- *Vasopressor/inotropic therapy* (Chapters 7, 12) aims to maintain MAP ≥ 65 mmHg if initial fluid administration is unsuccessful. These drugs should be given through central lines and require an arterial line for blood pressure monitoring. *In early sepsis*, widespread vasodilation (i.e. low systemic vascular resistance [SVR]) causes hypotension and relative hypovolaemia. Although cardiac output (CO) may be raised, inappropriate distribution can cause regional (i.e. splanchnic, renal) ischaemia. In these patients, a *vasopressor agent* (e.g. norepinephrine or vasopressin) increases blood pressure, SVR and organ perfusion. *In late sepsis*, toxic myocarditis impairs myocardial contractility and requires an *inotropic agent* (e.g. dopamine, dobutamine or, less commonly, epinephrine) to improve cardiac function and maintain CO. The specific properties of these drugs mean that they are often used in combination to achieve the best results (e.g. dobutamine with norepinephrine).
- *Low*-dose steroid therapy (e.g. hydrocortisone 8 mg/h) may be beneficial if hypotension is refractory to fluid and vasopressor support, because relative adrenocortical insufficiency occurs in severe sepsis.
- *Activated protein C* improves outcome in septic shock (APACHE II ≥ 25), if there are no contraindications to use (e.g. bleeding), by reducing microcirculatory thrombosis and organ ischaemia.

d. *Supportive therapy*
- *General measures* include oxygen therapy, ventilatory support, glycaemic control (i.e. blood sugar <7–9 mmol/L), renal support, nutrition and prophylaxis against peptic ulceration and thromboembolism.
- *Sepsis prevention* includes infection control (e.g. hand washing), microbiological monitoring, appropriate prophylactic antibiotics and prompt management of suspected infection.

Prognosis

Mortality is >40% in septic shock; 25–40% in Gram-negative sepsis and 10–20% in Gram-positive sepsis. Outcome deteriorates with age, lactic acidosis, low white cell count, cytokine elevation, reduced SVR and number of organ failures.

26 Hospital-acquired (nosocomial) infections

Figure 23a Organisms responsible for most nosocomial infections

Methicillin-resistant *Staphylococcus aureus* (MRSA)	Increasing prevalence. Colonizes and infects. Easily treated but glycopepide resistance increasing
Coagulase negative staphylococcus (CNS)	Frequent skin colonization. Low virulence organisms. Increasing cause of nosocomial infections
Enterococcus faecalis (e.g. vancomycin resistant enterococcus (VRE))	Emerge with 3rd generation cephalosporin use. Often sensitive to ampicillin but resistance to aminoglycosides, ampicillin and vancomycin increasing (e.g. VRE)
Pseudomonas aeruginosa	Very broad spectrum of antibiotic resistance. Common in ICU and chronic lung disease
Stenotrophomonas maltophilia	Environmental organism. Increasingly common. Very broad spectrum of antibiotic resistance
Acinetobacter baumanii	Increasingly common. Multi-resistant to antibiotics but may be sensistive to carbapenems
Klebsiella spp.	Extended β-lactam resistance ± multi-resistant to antibiotics
Enterobacter sp	Occur in normal intestinal flora and develop extended β-lactam resistance
E.coli	Variable resistance seems to correspond with use of quinolones
Others: *Proteus* spp, *Serratia marcescens*	Broad spectrums of antibiotic resistance
Clostridium difficile	Spore forming, multi-antibiotic resistant bacillus that colonizes intestine in hospital patients
Candida species	Overgrowth due to antibiotic pressures. Diagnosis suggested by growth in more than 2 sites

Figure 23b Risk factors for nosocmial infection

Patient factors
- Nutritional status, immunosuppression (e.g. steroids)
- Underlying disease (e.g. diabetes, SLE)
- Integrity of natural defences (e.g. burns, lines, open wounds)
- Multiple or prolonged antibiotic usage (i.e. resistant clone selection)

Environmental factors
- Inadequate infection control (e.g. hand washing, isolation)
- Inadequate staffing or inexperienced, new staff
- Transmission (e.g. overcrowding, frequent relocation, prolonged stay)
- Iatrogenic infection (e.g. during endotracheal tube or line insertion)

Organism factors
- Prevalence, resilience (e.g. spore formation, adherence), colonization
- Antibiotic resistance and selection
- Pathogenicity

Figure 23c Control of endemic nosocomial infection

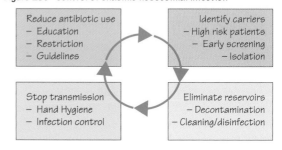

Reduce antibiotic use
- Education
- Restriction
- Guidelines

Identify carriers
- High risk patients
- Early screening
- Isolation

Stop transmission
- Hand Hygiene
- Infection control

Eliminate reservoirs
- Decontamination
- Cleaning/disinfection

Figure 23d Prevention of central venous catheter or intra-arterial line infection

Strict aseptic insertion technique
- Mask
- Sterile gown
- Sterile gloves
- Sterile drapes

Skin antisepsis
Use 2% aqueous chlorhexidine to clean skin and allow to dry

Insertion site
- Firmly secure cannulae as movement risks infection
- Transparent dressings to allow regular inspection
- Change line if signs of local infection / cellulitis

Type of cannulae
Antimicrobial or antiseptic impregnated CVC (e.g. silver) may reduce catheter associated bacteraemia

Environment
Cleaning and disinfection

Line Management
- Use closed systems
- Avoid 3-way tap contamination
- Clean access ports with 70% alcohol before use
- Give TPN through a dedicated lumen
- Replace administration sets at ≥72hrs unless used to administer lipid, blood or blood products when they should be changed at 24hrs

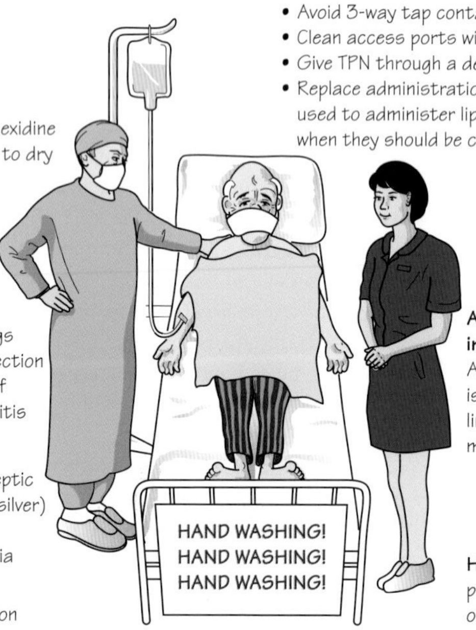

Assistance during line insertion
Always ensure an assistant is available when inserting lines. This helps with maintaining sterility

HAND WASHING!
HAND WASHING!
HAND WASHING!

HAND WASHING
prevents transmission of organisms between patients

Figure 23e Risk factors for line infection

- Non-sterile CVC insertion technique (e.g. emergency, skin preparation)
- Poor hand hygiene (i.e. peripheral catheters)
- >5 days since line insertion
- Iatrogenic (e.g. operator inexperience)
- Inadequate line-care
- Infection from distant sites (e.g. endocarditis)
- Contamination from infusions (e.g. propofol, TPN)
- Host risk factors (e.g. steroids, immunosuppression, diabetes)
- Catheter type (e.g. silver or antibiotic impregnation reduces risk, multilumen increases risk)
- Line material (e.g. silicone better than PVC or polyethylene lines)
- Line insertion site (e.g. subclavian at lower risk than femoral lines)

CVC=central venous catheter, TPN=total parenteral nutrition, PVC=polyvinyl chloride

Critical Care Medicine at a Glance, Third Edition. Richard Leach. © 2014 John Wiley & Sons, Ltd. Published 2014 by John Wiley & Sons, Ltd.

Hospital-acquired infections are an increasingly important cause of morbidity and mortality in hospitals and nursing homes. **Causative organisms** (Figure 26a) are often virulent, antibiotic resistant and spore forming, which impedes environmental eradication and encourages recurrent infection. Methicillin-resistant *Staphylococcus aureus* (MRSA), *Clostridium difficile* and multidrug-resistant (MDR) Gram-negative bacilli (e.g. pseudomonas) are typical. **Common infection sites** are the urinary tract ($\sim$40%; but less common in intensive care), surgical wounds ($\sim$15%), respiratory tract ($\sim$15%; Chapter 39), line-related bacteraemia ($\sim$10%) and colitis ($<$10%). **Risk factors** include host, environmental and pathogen-related factors (Figure 26b). **Prevention** requires identification of carriers of causative organisms, elimination of reservoirs, prevention of transmission and appropriate antibiotic usage (Figure 26c).

Line-related sepsis

Five days after insertion, $\sim$10–20% of central venous catheters (CVCs) are colonized and 2–5% develop bacteraemia. The average rate of CVC-associated bacteraemia is $\sim$5/1000 CVC days but varies between critical care units (CCUs), patient type (e.g. burns, surgical), severity of illness and CVC types (e.g. urgent, tunnelled, insertion site, antibiotic/silver-impregnation). Peripheral intra-arterial lines (e.g. radial) are colonized less frequently ($\sim$4–5% at day 5) and bacteraemia occurs on 2.9/1000 catheter days. Long, antecubital, peripheral venous catheters (PVCs; $>$12 cm) are associated with bacteraemia on 0.8/1000 catheter days and short PVC (i.e. $<$12 cm) even less, although local phlebitis is common. **Microbiology**: *Staphylococcus epidermidis* ($\sim$35%), *S. aureus* ($\sim$15%) and Gram-negative bacilli (e.g. *E. coli*; $\sim$15%) are the most common organisms. **Risk factors** for line infection are listed in Figure 26e and factors preventing infection in Figure 26d. **Line replacement**: resite short PVC at 72–96 hours. Scheduled CVC and arterial line replacement is not required because this does not reduce line-related bacteraemias in normally functioning catheters with no complications. Inspect lines daily, replace if infection is suspected and remove promptly when not needed. Always assess the risks of line replacement (e.g. pneumothorax). **Management**: if infection is suspected (i.e. sepsis, positive blood cultures), remove the line and send the tip for culture. If needed, new lines should be inserted at different sites. Start empiric antibiotic therapy while awaiting microbiology results, although fever and symptoms may resolve spontaneously after line removal.

Methicillin-resistant *Staphylococcus aureus*

MRSA infection has increased over the last 10 years. It is still largely associated with hospital and care homes but increasingly common in community settings, partly due to 'silent' healthcare acquisition in the preceding year. Once established within healthcare environments, it is difficult to eradicate. **Prevention** utilizes the strategies in Figure 26c. Unrecognized MRSA carriage is present in $\sim$3% of hospital and $\sim$30% of intensive care unit admissions (e.g. asymptomatic skin colonization), which constitutes the main source of hospital transmission. **Detection** requires active surveillance especially in high-risk patients (e.g. $>$75 years old, antibiotic use within $<$6 months, hospitalization within $<$1 year, urinary catheter at admission, CCU). **Decolonization** aims to reduce MRSA carriage. Although intranasal mupirocin and chlorhexidine-based skin cleaning are often used, evidence for benefit is limited. Environmental cleaning and disinfection may be more effective. **Early diagnosis** with rapid molecular screening

techniques and prompt patient isolation reduce MRSA acquisition. **Antibiotic restrictions** that limit usage and avoid certain antibiotics (e.g. quinolones, cephalosporins) decrease MRSA infection rates. **Antibiotic sensitivity**: MRSA resistance to fluoroquinolones occurs in $\sim$80%, macrolides $\sim$70%, trimethoprim $\sim$35%, gentamicin 12% and mupirocin 12%. Most isolates are susceptible to tetracycline, fusidic acid and rifampicin. **MRSA therapy**: vancomycin, teicoplanin and linezolid should be reserved for patients with severe line-related or neutropenic sepsis, burns, serious soft tissue infections and prosthetic valve infections. A treatment period of $\geq$14 days is required for bacteraemia and endocarditis. Monitor drug levels during vancomycin and teicoplanin therapy. Tetracyclines, trimethoprim and combinations of rifampicin and fusidic acid are effective in cellulitis, urinary and respiratory tract infections, and as part of eradication therapy. Inadequate therapy contributes to excess mortality in critically ill patients.

Clostridium difficile

C. difficile is a ubiquitous, Gram-positive, anaerobic, motile, spore-forming bacillus that colonizes the intestines of nursing home or long-stay hospital patients (i.e. 13% and 50% acquisition at 2 and $>$4 weeks respectively). It is resistant to most antibiotics, forms heat- and/or disinfectant-resistant spores and can survive for long periods in hospital environments. Fortunately, bleach-containing disinfectants destroy the organism. **Clinical features**: spores are transmitted by the faecal–oral route. After ingestion, they pass through the stomach because they are acid resistant, then change to their active form and multiply in the colon. In small numbers, *C. difficile* is not harmful but after disruption of normal intestinal flora by broad-spectrum antibiotics (especially quinolones, cephalosporins), overgrowth may cause a spectrum of symptoms ranging from asymptomatic to life-threatening diarrhoea and pseudomembranous colitis. Pathogenic *C. difficile* produces toxins responsible for diarrhoea and inflammation. The best characterized are toxins A and B. **Diagnosis** is based on clinical features (e.g. odorous diarrhoea, antibiotic exposure), toxin detection and characteristic CT scan features (e.g. colonic wall thickening $>$4 mm). Delayed diagnosis risks bowel perforation and increased mortality. **Treatment**: oral metronidazole is the initial drug of choice in symptomatic patients. Oral vancomycin, and occasionally linezolid, is used in severe or resistant cases. Asymptomatic patients may not require antibiotic therapy. Antidiarrhoeal drugs (e.g. loperamide) are contraindicated because they prolong toxin-induced colonic damage. Probiotics (i.e. 'good' intestinal flora) may be beneficial. **Prevention** includes avoiding inappropriate antibiotic therapy (especially in older people), use of gloves and appropriate infection control measures to reduce transmission. The value of prophylactic probiotics has not been established. **Mortality**: hospital outbreaks, often with virulent strains (e.g. Quebec strain), have caused many deaths, especially in older people or the immunocompromised.

Urinary tract infections

Catheterization introduces perineal organisms into the bladder causing urinary tract infections (UTIs). Although mortality rates are low, aseptic catheterization, closed unobstructed drainage and well-secured catheters prevent patient discomfort and reduce infection risk.

Pearl of wisdom

Good antibiotic stewardship and infection control policies reduce hospital-acquired infections

27 Fever in the returning traveller

Figure 27a Clinical features and associated infections

Delirium/confusion
- Malaria
- Viral enchephalitis
- Hepatic failure

Hepatomegally
- Hepatitis
- Typhoid
- Leptospirosis
- Amoebic liver abscess (may be tender)
- Malaria

Diarrhoea
- GI infections

Skin lesions
- Rose spots
  – typhoid
- Maculopapular
  – dengue, syphilis, typhus, HIV, leptospirosis, arboviruses
- Petechiae/haemorrhage
  – viral haemorrhagic fever, leptospirosis
- Eschar
  – anthrax, tick typhus
- Chancre
  – trypanosomiasis

Jaundice
- Malaria
- Hepatitis
- Leptospirosis
- Yellow fever

Vomiting
- Malaria
- GI pathogens

Chest signs
- Pneumococcus
- Tuberculosis
- Legionella

Splenomegaly
- Malaria
- Typhoid
- Visceral leishmaniasis (often marked)
- Brucellosis
- Rickettsial disease

Lymphadenopathy
- HIV
- Brucellosis
- Visceral leishmaniasis
- Rickettsial disease
- Filariasis
- Plague

GI = gastrointestinal infection

Pearl of wisdom

Most fevers in returning travellers are due to common viral, respiratory or urinary tract infections

Figure 27b Pathogenesis of malaria

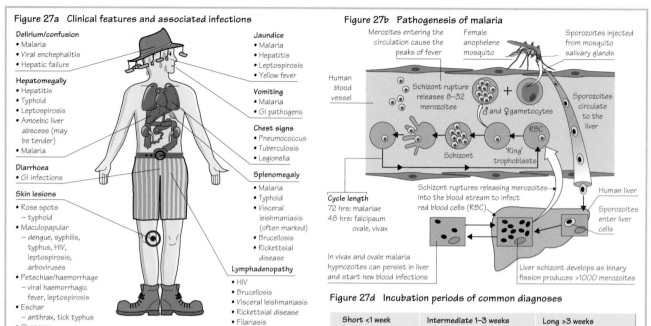

Merozites entering the circulation cause the peaks of fever

Female anophelene mosquito

Sporozoites injected from mosquito salivary glands

Human blood vessel

Schizont rupture releases 8–32 merozoites

♂ and ♀ gametocytes

Sporozoites circulate to the liver

RBC

Schizont

'Ring' trophoblasts

Cycle length
72 hrs: malariae
48 hrs: falcipaum ovale, vivax

Schizont ruptures releasing merozoites into the blood stream to infect red blood cells (RBC)

Human liver

Sporozoites enter liver cells

In vivax and ovale malaria hypnozoites can persist in liver and start new blood infections

Liver schizont develops as binary fission produces >1000 merozoites

Figure 27d Incubation periods of common diagnoses

Short <1 week	Intermediate 1–3 weeks	Long >3 weeks
Enteric infections	Malaria	Malaria
Dengue	Typhoid	Viral hepatitis
Other arboviruses	Typhus	HIV seroconversion
Relapsing fever	Leptospirosis	Acute schistosomiasis
Legionella	Brucellosis	Amoebic liver abscess
Plague	African trypanosomiasis	Brucellosis
	Haemorrhagic fever	Visceral leishmaniasis

Figure 27c Other tropical diseases (* = rare, + = common)

Disease	Incubation period	Cause and clinical features	Diagnosis and treatment
+ Typhoid	10–14 days	Follows ingestion of food/water infected with Gram-negative bacteria *Salmonella typhi* or *paratyphi*. It multiplies in gut mesenteric lymph nodes/macrophages before widespread blood transmission. Gradual onset of fever, headache, malaise and cough; 1st week abdominal pain with constipation or diarrhoea; 2nd week diarrhoea, hepatosplenomegally and rose spots (60%). Shock, AKI and confusion/coma occur in severe cases. Complications include ileal perforation/bleeding, myocarditis, biliary stasis and osteomyelitis (mainly in sickle cell disease). Relapse occurs after therapy in 10% and asymptomatic gallbladder carriage in 5% (i.e. risks transmission).	↓WCC (+), ↑ALT; culture (blood, urine, stool) is diagnostic, serology (Widal test) is helpful if non-immune. Fluoroquinolones for <7 days are the treatment of choice. Often resistant to co-trimoxazole, ampicillin and chloramphenicol. Sensitivity testing is helpful.
+ Dengue	3–8 days	Arbovirus transmitted by Aedes sp. mosquito. Dengue fever causes sudden onset of biphasic fever, rigors, headache, myalgia and backache. Dengue haemorrhagic fever/shock syndrome (DHF) occurs in children in endemic areas (i.e. rare in UK) due to an immunological reaction to a second infection. Causes shock, petechiae and bleeding and has a high mortality.	↓WCC, ↓plats (+), in DHF severe ↓plats, ↑hct, ↑ALT. Retrospective serology diagnostic. Treatment is supportive (i.e. no specific therapy) with fluids in DHF.
* Tick typhus (UKs commonest rickettsial disease)	7–14 days	Tick bite infection (many rickettsial species, wide geographical variation), often in travellers from southern Africa. Causes fever, headache, myalgia, an eschar (necrotic skin lesion) at the site of the tick bite, a maculopapular rash, lymphadenopathy and rarely severe systemic illness.	Retrospective serology is diagnostic. Treatment with tetracycline is very effective.
* Leptospirosis (can also be acquired in UK)	7–14 days	Contact with water (e.g. sewer workers) infected by animal (e.g. rat) urine containing leptospires which penetrate skin, multiply in blood and then localize in liver, CNS, muscle and kidneys. Spectrum of illness from fever, myalgia and headache to jaundice, AKI, conjunctivitis, haemorrhage and pneumonitis.	↓WCC, ↓plats (+), CK (if severe), ↑ALT +AKI. Blood/urine microscopy for leptospires. Retrospective serology is diagnostic. Treat with doxycycline or IV penicillin in severe cases.
Schistosomiasis Affects 200 million worldwide	>21 days	Schistosomal cercariae from freshwater snails penetrate skin during freshwater contact, migrate to blood vessels in the gut or bladder, where eggs are produced, cause local inflammation ± fibrosis (portal hypertension) and are released back into the gut. Often asymptomatic but may cause a transient rash 1–2 days after exposure (swimmer's itch) and occasionally a self-limiting acute fever, sweats, malaise, lymphadenopathy and hepatosplenomegally at 4–10 weeks (Katayama fever). Urinary (S.haematobium) and intestinal (S. mansoni/S. japonicum) schistosomiasis may be asymptomatic but can cause urinary symptoms, haematuria, vague abdominal features and portal hypertension (e.g. ascites is common worldwide).	↑eosinophils (+). Look for eggs in urine stool and rectal biopsies. Serology is useful but nay may not be positive for several months after exposure. Low level infection means travellers rarely seriously affected. Treatment with praziquantel is effective for all species.
* Viral haemorrhagic fever (VHF)	7–21 days	VHF, a group of acute RNA virus infections (e.g. Lassa fever, yellow fever, Hanta virus). Causes fever, myalgia, pharyngitis (in Lassa fever), petechiae, haemorrhage (many sites) and shock. Consider in returning travellers because of the risk of transmission and high mortality. Main differential diagnosis is malaria.	Viral serology or culture are diagnostic. Isolate patient until VHF excluded. Treatment supportive, but ribavirin may be useful (e.g. Lassa fever)
* African Trypanosomiasis	<7 days	Trypanosome infection transmitted by Tsetse flies. Initial painful chancre and local lympadenopathy, then relapsing flu-like illness (weeks) with progressive dementia, sleepiness ('sleeping sickness') and coma.	Suramin in early infection. Melasoprol required for established meningio-enchephalitis
* Brucellosis	14–28 days	Gram negative coccobacillus (Brucella abortus, B.melitensis, B.suis, B.canis) acquired from contact with animals and milk products. Most UK infection imported, but occupational in vets and farmers. Causes fever, malaise, nausea, hepatosplenomegally, meningitis, endocarditis and respiratory, bone and urinary infection.	Prolonged culture (blood) or serology diagnostic. Treat with doxycycline and rifampicin (or an aminoglycoside to prevent relapse) for >6 weeks
* Viseral Leishmaniasis	3–18 months	Also known as kala-azar. Protozoal infection (e.g. Leishmania donovanni in east Africa) transmitted by the female sandfly. Often asymptomatic or relapsing fever and remain well until advanced hepatosplenomegally.	Microscopy or serology often diagnostic. Treat with oral miltofosine or IV amphotericine B

WCC = white cell count, AKI = acute kidney injury, ALT= alanine transaminase, plats = platelets, IV = intravenous, CK = creatine kinase, CNS = central nervous system, HCT = haematocrit

Critical Care Medicine at a Glance, Third Edition. Richard Leach. © 2014 John Wiley & Sons, Ltd. Published 2014 by John Wiley & Sons, Ltd.

Fever is reported by ~2–3% of travellers returning from tropical and 1% from non-tropical (e.g. Greece) destinations. Most fevers are due to common viral, respiratory or urinary tract infections but tropical pathogens, especially malaria, should be excluded. Figures 27c and 27d list common imported infections and associated incubation periods.

Establishing a diagnosis

Essential history includes:

• **Travel history**: carefully establish geographical areas visited including previous trips (e.g. Lassa fever occurs in specific West African rural areas). Some diagnoses can be excluded by comparing symptom time course (±onset) and travel duration with incubation periods.

• **Type of travel**: (e.g. business trip, package holiday). Travellers living with local populations are at greatest risk.

• **Vaccination/prophylaxis**: vaccination is effective (e.g. hepatitis A, typhoid, yellow fever). Chemoprophylaxis is less reliable, partly because of poor compliance (e.g. malaria).

• **Contact history**: review illness in fellow travellers/natives.

• **Food and water history** (e.g. hepatitis, diarrhoea).

• **Activity**: review sexual (e.g. human immunodeficiency virus [HIV]), freshwater (e.g. schistosomiasis in African lake swimmers) and animal (e.g. brucellosis, histoplasmosis from cave bat) contact.

• **Bites**: eschars are distinctive and Tsetse fly bites painful (e.g. trypanosomiasis). Mosquito/fly bite history is usually unhelpful. Tick bites are painless and often unnoticed but removal of skin ticks may be remembered.

Physical signs/key investigations: signs are non-specific (Figure 27a). Confirm the pattern and presence of fever (i.e. biphasic in dengue). Examine for rashes, bites, ticks, lymphadenopathy, jaundice and hepatosplenomegally. Detection of lymphopaenia, thrombocytopaenia (e.g. dengue, typhoid) and eosinophilia (e.g. filariasis, liver flukes, schistosomiasis) are helpful. If malaria is suspected, perform at least three thick blood films. If indicated, arrange specific serology (or store serum for later use). Culture blood, sputum, urine (±dipstick) and stool. Examine stool for ova, cysts and parasites. Test for HIV if sexually active. Arrange a chest radiograph.

Management: exclude malaria (~30–50% of imported tropical infection) and determine if potential causes are transmissible requiring isolation (e.g. Lassa fever, although rare, is highly infectious and lethal). Treatment depends on the pathology (Figure 27c) and, in some cases, may be started on clinical suspicion alone because confirmatory serology can take weeks (e.g. treat fever, eschar and rash as African tick typhus in South African travellers).

Malaria

Epidemiology: Malaria is endemic in the tropics and sub-tropics causing a million deaths annually, mainly in sub-Saharan children. In the UK, it is the most common imported infection (1500–2000 cases/year) and occurs mainly in immigrant populations. Immunity modifies clinical severity because previous infection, some blood groups (e.g. Duffy negative) and haemoglobinopathies (e.g. HbS, thalassaemia) confer protection against severe disease. Children are at greatest risk. Most UK deaths (~10/year) occur in non-immune caucasian travellers.

Pathogenesis (Figure 27b): malaria, a protozoal infection caused by five species in humans (*P. falciparum*, *P. vivax*, *P. ovale*, *P. malariae* and *P. knowlesi*), is transmitted by the female anophelene mosquito. *P. vivax* and *P. ovale* form hypnozoites that can lie dormant in liver for years with relapsing infection. Transmission rates vary according to parasite burden, which is greatest in West Africa.

Clinical features: the incubation period is 10–14 days (occasionally, 3–6 weeks; rarely, several months). Clinical features are non-specific but fever is almost invariable and periodic in untreated cases. Drenching sweats, rigors, chills, headache and malaise are common. False localizing symptoms (e.g. cough, diarrhoea) can be misleading. In uncomplicated cases, physical signs are unusual, apart from fever, jaundice or hepatosplenomegaly. Rash is rare and suggests another cause. Helpful laboratory findings include thrombocytopaenia (~60%), mild normocytic anaemia with occasional leukopenia and raised bilirubin. **Severe malaria**, only caused by *P. falciparum*, is a medical emergency (~20% mortality rate). Third trimester pregnant women, Caucasians and patients >60 years old with asplenia, sickle cell disease or parasitaemia >2% are at greatest risk. It manifests as cerebral malaria (i.e. unrousable coma, seizures, inability to sit up and occasionally hemiplegia), severe anaemia (haemoglobin <5 g/dl); acute respiratory distress syndrome (ARDS, especially in children) and acute kidney injury (AKI; 'blackwater fever' is due to haemolysis, haemoglobinuria and jaundice). Shock, hypoglycaemia, metabolic acidosis, hepatosplenomegally and disseminated intravascular coagulation (DIC) are common. Jaundice and liver dysfunction are not good predictors of a poor outcome.

Diagnosis: thick (to screen for the presence of parasites) and thin (to determine species) blood films using Giemsa stains are the mainstay of parasitological diagnosis. Immunochromatographic tests detect *P. falciparum* accurately but are less reliable in other species. Three films are necessary to exclude malaria especially after self-treatment or partial chemo-prophylaxis.

Management: Severe malaria is managed in a critical care unit. Fluid management aims to avoid AKI and pulmonary oedema. Haemodynamic compromise due to fluid depletion is uncommon. Anticipate and prevent hypogycaemia. Species and antimicrobial resistance (a major issue in *P. falciparum* malaria, especially in South-East Asia) determines treatment and should be discussed with infectious disease teams.

• **Severe P. falciparum malaria** (parasitaemia >2–5%) is treated with intravenous quinine. A loading dose rapidly achieves therapeutic concentrations. Electrocardiogram (ECG) and blood sugar monitoring is required because quinine prolongs QT intervals, risking arrhythmia, and may cause hypoglycaemia. Parenteral artesunate, an alternative to quinine, may reduce mortality. Exchange transfusion for parasitaemia >10% is controversial.

• **Uncomplicated P. falciparum malaria** is treated with oral quinine for 7 days, combined with doxycycline (contraindicated in pregnancy) or clindamycin, because quinine compliance is poor because of side-effects. Chloroquine resistance is common. Alternative regimes include Atovaquone–proguanil or Artemether–lumefantrine.

• **Non-falciparum (benign) malaria** (e.g. *P. vivax*, *P. ovale*) is treated with chloroquine on 3 successive days to eliminate red blood cell infection. In *P. ovale* and *P. vivax*, a further 2 weeks of primaquine eliminates liver hypnozoites. Check glucose-6-phosphate deghydrogenase levels to avoid primaquine-induced haemolysis. These cases can be managed as outpatients.

Prevention: avoid mosquito bites (long-sleeve shirts, mosquito nets, insect repellents). Encourage public health programmes (e.g. control mosquito breeding grounds). Chemoprophylactic regimes depend on resistance patterns (South-East Asia requires specialist advice). Use doxycycline, mefloquine or atovaquone–proguanil in chloroquine-resistant areas.

Pearl of wisdom

Most fevers in returning travellers are due to common viral, respiratory or urinary tract infections

28 Fever (pyrexia) of unknown origin

Figure 28a Clinical examination and causes of fever of unknown origin

Neck pathology
• Thyroiditis (± thyrotoxicosis)

Raised jugular venous pressure
• Pulmonary embolus
• Pericarditis
• Endocarditis

Tender shoulder/hip muscles
• Polymyositis
• Polymyalgia rheumatica

Hepatomegaly
• Hepatitis
• Malignancy (secondaries)

Splinter haemorrhages
• Sepsis
• Endocarditis
• Vasculitis

Renal mass
• Abscess/cancer

Arthralgia/joint effusion
• Rheumatological disease
• Connective tissue disease
• Infection

Myalgia/bone pain
• Muscle pain (infection/inflammation)
• Bone pain (malignacy/infection)

Leg/calf swelling + tenderness
• Deep venous thrombosis

Tender temporal artery
• Temporal arteritis

Skin infection
• Cellulitis

Sinus-related disease
• Sinusitis
• Wegener's granulomatosis

Tooth infection
• Abscess
• Osteomyelitis

Lymphadenopathy
• Infections (e.g. viral, TB)
• Granulomatous disease
  (e.g. sarcoidosis)
• Malignancy

Splenomegaly
• Sepsis/tropical infection
• Lymphoma/leukaemia
• Cirrhosis/portal hypertension

Cardiac features
• Pericarditis
• Dressler's syndrome
• Infective endocarditis
• Atrial myxoma
• Pulmonary hypertension
  due to pulmonary emboli

Aortic aneurysm
• Mycotic
• Inflammatory

Gastrointestinal/perianal lesions
• Crohn's disease
• Abscesses (e.g. subphrenic, pelvic)

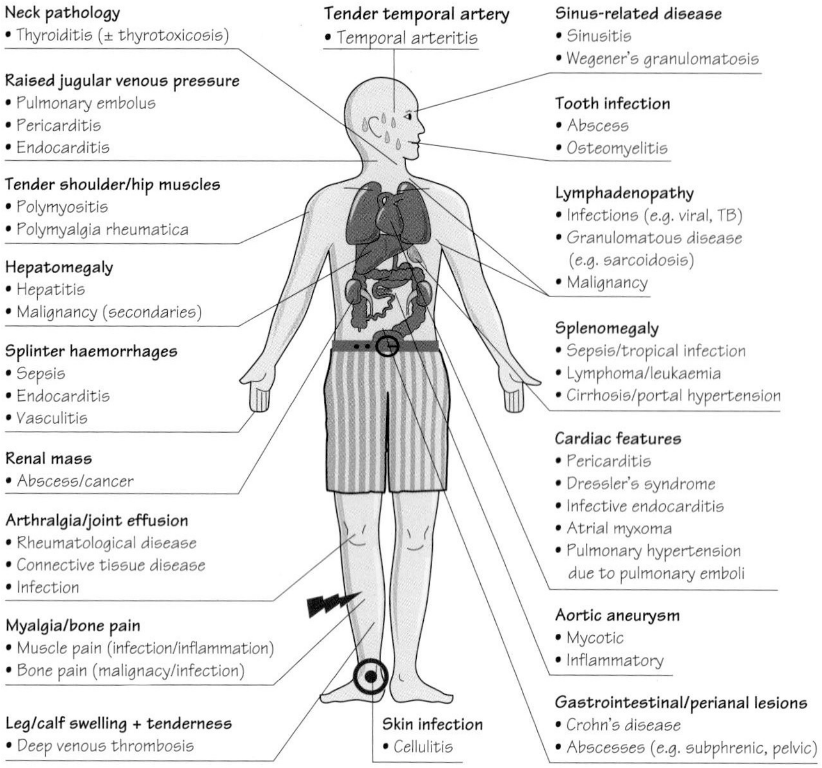

Figure 28c Hereditary periodic fever

Familial Mediterranean fever

A hereditary, autosomal recessive condition in patients with Jewish, Turkish or Arab ancestry. It presents before 20 years old. Episodic fevers, polyserositis (e.g. pleurisy, arthritis, pericarditis) and peritonitis are typical. Early appendicectomy often follows misdiagnosed abdominal pain. Attacks last hours to days. Between episodes the patient is well. Identification of the defective pyrin gene confirms the diagnosis. Renal failure due to amyloid deposition is the main complication and is prevented with colchicine therapy

Other rare hereditary periodic fevers

Include: hyper-IgD syndrome (autosomal recessive disease in French and Dutch families) and TNF receptor associated periodic syndrome (autosomal dominant disease) in Scottish and Irish families

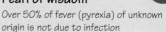

Pearl of wisdom
Over 50% of fever (pyrexia) of unknown origin is not due to infection

Figure 28b Causes of fever of unknown origin

Common causes of FUO	Less common and rare causes of FUO
Infections • **Localized abscesses** (e.g. subphrenic, hepatic, paracolic, pelvic) • **Endocarditis** (e.g. bacterial or culture negative due to prior antibiotics) • **Occult tuberculosis** (e.g. miliary, renal, peritoneal, spinal TB) • **Viral** (e.g. Epstein Barr Virus in glandular fever, cytomegalovirus)	**Infections** • **Endocarditis** (e.g. Q fever, brucellosis, chlamydia, bartonellosis, fungal) • **Atypical mycobacterial disease** (e.g. mycobacterium avian intracellulare) • **Whipples disease** due to infection with Tropheryma whippeli is rare. It occurs mainly in white middle-aged men from mid-Europe and presents with fever (50%), weight loss, watery diarrhoea, chronic migratory peripheral joint arthropathy, sacroileitis (33%), CNS disease, lymphadenopathy (±hyperpigmentation, murmurs, duodenal lesions). Untreated it can be fatal. Treatment is with co-trimoxazole for 1 year (preceded by 2 weeks of iv ceftriaxone if severe or CNS involvement)
Neoplasms • **Lymphomas/leukaemia** • **Solid tumours** (e.g. renal cell, ovary)	**Neoplasms** • **Atrial myxoma** resembles endocarditis with rash, arthralgia, anaemia, raised ESR and weight loss. A murmur may be absent but a tumour 'plop' can occur during diastole
Connective tissue diseases • **Temporal arteritis/polymyalgia rheumatica** • **Systemic lupus erythematosus** • **Polyarteritis nodosa**	**Connective tissue diseases** • **Adult Stills disease** presents with the triad of high fever (>39°C), transient rash and arthralgia, especially if sore throat is present. Cervical lymphadenopathy, pericarditis, splenomegally, anaemia, neutrophilia and raised ESR (and ferritin) are also typical but there is no definitive test
Miscellaneous • **Drug fever** develops 1–3 weeks after starting a new drug (e.g. anticonvulsants [phenytoin] and antibiotics [sulphonamides-lactams]) • **Crohn's disease** may present with fever, weight loss + anaemia but few gastrointestinal symptoms • **Haematoma** (e.g. retroperitoneal) • **Factitious fever** occurs in well-looking young often paramedical or female adults when fraudulent behaviour may cause fever (e.g. contaminating intravenous lines)	**Miscellaneous** • **Castleman's disease** presents with focal mediastinal or generalized lymphadenopathy. Localized disease occurs in young adults and is curable by surgery. The generalized form may undergo malignant transformation. • **Kikuchi's disease:** is an uncommon, idiopathic necrotising lympadenitis affecting young adults. It has a benign, self-limiting course (1–6 months) but may be recurrent. • **Sweets syndrome** is an acute onset dermatosis, characterized by fever, leukacytosis, arthralgia and tender erythematous papules and plaques, mainly affecting the face and upper body. Usually idiopathic but can occur with haematological malignancies and inflammatory disorders (e.g. rheumatoid arthritis, IBD). Treatment with steroids is usually effective. • **Hereditary periodic fevers** (Figure 27c; e.g. Familial Mediterranean fever)

TB = tuberculosis, CNS = central nervous system, ESR = erythrocyte sedimentation rate, IBD = inflammatory bowel disease

Fever is successfully treated or self-limiting (e.g. viral) in 95% of cases. Persisting fever, after initial negative investigations, is termed 'fever of unknown origin' (FUO; Figures 28a, 28b). It is defined as persisting fever ≥38.3 °C, without diagnosis, for ≥3 weeks despite (a) in-patient investigation for a week (classic definition) or (b) >3 days inpatient investigation or >2 outpatient visits (a new definition acknowledging modern diagnostics, admissions avoidance protocols and immunocompromised hosts). Practically, FUO is community-acquired (classical), hospital-acquired (Chapter 26) or due to immunosuppression (i.e. chemotherapy or human immunodeficiency virus [HIV; Chapter 68]).

Epidemiology

Community-acquired FUO is due to infectious (∼25–45%), neoplastic (∼10–20%), autoimmune, connective tissue disease (CTD; ∼15–40%) or miscellaneous causes (∼10–20%). It is undiagnosed in 10–20%. The distribution of causes depends on geographical location (i.e. more infection in developing countries), patient age (i.e. CTD, temporal arteritis and neoplasia in older people; systemic lupus erythematosus [SLE], Still's disease and factitious fever in the young), ethnicity (i.e. tuberculosis [TB] in immigrant populations) and immune status (i.e. HIV).

Pathology

• *Infectious* causes of FUO include: (a) localized, often occult, abscesses (e.g. subphrenic, pelvic) or conditions (e.g. endocarditis); (b) 'difficult-to-diagnose' systemic infections like brucellosis, culture negative endocarditis (e.g. prior antibiotics, Q-fever), viral illnesses (e.g. Epstein–Barr virus [EBV], cytomegalovirus [CMV]), miliary TB and atypical mycobacteria; and (c) rare causes like Whipple's disease.

• *Neoplastic* causes of FUO are often haematological. Lymphoma is most common and may be associated with fever, which can precede lymphadenopathy, sweats and weight loss. Classic 'Pel–Ebstein fever' with intermittent febrile episodes lasting several days is rare. Solid tumours, especially renal cell carcinoma, ovarian cancer, adenocarcinomas (e.g. pancreas, gastrointestinal [GI] tract), necrotic malignancies and liver metastases can cause FUO. Rarely, atrial myxomas present with fever.

• *Multisystem inflammatory disease*: adult Still's disease is the most common rheumatological cause of FUO. It occurs in young adults with the classic triad of fever, arthralgia and transient rash. In older patients, polymyalgia rheumatica is common, as is temporal arteritis, although temporal artery tenderness and an elevated erythrocyte sedimentation rate (ESR) are not always present. In the absence of an alternative cause, a 'blind' temporal artery biopsy may be required.

• *Miscellaneous causes* include drugs (e.g. phenytoin, sulphonamides, β-lactams), occult haematomas (e.g. retroperitoneal), recurrent pulmonary emboli (lactate dehydrogenase often raised), inflammatory bowel disease (e.g. Crohn's disease) and occult granulomatous liver disease (non-specific raised liver function tests, often steroid responsive). Factitious fevers (e.g. deliberate intravenous line contamination) is more common in paramedical professions and women.

• *Rare conditions* presenting with FUO (Figure 28b) include Castleman's disease (angiofollicular lymph node hyperplasia), Kikuchi disease (idiopathic necrotizing lymphadenitis), Sweets syndrome (neutrophilic dermatosis) and hereditary periodic fevers (Figure 28c).

Investigation

The most important diagnostic tools are a detailed clinical (e.g. duration, pattern, severity of illness), drug and travel history, and a careful examination. Confirm fever is present and establish whether the patient is unwell but stable or deteriorating. Stop all non-essential drugs. Intermittent febrile episodes suggest malaria, filariasis, autoimmune/vasculitic flares or hereditary periodic fever. Prolonged (>1 year) febrile illnesses are unlikely to be infective. Investigations include:

• *Blood tests*: white cell counts aid diagnosis (e.g. low neutrophil count in typhoid, brucellosis or ricketsial infection; high eosinophil counts in schistosomiasis and parasitic infections, very high counts (>3 × 10⁹/L) suggest malignancy, Churg–Strauss or drug reactions). High ESR or C-reactive protein (CRP) levels indicate major systemic illnesses (e.g. temporal arteritis, Still's disease, myeloma, malignancy) or infection (e.g. endocarditis) and make 'factitious fever' less likely. Raised liver function tests occur in viral illness, Still's disease, Q fever, brucellosis and drug fever. An isolated rise in alkaline phosphatase may suggest TB or, in advanced HIV disease, crytospordiosis or *Mycobacterium avian intracellulare (MAI)*. Serum angiotensin-converting enzyme is raised in sarcoidosis or TB and an elevated antinuclear antibody (ANA), antineutrophil cytoplasmic antibody (ANCA) or rheumatoid factor suggests CTD.

• *Routine tests*: urinalysis may indicate a renal cause, endocarditis or a vasculitis. Take blood cultures and send (or save) serum for appropriate serological testing. However, 'blind' serology/autoimmune tests have low diagnostic yields in FUO. A Paul Bunnell test provides a rapid result compared with EBV or CMV serology. HIV testing may be appropriate. A Mantoux test excludes TB. Early morning urine samples are only sent if renal TB is suspected. Chest CT scans reveal intrathoracic lymphadenopathy, pulmonary emboli or tuberculous 'miliary' shadowing that may not be seen on chest radiographs. Ultrasonography or abdominal CT scans detect occult infections (e.g. abscesses, peritoneal thickening suggestive of TB) malignancy or lymphadenopathy.

• *Specific investigations* should focus on clinical abnormalities. Consider echocardiograms in suspected endocarditis, extended blood cultures (e.g. brucellosis, *MAI*) and specific tissue biopsies of lymph nodes (e.g. lymphoma), liver (e.g. miliary TB), temporal artery or bone marrow (e.g. histoplasmosis, leishmaniasis).

Management

FUO remits spontaneously, with a good outcome in many stable, undiagnosed patients following simple observation. Empiric treatment is avoided unless the patient is unwell or severely immunocompromised, and only after appropriate culture and diagnostic tissue samples have been obtained:

• *Broad spectrum antibiotics* (±antifungals, ±antivirals) may be indicated if the patient is unwell, immunocompromised or if culture negative endocarditis is suspected (i.e. prior antibiotic therapy). Antituberculous therapy is justified if clinical suspicion is high, because microbiological confirmation can take weeks. A full course of treatment is required unless an alternative diagnosis is established or significant adverse drug effects occur.

• *Corticosteroids* may be given empirically in older patients with suspected temporal arteritis/polymyalgia rheumatica or in young patients with Still's disease. As far as possible, exclude potential infections and lymphoma and monitor fever, CRP and ESR response to treatment. However, be aware that steroids blunt infectious fevers and may improve symptoms due to malignancy.

29 End of life issues

Figure 29a Brainstem death can only be diagnosed if all the following preconditions and exclusion criteria are met

Essential preconditions include:
1. Apnoeic coma requiring mechanical ventilation
2. An established cause for the irreversible brain damage

Factors that must be excluded:
a) Sedative drugs, neuromuscular blocking agents + poisons
  • Test blood and urine for drugs if doubt exists
b) Significant metabolic, acid-base or endocrine abnormalities:
  • metabolic (e.g.uraemia, hyponatraemia, liver encephalopathy)
  • acid-base (e.g. acidosis, CO_2 retention)
  • endocrine (e.g. diabetic, thyroid, Addisonian crisis)
c) Hypothermia (temperature <35 °C)
d) Severe hypotension

Figure 29b Potential complications during the period before operative organ harvesting

Cardiovascular instability
• Hypotension; due to myocardial depression + vasodilation
• Autonomic instability; arrhythmias + bradycardia

Endocrine disorders
• Diabetes insipidus; diuresis, hypovolaemia, hypernatraemia
• Thyroid hormone deficiency
• Adrenal (cortisol) deficiency
• Pancreatic (insulin) deficiency; hyperglycaemia

Temperature control
• Hypothermia; due to ↓ metabolic rate + ↓ muscle activity

Pulmonary oedema + hypoxaemia
Coagulopathy
Acid-base disorders + electrolyte imbalance

Figure 29c Brainstem function testing: Criteria required to establish brainstem death (BSD) in the UK

The following 6 reflexes/responses must be absent to establish BSD

1. Pupillary responses:
Pupils must be fixed and unresponsive to light. Absent direct and consensual reactions confirm midbrain dysfunction. Pupillary size is irrelevant

2. Corneal reflex:
The reflex is absent if there is no blinking response to firmly touching the cornea with a piece of tissue paper

3. Vestibulo-ocular reflex (caloric testing): 30 mL of ice-cold water is slowly injected into each external auditory meatus after visualization of the ear-drums and removal of any obstructing wax

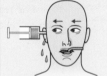 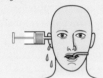

Normal reflex/response:
Conjugate eye deviation and nystagmus within ~20s

Absent reflex:
No eye response. Confirms loss of pontine function

4. 'Gag' and cough (tracheal) reflexes:
Pharyngeal/laryngeal stimulation (i.e. by endotracheal tube movement) normally causes 'gag'. Tracheal stimulation with a suction catheter normally causes cough. Absence of these reflexes indicates medullary dysfunction

5. Motor response to painful stimuli:
Central (e.g. pressure between the eyes* or behind the ears**) or peripheral (e.g. limbs) painful stimuli cause no motor responses in cranial nerves. Normally grimacing occurs

6. Apnoea test:
Demonstrates absent respiratory effort despite a P_aCO_2 >6.7–8kPa off the ventilator

After ventilation with 100% O_2 + whilst O_2 therapy is maintained through a tracheal catheter, the patient is disconnected from the ventilator and observed for respiratory effort. Apnoea confirms medullary dysfunction

Apnoea should continue until the P_aCO_2 is >6.7–8kPa on blood gas examination, which confirms adequate respiratory stimulation

Testing is discontinued if S_aO_2 falls <90% or haemodynamic instability develops

Oculocephalic reflexes; are also absent, but not a legal requirement for BSD diagnosis. Normally when the head is rotated the eyes move in the opposite direction in the orbit. In BSD, when the head is rotated the eyes remain stationary within the orbit (i.e move with the head)

The normal oculocephalic reflex (eyes appear fixed on a distant object)

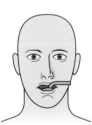 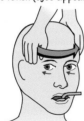 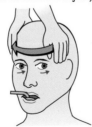

Neutral head position Eyes look forward at a fixed point

When head turned left Eyes move rightwards + continue to look at the same fixed point

When head turned right Eyes move leftwards + continue to look at the same fixed point

Absent oculocephalic reflex (eyes appear immobile within the orbits)

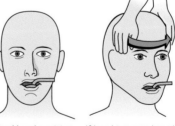 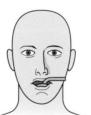 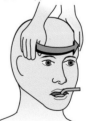

Neutral head position Eyeys look forward at a fixed point

If head is turned to the left or right, eyes do not move in the orbit (i.e. stare directly forward and away from the initial fixed point)

Critical Care Medicine at a Glance, Third Edition. Richard Leach. © 2014 John Wiley & Sons, Ltd. Published 2014 by John Wiley & Sons, Ltd.

Critical care medicine is often life-saving and many patients make a complete recovery or achieve a quality of life (QOL) which, although impaired, is tolerable for the patient. However, treatment that prolongs the dying process or results in an unacceptable QOL may cause unnecessary suffering, loss of dignity and undue emotional distress. Unfortunately, in emergency situations, it is often impossible to identify those individuals who will not benefit from therapy. In these patients, humane and cost-effective management requires a willingness to limit or withdraw treatment when it becomes clear that the prognosis is poor and that ongoing therapy is not in their best interests.

Decisions about end of life care are often difficult and based on accepted **ethical and moral principles**, including: (a) **beneficence**: the preservation of life, moderated by the need to relieve suffering; (b) **non-maleficence**: the duty to do no harm; (c) **respect for autonomy**: the right to make informed choices; (d) **justice**: fair allocation of medical resources; and (e) **professional virtue**: including compassion and integrity. The **'duty of care'** expected from medical professionals has been documented by many statutory bodies including the American Medical Association and the General Medical Council (UK).

Brainstem death

Brainstem death (BSD) is defined as irreversible loss of brainstem function with associated unconsciousness and cessation of spontaneous respiration. In many countries, BSD is considered to be a definition of death itself (i.e. despite a beating heart) because cardiac arrest (i.e. 'normal' death) always follows within ~1–21 days irrespective of ongoing mechanical ventilation. The purpose of establishing BSD is to demonstrate that continuing life support is futile, and to meet the legal requirements for organ donation (see later).

The following criteria for BSD are used in the UK, although there are international variations:
• **Diagnosis** requires that certain preconditions and exclusions are fulfilled (Figure 29a).
• **Brainstem function tests (BSFTs)**: are performed >6–24 hours after the precipitating event. Two doctors who are not part of the transplant team, one a consultant and both registered for >5 years, must complete two sets of BSFTs either separately or together. The six legally required findings that establish BSD are illustrated in Figure 29c. These are absent **pupillary**, **corneal**, **vestibulo-ocular** and **gag/cough reflexes**, **no cranial nerve motor responses** to painful stimuli and **apnoea** following disconnection from the ventilator despite a $P_a\text{co}_2$ >6.7–8 kPa. Although not a legal requirement, **oculocephalic reflexes** are also absent. Seizure activity and decerebrate or decorticate posturing are inconsistent with BSD but spinal reflexes may occur.
• Some countries require an **electroencephalogram**, **radioisotope scan** or **cerebral angiography** to confirm BSD. Although there is no evidence that these increase diagnostic accuracy, they are useful when cranial nerve injuries or severe hypoxia prevent normal BSFTs.

Withdrawal of treatment

The prognostic certainty of death associated with BSD relieves the anxiety associated with discontinuation of therapy. However, prolonged self-ventilated survival without cognitive function is possible when the brainstem is intact but cortical function impaired due to ischaemic damage (e.g. cardiac arrest) or diffuse cerebral injury (e.g. head trauma). This situation is termed **persistent vegetative state (PVS)**. In these patients, withdrawal of treatment (WOT) decisions are difficult because there is often prognostic uncertainty. Previous ethical and medico-legal deliberations recommend that decision making should focus on 'the likelihood of return to cognitive function' and that life-sustaining therapy should be withdrawn when it is clear that the patient is 'unlikely to regain cognitive behaviour, the ability to communicate or purposeful interaction'. In these circumstances, it is generally agreed that treatment other than basic medical and nursing care is inappropriate.

In '**severely disabled patients**', ethical dilemmas are particularly complicated. It is important to appreciate that rational patients or legal surrogates have the right to refuse treatment even if this includes discontinuation of mechanical ventilation. Conversely, patients cannot demand life-saving therapy when clinicians consider it inappropriate. In practice, many patients cannot discuss treatment. Responsibility for WOT lies with the senior physician, who must review any such decisions made by other staff. These assessments are usually made in consultation with the family, taking into account prognosis, expected QOL, opinions of the wider medical team (e.g. nursing staff) and the patient's previously expressed views (e.g. advance directives). It should be recognized that medical staff often underestimate a patient's willingness to undergo treatment independent of age or poor prognosis.

Once a WOT decision is made, **protocols** ensure patient comfort and dignity, reduce stress and highlight the support required by relatives and junior staff. Physicians must decide which interventions to withdraw, recognizing that this will influence the rapidity, comfort and dignity of the patient's death. The usual preference for the order of WOT is renal replacement therapy, inotropic support, antibiotics, mechanical ventilation, feeding and, finally, intravenous fluids. Unfortunately, these biases can prolong dying, causing unnecessary suffering. To prevent this, WOT plans must be regularly updated. Liberal opiate therapy may be required to relieve discomfort, particularly when ventilation is discontinued.

Organ donation

Organ donation is a successful treatment for end-stage organ failure, limited only by the shortfall of organs for transplantation. Organ retrieval from suitable BSD patients must be maximized but dying patients should not be ventilated simply to allow organ donation. The question of organ donation is usually raised with relatives at the time of BSFT. The decision should be autonomous and 'unpressured'. The process is easier if the patient is a registered organ donor. Following consent, blood is sent for tissue typing, human immunodeficiency virus (HIV), hepatitis and cytomegalovirus (CMV) testing. In the UK, each region has a transplant coordinator who, when contacted, will arrange retrieval and allocation of donated organs. Figure 29b lists **potential complications** before organ retrieval in the operating theatre. Graft survival is improved by maintaining pre-operative organ perfusion (e.g. fluids, inotropes, monitoring) and oxygenation (i.e. $P_a\text{o}_2$ >10 kPa). Inotropes are selected to minimize organ dysfunction. Spinal reflexes and autonomic haemodynamic responses are controlled with neuromuscular blockers and opioids. Continuing emotional support for relatives and staff is essential.

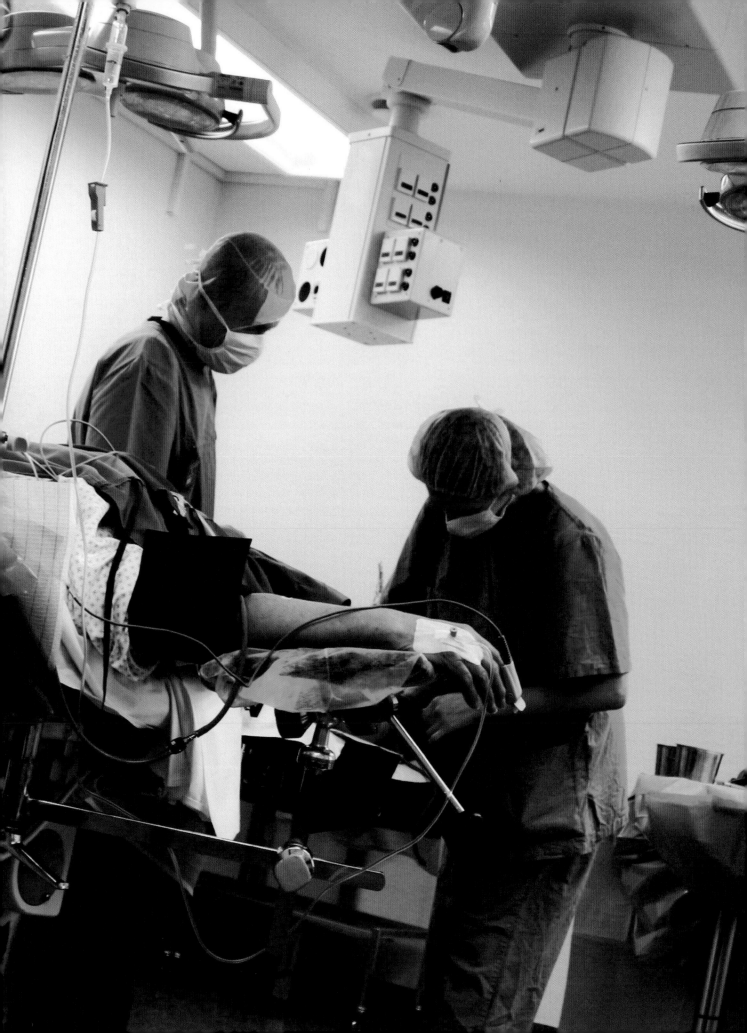

Medical

Part 2

30 Acute coronary syndromes I: clinical pathophysiology

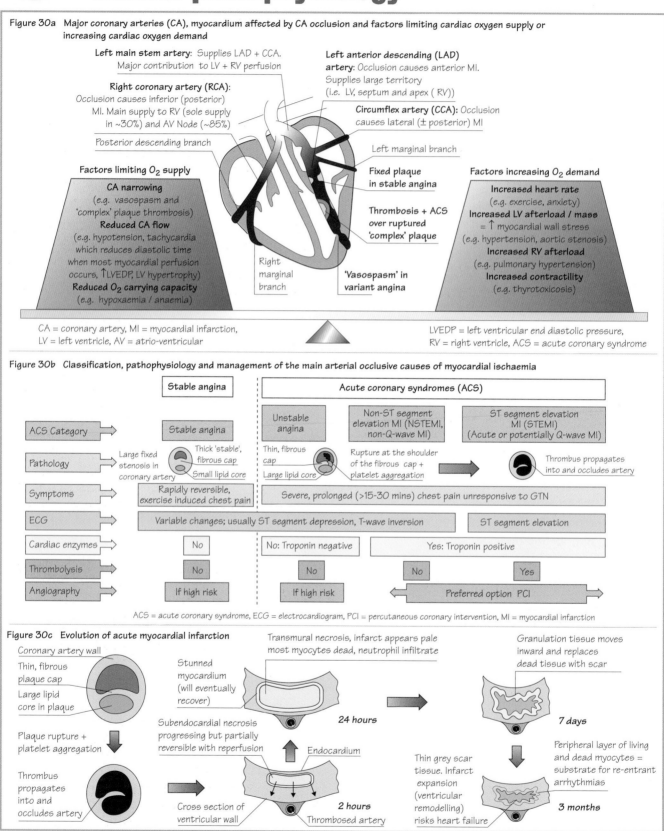

Figure 30a Major coronary arteries (CA), myocardium affected by CA occlusion and factors limiting cardiac oxygen supply or increasing cardiac oxygen demand

Left main stem artery: Supplies LAD + CCA. Major contribution to LV + RV perfusion

Left anterior descending (LAD) artery: Occlusion causes anterior MI. Supplies large territory (i.e. LV, septum and apex (RV))

Right coronary artery (RCA): Occlusion causes inferior (posterior) MI. Main supply to RV (sole supply in ~30%) and AV Node (~85%)

Circumflex artery (CCA): Occlusion causes lateral (± posterior) MI

Posterior descending branch

Left marginal branch

Factors limiting O₂ supply

Fixed plaque in stable angina

Factors increasing O₂ demand

CA narrowing (e.g. vasospasm and 'complex' plaque thrombosis)
Reduced CA flow (e.g. hypotension, tachycardia which reduces diastolic time when most myocardial perfusion occurs, ↑LVEDP, LV hypertrophy)
Reduced O₂ carrying capacity (e.g. hypoxaemia / anaemia)

Thrombosis + ACS over ruptured 'complex' plaque

Increased heart rate (e.g. exercise, anxiety)
Increased LV afterload / mass = ↑ myocardial wall stress (e.g. hypertension, aortic stenosis)
Increased RV afterload (e.g. pulmonary hypertension)
Increased contractility (e.g. thyrotoxicosis)

Right marginal branch

'Vasospasm' in variant angina

CA = coronary artery, MI = myocardial infarction, LV = left ventricle, AV = atrio-ventricular

LVEDP = left ventricular end diastolic pressure, RV = right ventricle, ACS = acute coronary syndrome

Figure 30b Classification, pathophysiology and management of the main arterial occlusive causes of myocardial ischaemia

	Stable angina	Acute coronary syndromes (ACS)		
ACS Category	Stable angina	Unstable angina	Non-ST segment elevation MI (NSTEMI, non-Q-wave MI)	ST segment elevation MI (STEMI) (Acute or potentially Q-wave MI)
Pathology	Large fixed stenosis in coronary artery. Thick 'stable', fibrous cap. Small lipid core	Thin, fibrous cap. Large lipid core	Rupture at the shoulder of the fibrous cap + platelet aggregation	Thrombus propagates into and occludes artery
Symptoms	Rapidly reversible, exercise induced chest pain	Severe, prolonged (>15-30 mins) chest pain unresponsive to GTN		
ECG	Variable changes; usually ST segment depression, T-wave inversion			ST segment elevation
Cardiac enzymes	No	No: Troponin negative	Yes: Troponin positive	
Thrombolysis	No	No	No	Yes
Angiography	If high risk	If high risk	Preferred option PCI	

ACS = acute coronary syndrome, ECG = electrocardiogram, PCI = percutaneous coronary intervention, MI = myocardial infarction

Figure 30c Evolution of acute myocardial infarction

Coronary artery wall
Thin, fibrous plaque cap
Large lipid core in plaque
Plaque rupture + platelet aggregation
Thrombus propagates into and occludes artery

Stunned myocardium (will eventually recover)
Subendocardial necrosis progressing but partially reversible with reperfusion
Cross section of ventricular wall
Thrombosed artery
2 hours
Endocardium

Transmural necrosis, infarct appears pale most myocytes dead, neutrophil infiltrate
24 hours

Granulation tissue moves inward and replaces dead tissue with scar
7 days
Thin grey scar tissue. Infarct expansion (ventricular remodelling) risks heart failure
Peripheral layer of living and dead myocytes = substrate for re-entrant arrhythmias
3 months

Critical Care Medicine at a Glance, Third Edition. Richard Leach. © 2014 John Wiley & Sons, Ltd. Published 2014 by John Wiley & Sons, Ltd.

Epidemiology

Prevalence: ischaemic heart disease (IHD) affects ~5% of the population in developed countries (~2.7 and ~18.5 million people in the UK and USA respectively). In the UK, ~1.5 million people experience angina and 275,000 develop a myocardial infarction (MI) annually. **Incidence** increases with age, male sex and the menopause in women. **Risk factors** include smoking, hypertension, diabetes, hypercholesterolaemia and family history. **Mortality**: IHD accounts for ~0.11, 0.53 and 0.75 million deaths annually in the UK, USA and EU respectively (i.e. ~20% of male and ~16% of female deaths). Following MI, 33–66% of deaths occur before hospital admission, ~10% during admission and ~20% within 2 years due to heart failure or further MI.

Pathophysiology

Figure 30a illustrates the effects of coronary artery occlusion and factors that cause myocardial ischaemia. Figure 30b illustrates the classification, characteristics and management of myocardial ischaemia.

1 Chronic stable (exertional) angina (SA) occurs when fixed, stable coronary artery occlusions (>70%) limit blood flow causing 'predictable', reversible cardiac ischaemia during exercise. These stenoses are due to smooth, often circumferential atherosclerotic plaques with thick fibrous caps that are unlikely to rupture. Resulting ischaemia is usually subendocardial because systolic compression mainly affects endocardial arterioles. **Variant (Prinzmetal's) angina** is uncommon and caused by transient coronary artery vasospasm or impaired vasodilation. It often occurs in the vicinity of atherosclerotic plaques, but there may be no association with atherosclerosis.

2 Acute coronary syndrome (ACS) describes a spectrum of ischaemic events, of varying severity, that follow sudden coronary artery occlusion (±vasoconstriction). ACS is initiated by stress-induced rupture of small, eccentric (i.e. non-circumferential), non-occlusive (i.e. <50%), 'complex' atherosclerotic plaques with lipid-rich cores and thin fibrous caps. Plaque rupture stimulates thrombus formation, vasospasm and arterial occlusion. The duration and degree of occlusion determine the severity of the ischaemia, which defines the clinical syndrome, associated symptoms, electrocardiogram (ECG) changes and extent of myocardial necrosis as indicated by cardiac enzyme (CE) release (Figure 30b).

- **Unstable angina (UA)** describes occlusions of limited extent and duration (<20 min) that cause ischaemia but not necrosis. Symptoms occur but neither CE nor ST segments are elevated.
- **Non-ST segment elevation MI (NSTEMI, non-Q wave MI)** describes occlusions which are temporary, incomplete or alleviated by collateral vessels. This limits ischaemia and necrosis to the subendocardium causing CE release but not ST elevation.
- **ST segment elevation MI (STEMI; Q-wave MI; acute MI)** describes occlusions that cause transmural cardiac ischaemia (i.e. immediate ST elevation on ECG and development of Q-waves in the absence of treatment). Figure 30c illustrates MI evolution. Coronary angiography reveals complete occlusion in ~85% of infarct-related arteries within 4 hours of symptom onset and ECG ST elevation. MI with normal coronary arteries is rare but may follow embolic occlusion (e.g. endocarditis), non-thrombotic vasospasm or cocaine abuse. Therapy aims to minimize infarct size and prevent transmural wall death (i.e. development of Q-waves on ECG).

Clinical features

Myocardial ischaemia causes 'crushing, heavy' retrosternal chest pain radiating to the neck, medial aspect of the left arm and occasionally the right chest or shoulder blades. Pain may be atypical (i.e. burning), localized (i.e. jaw only) or absent in ~20% (e.g. people with diabetes, older people). Pain severity, duration, relationship to exercise and the response to nitrates defines clinical subgroups but UA/NSTEMI and NSTEMI/STEMI show overlap:

- **Stable 'exercise-induced' angina (SA)** is 'predictably' precipitated by exercise or anxiety, is short-lived and relieved in <5 minutes by rest and sublingual nitrates.

- **Unstable angina and NSTEMI (UA/NSTEMI)** have clinical similarities and **do not** benefit from thrombolytic therapy. Symptoms are 'unpredictable', frequent, prolonged (>15 min) and unlikely to respond to nitrates. 'Altered SA pattern' (i.e. with less exercise), autonomic features (e.g. nausea, sweating) and radiation to 'new' sites (e.g. jaw) indicate UA/NSTEMI and increasing coronary artery occlusion. Typical presentations include angina at rest or on minimal exertion, crescendo angina (i.e. increasingly frequent, prolonged, severe angina) and post-MI angina. Both UA and NSTEMI may present with ST depression and/or T-wave inversion on ECG. The occurrence of UA/NSTEMI indicates a high risk of imminent coronary artery occlusion and death (i.e. within 4–6 weeks). About 3–5% of hospitalized UA/NSTEMI patients die within 30 days and ~8% reinfarct. **Risk assessment**: factors associated with increased risk of future cardiac events include ST depression, elevated troponin levels, recurrent angina, diabetes, previous STEMI, impaired left ventricular (LV) function and heart failure. High-risk patients require early cardiac angiography. Pain-free patients, without risk factors, need an exercise ECG: ischaemia at low workloads indicates high risk and the need for angiography.

- **MI** includes both NSTEMI and STEMI (i.e. 'troponin/CE positive' events). However, they are managed differently in that thrombolytic therapy is only beneficial in STEMI. MI is characterized by sudden, severe, prolonged pain unrelieved by nitrates, autonomic symptoms (e.g. 'cold, clammy appearance', sweating, nausea, vomiting), dyspnoea and anxiety. Most cases have known IHD or risk factors but only 25% have preceding UA. Tachycardia often accompanies anterior MI whereas bradycardia (±heart block) is more common after inferior MI due to conducting tissue damage (Figure 30a). Hypotension (systolic BP <90 mmHg) suggests a large MI (>40% LV damage) and heralds cardiogenic shock (Chapters 7, 34). Auscultation may reveal a third or fourth heart sound (i.e. gallop rhythm) and a systolic murmur. **Early MI complications (<7 days)** include arrhythmias (Chapters 32, 33), pericarditis, papillary muscle or free wall rupture (days 4–7) and ventricular septal defects. Heart failure occurs with >20% LV damage. **Late MI complications (>7 days)** include (a) mural thrombus over damaged myocardium (±thromboembolism) and (b) autoimmune pericarditis (Dressler's syndrome), which may require treatment with NSAIDs (±steroids).

Pearl of wisdom

Myocardial infarction (MI) may present as falls, confusion, heart failure or metabolic dysfunction, rather than chest pain, in elderly or diabetic patients

31 Acute coronary syndromes II: investigations and management

Figure 31a ECG changes in acute coronary syndrome (ACS) including unstable angina (UA) and myocardial infarction (MI)

Serial ECG are required to establish a diagnosis (i.e. UA, MI) as changes may be delayed, obscured (e.g. LBBB) or evolve gradually

Unstable angina: with reversible ischaemia causes:

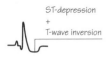
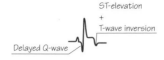

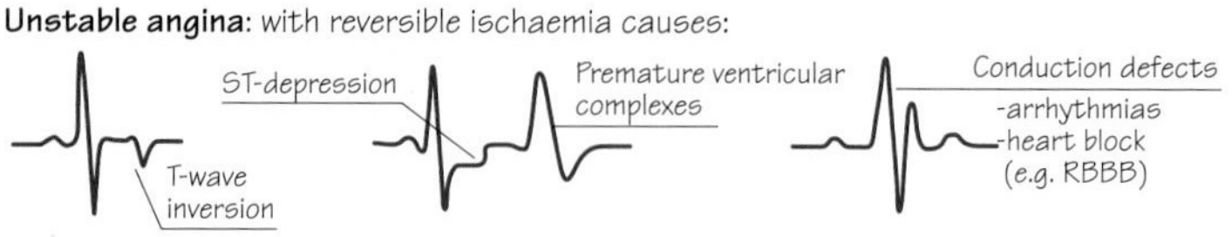

ST-depression
T-wave inversion
Premature ventricular complexes
Conduction defects -arrhythmias -heart block (e.g. RBBB)

Myocardial infarction: proceeds from the endocardial to epicardial surfaces

Non-ST elevation MI (NSTEMI or subendocardial MI) occurs if damage does not extend to the epicardial surface

A 'transmural MI' with epicardial damage produces ECG changes in leads over infarcted regions (Table b)

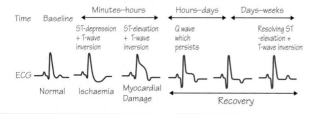

ST-depression + T-wave inversion

ST-elevation + T-wave inversion

Delayed Q-wave

Phases of ECG evolution during a myocardial infarction

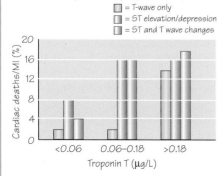

Time	Baseline	Minutes–hours		Hours–days	Days–weeks
		ST-depression + T-wave inversion	ST-elevation + T-wave inversion	Q wave which persists	Resolving ST -elevation + T-wave inversion
ECG	Normal	Ischaemia	Myocardial Damage	Recovery	

Figure 31d Association between ECG changes, trophin T and prognosis

- ☐ = T-wave only
- ☐ = ST elevation/depression
- ☐ = ST and T wave changes

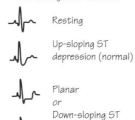

Cardiac deaths/MI (%) vs Troponin T (µg/L): <0.06, 0.06–0.18, >0.18

Figure 31e Exercise testing

Bruce Protocol

Stage	I	II	III	IV
Time (mins)	0–3	3–6	6–9	9–12
Gradient (%)	10	12	14	16
Walk speed (mph)	1.7 Slow	2.5 Normal	3.4 Brisk	4.2 Fast

Failure of HR + BP to gradually increase is an abnormal response suggesting ischaemia

ECG changes on exercise

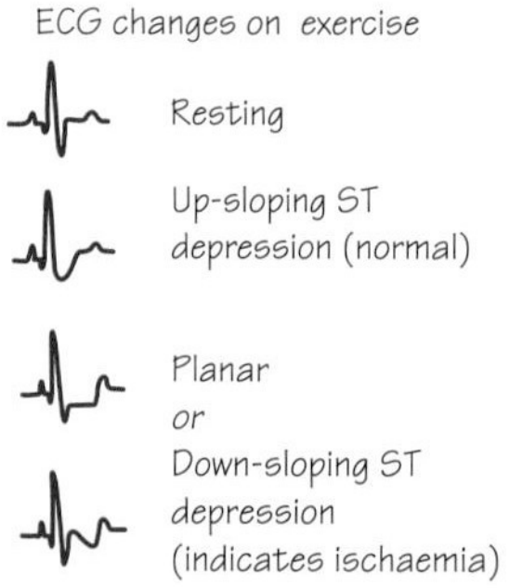

Resting

Up-sloping ST depression (normal)

Planar or Down-sloping ST depression (indicates ischaemia)

Figure 31b Myocardial injury patterns

Location of ischaemia/MI	Artery occluded	Leads showing ECG changes
Inferior	Right (mainly)	II, III, aVF
Anterior Anteroseptal Anterolateral Apical	Left Anterior Descending Artery	I, aVL, V2-5 V2-4 V3-5 II, III, aVF, V5-6
Lateral	Circumflex or diagonal	I, aVL, ±V6
Posterior	Right or circumflex	R wave in V1-2 with ST depression

Figure 31c Cardiac enzymes (CE) profiles

Myocardial necrosis releases CE into plasma with specific concentration profiles including:
- creatine kinase-MB (CK-MB)
- lactate dehydrogenase-1 (LDH-1)
- cardiac troponin T (CTT)

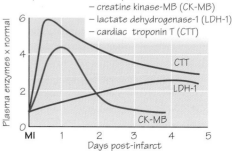

Plasma enzymes × normal vs Days post-infarct (MI, 1, 2, 3, 4, 5): CTT, LDH-1, CK-MB

Diagnosis is best established by raised CTT at 12hrs. Serial CK-MB, with doubling of baseline levels also confirms MI. Elevated LDH-1 (or CTT) confirms late presentation MI

Figure 31f Contraindication to thrombolytic therapy

Absolute contraindications	Relative contraindications
• Active bleeding (e.g GI haemorrhage) • Aortic dissection • Neurosurgery, head injury • Recent (<6 months) CNS disease (e.g. tumour) • CVA (<2 months) • Recent operation (<4 weeks) • Recent trauma (<4 weeks) • Diastolic hypertension (>130 mm/Hg) • Coagulopathy (e.g. ↓ platelets)	• Previous CVA or TIA (at any time) • Recent prolonged (>10 mins) CPR • Systolic hypertension (>180 mm/Hg) • Recent non-compressible central lines (e.g subclavian) • Intracardiac thrombus • Abdominal aortic aneurysm

Figure 31g Myocardial perfusion scans

1. Technetium pyrophosphate: concentrates in areas of myocardial damage (i.e useful when baseline ECG abnormal (e.g. LBBB) or after cardiac surgery)

2. Thallium scans: show 'cold' spots in non-perfused myocardium and demonstrate areas of reversible ischaemia

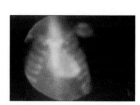

Technetium uptake in inferior myocardial infarction

Critical Care Medicine at a Glance, Third Edition. Richard Leach. © 2014 John Wiley & Sons, Ltd. Published 2014 by John Wiley & Sons, Ltd.

Chest pain accounts for ~15% of medical admissions. The initial diagnostic challenge is to differentiate acute coronary syndrome (ACS) and other life-threatening conditions (e.g. aortic dissection) from benign causes of chest discomfort (e.g. gastro-oesophageal reflux, musculoskeletal).

Investigations

Serial electrocardiogram (ECG) (Chapter 4) and cardiac enzymes (CE) establish the diagnosis and have prognostic significance (Figures 31a, 31c, 31d).

• **ECG** provides the earliest evidence of myocardial ischaemia, informs initial management and indicates the site and size of an infarct. Figures 31a and 31b illustrate ECG changes in ACS. ST segment elevation (ST↑; >0.1 mV in two chest leads or >0.2 mV in two limb leads) is diagnostic of acute myocardial infarction (MI) (Chapter 4) and suggests the need for immediate revascularization. However, ST segment depression (ST↓) and T-wave inversion occur in ~20% of MIs with raised CE. Patients with non-ST segment elevation MI (NSTEMI) do not benefit from thrombolysis. ACS patients with ST↓ have lower early mortality than those with ST↑ but survival at >6 months is similar.

• **Cardiac enzymes**: a ≥2-fold increase in plasma CE concentration indicates myocardial damage (Figure 31c). Cardiac troponins (CTs) measured at 12 hours are sensitive, specific markers of myocardial necrosis and can detect MI after surgery or when the ECG is non-specific (e.g. left bundle branch block [LBBB]).

• **Chest radiography** detects heart failure and aortic dissection.

• **Echocardiography** assesses contractility and reveals dyskinesia, thrombus, septal defects and papillary muscle rupture.

• **Incremental exercise stress tests** (EST) reveal cardiac ischaemia as angina, ECG changes (i.e. >2 mm ST↓, arrhythmias) or inappropriate heart rate or BP responses (Figure 31e).

• **Myocardial perfusion scans** (MPS) detect reduced isotope uptake in underperfused myocardium using a gamma camera (Figure 31g). It is an alternative to EST in the immobile or those with LBBB.

• **Coronary angiography** provides radiographic imaging and assessment of coronary artery disease severity.

Management

Treatment aims to reduce **myocardial oxygen consumption (MOC)** by decreasing heart rate (e.g. beta-blockers) and afterload (e.g. antihypertensives) while increasing **myocardial oxygen supply** with pharmacotherapy (±oxygen). Essential risk factor reduction includes smoking cessation, low fat diet, weight loss, exercise and control of diabetes or hypertension. Most patients require anti-platelet agents (e.g. aspirin), lipid-lowering drugs (e.g. statins to reduce low-density lipoprotein [LDL] to <2.6 mmol) and angiotensin-converting enzyme (ACE) inhibitors, which improve prognosis and reduce atherosclerosis.

Stable angina

The following therapies improve symptoms:

• **Nitrovasodilators** are effective but tolerance develops without nitrate-free periods (~6 hours/day).

• **Beta-blockers** improve prognosis and are first-line therapy. They enhance diastolic myocardial perfusion by slowing heart rate and lower heart wall tension by reducing preload (±afterload). Sublingual, oral and intravenous routes are effective.

• **Calcium channel antagonists (CCAs)** are useful if beta-blockers are contraindicated. They relieve coronary vasospasm but some cause tachycardia (e.g. nifedipine) and are negative inotropes (i.e. risk heart failure). Only CCAs that slow heart rate (e.g. diltiazem) are given as monotherapy.

• **Revascularization** is required if symptoms deteriorate, the EST is positive or angiography reveals >70% stenoses in all three main, left main or proximal left anterior descending (LAD) coronary arteries.

Unstable angina/NSTEMI

In UA/NSTEMI thrombolytic therapy (TT) is not beneficial. As in stable angina (SA), therapy includes nitrates, beta-blockers (±CCA) and additional:

• **Antiplatelet therapy**: give all patients 300 mg **aspirin** immediately and continue 75 mg/day indefinitely. Irreversible cyclo-oxygenase inhibition prevents platelet aggregation <15 min after chewing an aspirin, reducing MI and sudden death by 50%. Clopidogrel inhibits ADP-stimulated platelet aggregation, reduces mortality by ~20%, and is combined with aspirin for ≥30 days. Glycoprotein IIb/IIIa antagonists are effective platelet inhibitors that prevent stent-induced thrombosis after percutaneous coronary interventions (PCIs).

• **Anticoagulant therapy**: intravenous **unfractionated heparin (UFH)** or subcutaneous **low molecular weight heparin (LMWH)** prevent thromb-embolic complications in immobile patients.

• **Consider PCI** after 48 hours if medical therapy fails.

Myocardial infarction/STEMI

Early reperfusion after MI limits infarct size and reduces hospital mortality from 13% to <10%.

• **Immediate management** includes pain relief, monitoring and oxygen therapy. Patients without contraindications are given aspirin, clopidogrel and beta-blockers (±heparin). Do not delay revascularization with PCI or TT.

• **Pharmacological therapies**: **opiates** (e.g. morphine) relieve pain, reduce preload, lower MOC and lower anxiety-induced catecholamine release. **Aspirin** reduces 35-day mortality by 23% (42% when combined with TT). Immediate **beta-blockade** (e.g. metoprolol) reduces infarct size, arrhythmias and mortality, especially in hypertensive or tachycardic patients. Contraindications include asthma, heart failure and bradycardia. Early **nitrates** (<24 hours) reduce pain, infarct size and heart failure. **ACE inhibitors** reduce heart failure and improve 'remodelling' in high-risk patients. **Inotropic support** is required in cardiogenic shock (Chapters 7, 34). Prophylactic antiarrhythmic therapy is not recommended.

• **PCI** within ≤90 min of onset is the 'preferred' post-MI revascularization technique if facilities are available. Primary PCI (<6 hours) reopens >90% of occluded coronary arteries with few complications. Consider rescue PCI if TT fails, but mortality is significant if unsuccessful.

• **Thrombolytic therapy** dissipates thrombus, reverses ischaemia and limits myocardial injury and complications (e.g. heart failure). TT is most effective within 2 hours of symptom onset but benefit persists to 12 hours. It reduces mortality by ~25%. The main agents, **streptokinase** (SK) and **tissue plasminogen activator** (tPA), are given by infusion. SK is cheap but allergenic (i.e. single use). tPA has slight survival benefits and is given if SK has been used previously. Intravenous heparin is required for 48–72 hours after tPA. Newer agents (e.g. tenecteplase) may be as effective as PCI. The main risk of TT is haemorrhage (e.g. ~1% stroke). Contraindications (Figure 31f) prevent use in 50% of cases.

• **Follow-up** includes EST, risk factor reduction, anticoagulation after large MI and referral of high-risk patients for angiography.

Pearl of wisdom

Chewing an aspirin at the onset of chest pain/angina reduces myocardial infarction (MI) and sudden death by 50%

Arrhythmias: tachyarrhythmias

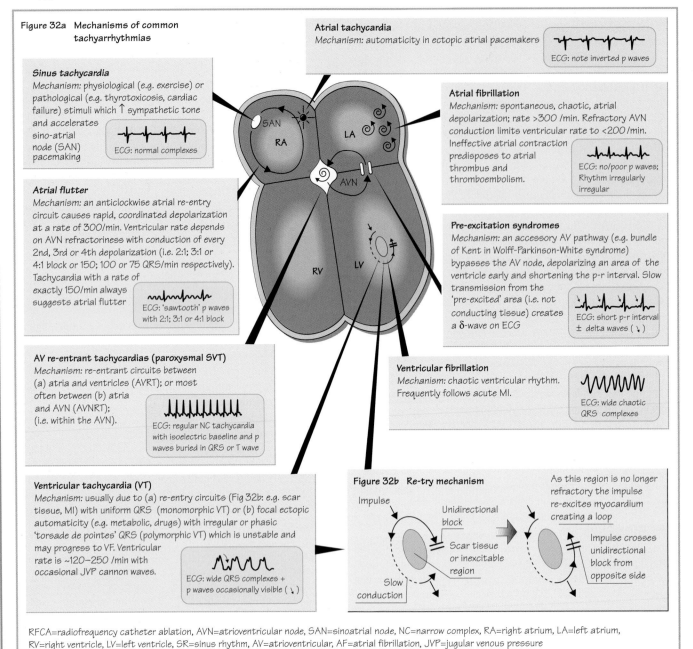

Figure 32a Mechanisms of common tachyarrhythmias

Atrial tachycardia
Mechanism: automaticity in ectopic atrial pacemakers
ECG: note inverted p waves

Sinus tachycardia
Mechanism: physiological (e.g. exercise) or pathological (e.g. thyrotoxicosis, cardiac failure) stimuli which ↑ sympathetic tone and accelerates sino-atrial node (SAN) pacemaking
ECG: normal complexes

Atrial fibrillation
Mechanism: spontaneous, chaotic, atrial depolarization; rate >300 /min. Refractory AVN conduction limits ventricular rate to <200 /min. Ineffective atrial contraction predisposes to atrial thrombus and thromboembolism.
ECG: no/poor p waves; Rhythm irregularly irregular

Atrial flutter
Mechanism: an anticlockwise atrial re-entry circuit causes rapid, coordinated depolarization at a rate of 300/min. Ventricular rate depends on AVN refractoriness with conduction of every 2nd, 3rd or 4th depolarization (i.e. 2:1; 3:1 or 4:1 block or 150; 100 or 75 QRS/min respectively). Tachycardia with a rate of exactly 150/min always suggests atrial flutter
ECG: 'sawtooth' p waves with 2:1; 3:1 or 4:1 block

Pre-excitation syndromes
Mechanism: an accessory AV pathway (e.g. bundle of Kent in Wolff-Parkinson-White syndrome) bypasses the AV node, depolarizing an area of the ventricle early and shortening the p-r interval. Slow transmission from the 'pre-excited' area (i.e. not conducting tissue) creates a δ-wave on ECG
ECG: short p-r interval ± delta waves (↘)

AV re-entrant tachycardias (paroxysmal SVT)
Mechanism: re-entrant circuits between (a) atria and ventricles (AVRT); or most often between (b) atria and AVN (AVNRT); (i.e. within the AVN).
ECG: regular NC tachycardia with isoelectric baseline and p waves buried in QRS or T wave

Ventricular fibrillation
Mechanism: chaotic ventricular rhythm. Frequently follows acute MI.
ECG: wide chaotic QRS complexes

Ventricular tachycardia (VT)
Mechanism: usually due to (a) re-entry circuits (Fig 32b: e.g. scar tissue, MI) with uniform QRS (monomorphic VT) or (b) focal ectopic automaticity (e.g. metabolic, drugs) with irregular or phasic 'torsade de pointes' QRS (polymorphic VT) which is unstable and may progress to VF. Ventricular rate is ~120–250 /min with occasional JVP cannon waves.
ECG: wide QRS complexes + p waves occasionally visible (↘)

Figure 32b Re-try mechanism
Impulse
Unidirectional block
Scar tissue or inexcitable region
Slow conduction
As this region is no longer refractory the impulse re-excites myocardium creating a loop
Impulse crosses unidirectional block from opposite side

RFCA=radiofrequency catheter ablation, AVN=atrioventricular node, SAN=sinoatrial node, NC=narrow complex, RA=right atrium, LA=left atrium, RV=right ventricle, LV=left ventricle, SR=sinus rhythm, AV=atrioventricular, AF=atrial fibrillation, JVP=jugular venous pressure

Tachycardia is a heart rate (HR) > 100 beats/min. Arrhythmias are abnormalities in the origin, timing and sequence of cardiac depolarization. They may be fast (HR > 100/min; tachyarrhythmias) or slow (HR < 60/min; bradyarrhythmias; Chapter 33). Atrial fibrillation (AF), the most common tachyarrhythmia, affects ~1% and ~10% of people >50 and >75 years old respectively. Ventricular arrhythmias cause 15–40% of deaths from ischaemic heart disease (IHD).

Automaticity describes the normal diastolic membrane depolarization in heart cells that triggers an electrical discharge (i.e. action potential [APo]) at a threshold voltage. HR is determined by the fastest pacemaker, usually the sinoatrial node (SAN). Tachyarrhythmias (Figure 32a) suppress SAN pacemaker activity and are caused by:

- **Ectopic pacemakers**: increased automaticity due to faster spontaneous membrane depolarization, lower threshold potentials or repolarization oscillations (e.g. digoxin toxicity) triggers early APo. They often arise in damaged tissue (e.g. myocardial infarction [MI] scars).
- **Re-entry circuits** (Figure 32b): a depolarization wave travels around a circuit of abnormal myocardial tissue; if the initiating tissue is not refractory when the impulse returns, it will depolarize again, creating a recurring circuit and a faster pacemaker. Re-entry circuits cause most paroxysmal tachycardia. They develop in scar tissue, the atrioventricular node (AVN) and abnormal 'accessory/ AVN' or 'atrial/AVN' pathways. The AVN is normally the only atrioventricular (AV) connection. Accessory pathways are

Figure 32c Vaughan Williams classification of anti-arrhythmic drugs, mechanism of action and uses

Vaughan Williams Class	Effect on action potential	Mechanism of action	Use
Class Ia Dysopyramide, quinidine	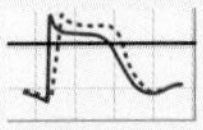	Limit cardiac cell Na⁺ entry and reduce spontaneous discharge rate. Class 1a lengthen the AP of the cell	SVT + VT but must block AVN (e.g. digoxin) in AF
Class Ib Lignocaine (lidocaine)	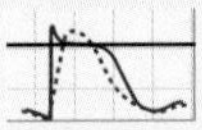	Shorten the AP	VT especially after MI
Class Ic Flecanide	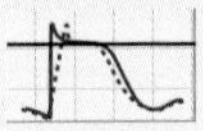	Reduce conduction, slowing the initial upstroke of the AP (phase 0) but with no effect on AP duration	VT + some SVT (e.g. WPW syndrome)
Class II β-blockers	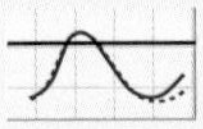	Slow spontaneous depolarization and act mainly on the sino-atrial node	SVT + VT especially after MI
Class III Amiodarone, sotalol	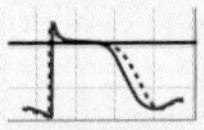	Block K⁺ channels. Increase AP duration by reducing repolarization. Prolonged QT interval risks arrhythmias	SVT + VT. Most effective in re-entry tachycardias
Class IV Diltiazem, verapamil	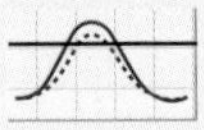	Block Ca²⁺ slow channels and reduce AVN conduction	SVT especially AVN re-entry tachycardias

AVN = atrioventricular node, AP = action potential, AV = atrioventricular, AF = atrial fibrillation, VT = ventricular tachycardia, SVT = supraventricular tachycardia, Na⁺ = sodium, Ca²⁺ = calcium, K⁺ = potassium, MI = myocardial infarction, WPW = Wolfe-Parkinson-White syndrome

Figure 32d Arrhythmias causing sudden cardiac death

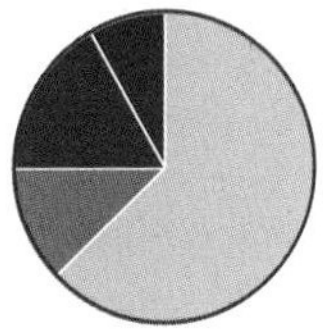

- Monomorphic VT
- Torsade des pointes
- Primary bradycardia
- Primary VF

Pearl of wisdom
Not all arrhythmias need immediate intervention. Some asymptomatic rhythms (e.g. SVT) can be observed whilst the cause (e.g. hypokalaemia) is corrected

---

common, additional tracts of abnormal AV conducting tissue, which, with the AVN, form re-entry circuits.

Tachyarrhythmias are classified as:
- *Supraventricular tachycardia* (SVT) if they originate in the atria or AVN. Ventricular rate is determined by the arrhythmia, AVN conduction and/or prolonged post-depolarization refractory periods.
- *Ventricular tachycardia* (VT) if they start in the ventricles.

Mechanisms and electrocardiograms (ECGs) are illustrated in Figure 32a.

Clinical features
Tachyarrhythmias may be asymptomatic or cause intermittent palpitations, cardiovascular failure, 'blackouts' or cardiac arrests. *Diagnosis* can be difficult. ECG interpretation is complicated by electrical artifacts, shivering, seizures and tremor. Oesophageal or right-sided ECG leads occasionally aid diagnosis.
- *Narrow QRS complex (NC) tachycardias* are usually SVTs. Intravenous (i.v.) adenosine boluses transiently (but sometimes permanently) terminate SVTs and confirm the diagnosis.
- *Wide QRS complex (WC) tachycardias* are usually due to VT but can be difficult to differentiate from SVT with abnormal conduction (SVT/AbC). After excluding AVN block, treat SVT/AbC as VT if haemodynamic instability co-exists. Lack of response to direct current (DC) cardioversion and/or i.v. lignocaine suggests an SVT/AbC, which is confirmed (±cardioverted) with i.v. adenosine. Treatment failure is managed with i.v. amiodarone (Figure 32c; Appendix 1) and repeated cardioversion.

General management
Rapid assessment is essential but not all arrhythmias need immediate intervention. Asymptomatic or stable rhythms (e.g. AF, SVT) can be observed while the cause (e.g. hypokalaemia) is corrected. Symptomatic tachyarrhythmias with hypotension, pulmonary oedema or tissue hypoperfusion (e.g. angina) are detrimental and require immediate termination (i.e. cardioversion, drugs).

Prevention: correct hypoxaemia, electrolyte disturbances (e.g. hypokalaemia, hypomagnesaemia), acid–base imbalance, cardiac ischaemia and arrhythmogenic factors including vagal stimulation (e.g. suctioning, pain), drugs (e.g. theophylline) or cardiac irritants

(e.g. central lines). **Prophylaxis**: β-blockers reduce IHD mortality but anti-arrrhythmics do not always improve outcome (e.g. lignocaine after MI).

Treatment options include:
- *Vagal stimulation* (e.g. carotid sinus massage): slows HR, aids diagnosis and may cardiovert some SVT.
- *Antiarrhythmic drugs*: classified by mechanism and site of action (Figure 32c; Appendix 1) and selected according to rhythm and pathophysiology. Therapeutic windows are often narrow, side-effects common and therapy is frequently ineffective (e.g. ~50% of VT). Paradoxically, treatment causes new arrhythmias in ~20%. '*Proarrrhythmic*' effects are common. Class 1a and III drugs prolong duration (i.e. QT interval), trigger automaticity and can precipitate VT (e.g. 'Torsade de pointes').
- *Non-pharmacological therapies* are often more successful than drugs and may be required in emergencies. In haemodynamically unstable VT or SVT, *DC cardioversion* using 50–360J shocks delivered through sternal and cardiac apex electrodes, in anaesthetized patients, achieves rapid cardioversion (Chapter 6). In recurrent VT, *implantable defibrillators* improve survival by >30% compared with drug therapy. *Radiofrequency catheter ablation* (RFCA) delivers radiofrequency energy through a catheter tip and safely destroys >90% of treatable accessory pathways or ectopic pacemakers. In refractory SVT, *overdrive atrial pacing* may restore sinus rhythm (SR).

Types of tachyarrhythmia
1 *Premature ectopic beats* may be:
- *Supraventricular*: with abnormal P waves (i.e. inverted or absent if the ectopic focus is near the AVN) that do not arise from the SAN but normal QRS complexes (i.e. normal ventricular conduction). They are benign and often followed by a 'sinus' pause before SR is reasserted.
- *Ventricular*: with wide QRS complexes (i.e. abnormal and/or slow ventricular conduction route). They occur randomly or follow every (bigeminy), or every second (trigeminy), normal beat. Although usually benign, they predispose to arrhythmias after MI and if they occur during the T wave of preceding beats.

2 Supraventricular tachyarrythmias

SVT originates above or within the AVN and presents with dizziness, palpitations and dyspnoea. Although rarely life-threatening, sudden death can occur.

- **Sinus tachycardia** (i.e. SR with a HR > 100/min) is a normal SAN physiological response to stress (e.g. exercise, emotion) or disease (e.g. fever, hypovolaemia).

- **Atrial tachycardia** (AT; HR 120–240/min) occurs in chronic cardiorespiratory disease due to ectopic atrial pacemaker activity caused by atrial surgery and metabolic, acid–base or drug (e.g. digoxin) toxicity. **Treatment**: use adenosine to terminate the AT, followed by class 1c (e.g. flecanide) or III (e.g. sotalol) drugs to prevent recurrence. Correct the underlying metabolic defects and/or consider RFCA.

- **Atrial fibrillation** may occur in isolation but is common in cardiac disease (e.g. heart failure), pneumonia, thyrotoxicosis and thromboembolism. Spontaneous, chaotic, atrial depolarization produces an irregular atrial rate >300/min, but refractory AVN conduction limits ventricular rate to <200/min. Ineffective atrial contraction predisposes to atrial thrombus and thromboembolism. **Treatment**: initially correct the underlying cause (e.g. hypokalaemia), which may restore spontaneous SR. **Drug therapy**: with β-blockers, digoxin or class VI drugs (e.g. diltiazem) controls ventricular rate by inhibiting AVN conduction. Cardiospecific β-blockers (e.g. bisoprolol) are preferred because they control resting and exercise-related HR. Cardioversion to SR may occur with class 1c (e.g flecanide) and class III (e.g. amiodarone) drugs. DC cardioversion restores SR in structurally normal hearts if AF has been present for <1 year. **Anticoagulation** (e.g. warfarin) prevents strokes and emboli from AF-induced left atrial thrombi and should be considered in all patients but especially those with paroxysmal AF, structural heart disease, enlarged atria (>4.5 cm on echocardiography) or requiring elective DC cardioversion.

- **Atrial flutter**: an anticlockwise atrial re-entry circuit causes rapid, co-ordinated depolarizations at a rate of 300/min. Ventricular rate depends on AVN refractoriness with conduction of every second (most frequently), third or fourth depolarization (i.e. 2:1; 3:1 or 4:1 block; HR 150, 100 or 75 beats[i.e. QRS complexes]/min respectively). The ECG shows a baseline 'sawtooth' appearance (best seen in leads III, aVf and V_1) due to rapid atrial depolarization. It is more obvious after i.v. adenosine, which inhibits AVN conduction. **Treatment** is similar to AF. Atrial RFCA breaks the re-entry circuit and may be curative. Low voltage (i.e. 50J) DC cardioversion is also effective.

- **Paroxysmal supraventricular tachycardias** cause episodic, sudden onset, regular, narrow QRS complex tachycardia (HR 150–250/min) interspersed with p waves lasting minutes to days. There are two types:
  - **Atrioventricular nodal re-entrant tachycardia** (AVNRT) is due to slowly conducting AVN accessory (β) pathways with short refractory periods. AVNRTs occur when a premature atrial ectopic is conducted slowly down the accessory pathway while the normal AVN (α) pathway is refractory. This impulse initiates a normal ventricular QRS contraction but also activates the distal end of the normal AVN (α) pathway, which is no longer refractory. A retrograde impulse returns to the atrium, initiating depolarization and a repeating circuit. Abnormal p waves follow the QRS complex on ECG.
  - **Atrio-ventricular re-entrant tachycardia** (AVRT) occurs when atrial impulses are conducted to the ventricle faster than in the AVN by accessory pathways (e.g. bundle of Kent in Wolff–Parkinson–White [WPW] syndrome) anatomically separated from the AVN. An area of ventricle is depolarized early (pre-excited), shortening the 'p-r' interval. Slow propagation (in non-conducting tissue) from the 'pre-excited' area creates a characteristic δ-wave on ECG. In AF, slow AVN conduction prevents excessive ventricular rates, whereas accessory pathways allow rapid conduction (≥250 beats/min) impairing ventricular filling and causing haemodynamic collapse or progression to ventricular fibrillation (VF). Pre-excited AF has wide QRS complexes because ventricular depolarization is largely from the accessory pathway impulse and requires immediate DC cardioversion. All patients with WPW syndrome need electrophysiological studies to determine conducting capacity and RFCA if it is high.

Treatment aims to impede AVN conduction to terminate the tachycardia. Options include: (a) vagal stimulation (e.g. carotid sinus massage, Valsalva manoeuvre) or (b) drug therapy. Adenosine (i.v.) transiently blocks (<5 secs) AV conduction and terminates AVNRT and AVRT tachycardias. Class Ic (e.g. flecanide), II (e.g. β-blockers), III (e.g. sotolol) and IV (e.g. diltiazem) drugs are useful for intermittent therapy and prophylaxis. RFCA is curative because it destroys the accessory pathway and is preferred if symptoms are severe or require long-term medication.

3 Ventricular tachyarrhythmia

3 Ventricular tachyarrhythmia (e.g. VT/VF) arise in the ventricles of patients with IHD, heart failure, cardiomyopathy or congenital heart disease. The risk of death due to VT/VF increases by 65% for each 10% decrease in ejection fraction following myocardial damage. VT and VF are generally more serious than SVT and are the most common causes of sudden death, which accounts for 10% of all mortality (Figure 32d).

- **VT** can be well tolerated but usually causes haemodynamic instability or degenerates into VF. Ventricular rate is ~120–250/min with occasional jugular venous pressure (JVP) cannon waves. **Monomorphic VT** is usually due to a stable re-entry circuit, typically in MI scar tissue (Figure 32b) with broad but uniform QRS complexes. **Polymorphic VT** is due to multiple foci of ectopic automaticity caused by metabolic or electrophysiological disturbances that prolong the QT interval (e.g. acute ischaemia, hypokalaemia, hypocalaemia, drugs, bradycardias). The ECG shows irregular or phasic 'Torsade de pointes' QRS complexes that are unstable and often progress to VF. **Treatment**: correct the underlying cause (e.g. hypokalaemia). Pulseless VT with cardiovascular collapse requires immediate DC cardioversion. Haemodynamically stable VT can be treated with class 1b (e.g. lignocaine) or 1a (e.g. disopyramide) drugs. Prophylaxis with class II (e.g. β-blockers) or III (e.g. amiodarone) drugs prevent initial recurrence. Angiotensin-converting enzyme (ACE) inhibitors improve heart failure and spironolactone maintains serum K^+. Slow heart rates prolong the QT interval and worsen polymorphic VT. Consequently, increasing the heart rate by pacing prevents the incidence of polymorphic VT. Implantable defibrillators are required for ongoing recurrence.

- **VF** results in rapid loss of cardiac output (CO) and unconsciousness. Death follows without resuscitation and DC cardioversion (Chapter 6). It is associated with severe heart disease and frequently follows acute MI. Ventricular rhythm is chaotic. **Treatment**: requires immediate DC cardioversion. Prophylaxis utilizes class II (e.g.β-blockers) or III (e.g. amiodarone) drugs and consideration of an implantable defibrillator.

33 Arrhythmias: bradyarrhythmias

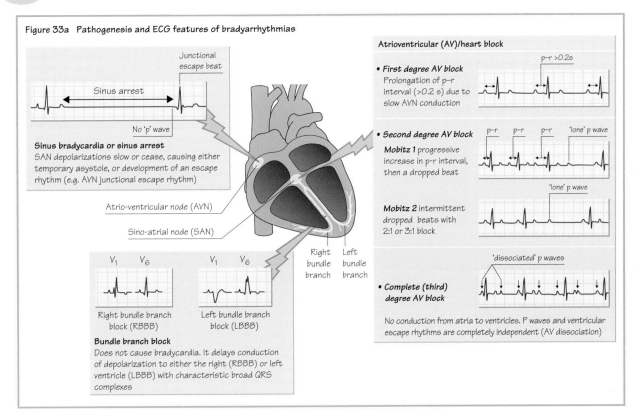

Figure 33a   Pathogenesis and ECG features of bradyarrhythmias

Sinus bradycardia or sinus arrest
SAN depolarizations slow or cease, causing either temporary asystole, or development of an escape rhythm (e.g. AVN junctional escape rhythm)

Atrio-ventricular node (AVN)

Sino-atrial node (SAN)

Bundle branch block
Does not cause bradycardia. It delays conduction of depolarization to either the right (RBBB) or left ventricle (LBBB) with characteristic broad QRS complexes

Right bundle branch block (RBBB)

Left bundle branch block (LBBB)

Atrioventricular (AV)/heart block

• *First degree AV block*
Prolongation of p–r interval (>0.2 s) due to slow AVN conduction

• *Second degree AV block*
Mobitz 1 progressive increase in p–r interval, then a dropped beat

Mobitz 2 intermittent dropped beats with 2:1 or 3:1 block

• *Complete (third) degree AV block*
No conduction from atria to ventricles. P waves and ventricular escape rhythms are completely independent (AV dissociation)

Bradycardia is a heart rate (HR) < 60 beats/min. **Bradyarrhythmias** are due to failure of the sinoatrial node (SAN) to produce regular depolarizations or abnormal atrioventricular node (AVN) conduction of atrial impulses to the ventricles (Figure 33a). Asystole (i.e. no depolarizations) is prevented by rapid emergence of escape rhythms in the next most active intrinsic cardiac pacemaker. This is usually the AVN if the SAN fails or the His–Purkinje conducting (HPC) or ventricular tissue in AVN block. Escape rhythm rates decrease with increasing distance from the SAN.

Clinical features: physiological or transient bradycardias are often asymptomatic or well tolerated. Symptomatic bradyarrhythmias cause faintness, fatigue, syncope or heart failure. Syncope ('Stokes–Adams' attack) is characterized by pallor and sudden, unheralded loss of consciousness and collapse lasting ~2–120 secs. Recovery is rapid with no residual focal neurology. The history, especially of witnessed attacks, is vital because differentiation from other causes of syncope (e.g. fits) can be difficult. **Diagnosis**: electrocardiograms (ECG) indicate the risk of developing, and type of bradyarrhythmia. Holter monitors (24hr ECG) detect both tachyarrhythmias and bradyarrhythmias.

Sinoatrial node disease presents as **sinus bradycardia** (i.e. normal ECG p-waves and AVN conduction) or **sinus arrest** with prolonged pauses (e.g. as atrial fibrillation terminates) that cause dizziness or fainting. '**Sick sinus syndrome**' is associated with both bradycardia and tachycardia (e.g. AF). Drugs (e.g. β-blockers) used to control tachyarrhythmia may aggravate the bradycardia. **Treatment** is only required in symptomatic SAN disease. Correct potential causes including pain and drug-toxicity (e.g. β-blockers).

Consider atropine, β-agonists (e.g. isoprenaline) or drug antidotes (e.g. digoxin antibodies) if symptoms persist.

Atrioventricular heart block (HB) impairs atrial 'p' wave conduction to the ventricles. It is due to AVN or HPC tissue disease/ischaemia. The right coronary artery supplies the AVN and transient HB often follows inferior myocardial infarction (MI) but rarely requires intervention. In contrast, HB after an anterior MI indicates a large infarct and needs early pacing. The left bundle of the HPC system is larger than the right and isolated left bundle branch block (BBB) is more likely to be associated with HB than right BBB.

• **First-degree HB** (1°HB) slows AVN conduction, prolonging the ECG pr interval (>0.2 secs). Bradycardia does not occur. Causes include pain (e.g. vagal) and drugs. It may precede higher degrees of HB. Neither 1°HB nor isolated BBB need therapy.

• **Second-degree HB** prevents conduction of atrial beats to the ventricles. *Mobitz 1 AVN block* (Wenkebach) causes progressive pr interval lengthening, then failure to transmit an impulse and a 'dropped' beat. It is often functional (i.e. drugs) and rarely requires pacing. *Mobitz II block* originates below the AVN in the HPC system. Every second or third atrial impulse initiates ventricular contraction (2:1; 3:1 block). Pacemaker insertion is required (e.g. after anterior MI) as complete HB often follows.

• **Complete HB**: conduction between atria and ventricles ceases. Subsequent AVN pacemaker activity produces 'junctional' escape rhythms (HR ~50/min) that are often transient and asymptomatic. Infranodal (ventricular) pacemaker escape rhythms are unstable, slower (HR ~35/min) and symptomatic, requiring urgent pacemaker insertion. Appendix 2 reports types and classifications of pacemakers.

Critical Care Medicine at a Glance, Third Edition. Richard Leach. © 2014 John Wiley & Sons, Ltd. Published 2014 by John Wiley & Sons, Ltd.

34 Heart failure and pulmonary oedema

Figure 34a Causes of heart failure and pulmonary oedema

Myocardial dysfunction	Ischaemic heart disease, cardiomyopathies, pregnancy and myocardial disease (e.g. amyloidosis). Isolated RVF follows ~33% of inferior MI as the RV blood supply is mainly from the right coronary artery
Pressure overload	*Left heart:* hypertension and aortic stenosis. Mitral stenosis does not often cause LVF. *Right heart:* pulmonary hypertension due to chronic lung disease (cor pulmonale), pulmonary stenosis
Volume overload	Excessive fluid administration or retention (e.g. renal failure). Aortic or mitral valve regurgitation causes LVF. Tricuspid regurgitation causes RVF
Impaired filling	Constrictive pericarditis (e.g. TB; rheumatic heart disease) or cardiac tamponade (e.g. pericardial effusion)
Arrhythmias Tachycardia	Impair ventricular filling causing atrial hypertension. Cause myocardial ischaemia by reducing diastole (e.g. atrial fibrillation, supraventricular tachycardia)
High output	Thyrotoxicosis, arteriovenous shunts, anaemia, Paget's disease, beriberi (vitamin B deficiency), sepsis

Figure 34b Cardiac output response of normal and failing hearts to loading conditions. Failing hearts respond well to afterload reduction but not preload increases

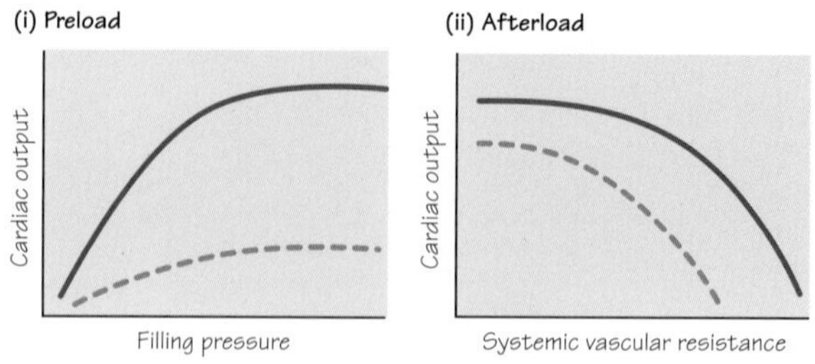

(i) Preload — Cardiac output vs Filling pressure

(ii) Afterload — Cardiac output vs Systemic vascular resistance

— Normal heart
- - - Failing heart

Figure 34c Cardiovascular compensatory mechanisms and the detrimental positive feedback effects they exert in heart failure. The location of action of key drugs is shown

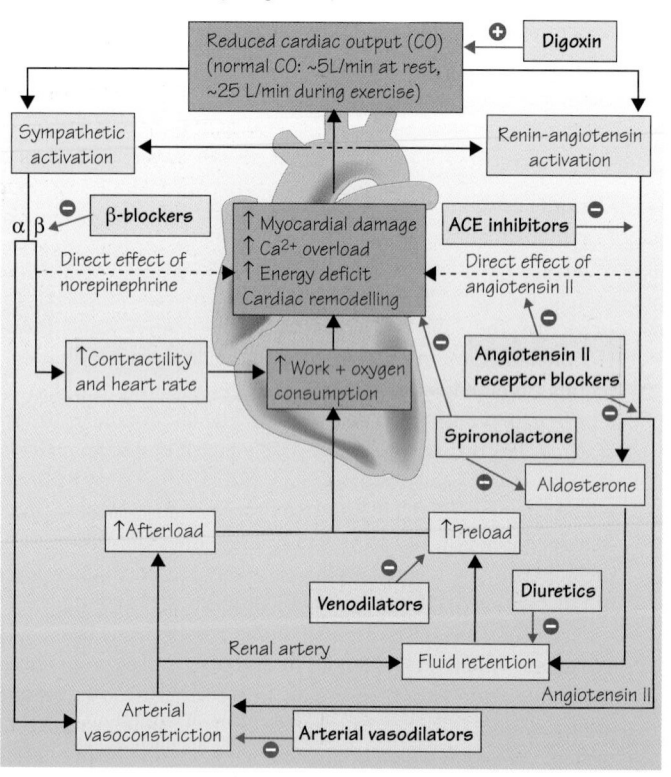

Figure 34d New York Heart Association (NYHA) classification of heart failure

- **Class I (mild):** No limitation of physical activity. No symptoms (e.g. fatigue, dyspnoea, palpitations) from ordinary activity
- **Class II (mild):** Slight limitation of physical activity. Comfortable at rest but ordinary activity causes symptoms
- **Class III (moderate):** Marked limitation of physical activity. Only comfortable at rest; minimal activity causes symptoms
- **Class IV (severe):** Unable to carry out any physical activity without discomfort. Symptoms at rest

Figure 34e The chest radiograph in heart failure shows an enlarged heart, pulmonary oedema with hilar 'bat's wing' shadowing, pleural effusions (usually right-sided) and upper lobe vein dilation due to increased venous pressure

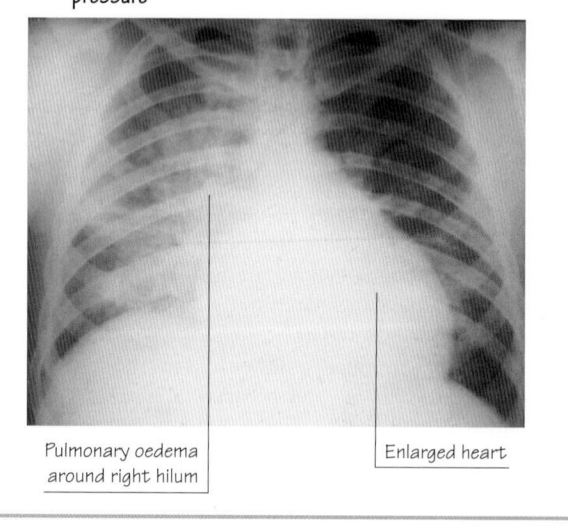

Pulmonary oedema around right hilum

Enlarged heart

Heart failure (HF) occurs when cardiac output (CO) is insufficient to meet the metabolic needs of the body, or if CO can only be maintained with elevated filling pressures (**preload**; Chapter 8). Initially, compensatory mechanisms maintain CO at rest, but, as HF (and CO) deteriorate, exercise tolerance falls and 'downstream'

hydrostatic pressures increase. The left, right or both sides of the heart can fail.
- **Left ventricular failure** (LVF) is most common. If the 'downstream' pulmonary capillary ('wedge') pressure (PCWP, Chapters 3, 8) rises to >20–25 mmHg, fluid filters into alveolar spaces

Critical Care Medicine at a Glance, Third Edition. Richard Leach. © 2014 John Wiley & Sons, Ltd. Published 2014 by John Wiley & Sons, Ltd.

causing **pulmonary oedema** and breathlessness. Hypoalbuminae-mia or increased membrane permeability (e.g. inflammation) can cause pulmonary oedema at lower PCWP.

- **Right ventricular failure** (RVF) causes systemic congestion (e.g. ankle oedema, hepatomegaly) and often occurs with LVF. Resulting biventricular failure is termed **congestive cardiac failure**.
- 'Cor pulmonale' describes RVF due to chronic lung disease.

Epidemiology

HF affects 2–3% of the population and >10% of people >65 years old. It is more common in men. **Causes** are listed in Figure 34a; most common are ischaemic heart disease (IHD) and hypertension. Volume overload can cause pulmonary oedema in normal hearts. **Prognosis**: 5-year survival is <50%.

Pathophysiology

- **Systolic failure**, with reduced myocardial contractility and ejection fraction (EF; <50%), causes 70% of HF. It is often due to IHD, cardiomyopathy, metabolic toxicity, valve defects or arrhythmias. Initially CO is maintained by compensatory mechanisms including: (i) *increased sympathetic drive*; (ii) *raised circulating volume* (i.e. salt and water retention due to renin-angiotensin system activation); (iii) *raised filling pressures* (Figure 34b(i); Chapter 8). Unfortunately, failing hearts respond poorly to preload (Figure 34b[i]) with subsequent pulmonary and peripheral congestion, while large ventricular volumes increase cardiac work and impair function (Figure 34c). In pressure overload (e.g. aortic stenosis), compensatory hypertrophy initially improves ventricular EF but reduced compliance eventually decreases blood flow and contractility.
- **Diastolic dysfunction** (DD) occurs when LV relaxation (i.e. filling), an energy-dependent process, is impaired by myocardial ischaemia, fibrosis, LV hypertrophy and associated poor diastolic LV perfusion. Reduced LV compliance (i.e. 'stiff' LV) increases PCWP and can precipitate pulmonary oedema despite normal contractility (i.e. EF >50%). DD affects ∼30% of HF patients. It is precipitated by tachycardia (short diastolic perfusion times) or impaired LV filling (e.g. atrial fibrillation [AF]).

Clinical features

Presentation of HF depends on speed of onset and underlying cause. It can be precipitated or aggravated by stress, acute illness, arrhythmias, pregnancy or drugs. Severity is often classified as in Figure 34d. Whatever the cause, reduced CO causes fatigue, anorexia and exercise limitation.

- **LVF** is characterized by breathlessness, hypoxaemia, orthopnoea, paroxysmal nocturnal dyspnoea and cough productive of frothy 'pink' sputum. Auscultation may reveal a gallop rhythm (S₃/S₄ added sounds) and coarse crepitations at the lung bases.
- **RVF** causes systemic congestion with raised jugular venous pressure (JVP), hepatomegaly, ascites and ankle oedema.

Onset may be **acute** (e.g. myocardial infarction [MI]) with cardiogenic shock (Chapter 7) or pulmonary oedema, or **chronic** with fatigue and fluid retention.

Diagnostic investigations

Investigations include cardiac enzymes, electrocardiogram (ECG) and chest radiograph (CXR) (Figure 34e). Serum b-type natriuretic peptide (BNP) increases with heart wall stress and is sensitive and specific for HF. Echocardiography demonstrates wall hypokinesia and ventricular enlargement. Ejection fraction is reduced in

HF although CO and blood pressure (BP) may be normal (see earlier). Cardiac catheterization is often required.

Management

The cause (e.g. IHD), underlying pathophysiology (e.g. DD) and precipitating events (e.g. arrhythmias) must be treated. In general, **afterload reduction** rapidly improves LV function and CO in the failing heart (Figure 34b[ii]) but may cause hypotension. By contrast, **preload reduction** relieves symptoms (e.g. pulmonary oedema) but CO is not increased (Figure 34b[i]), except when afterload is indirectly reduced (e.g. decreased LV size). Measurement of filling pressures, CO and vascular resistance (Chapters 3, 8) may be required to optimize HF treatment.

Acute left ventricular failure

Immediate relief of breathlessness due to pulmonary oedema is a priority. The **sitting position** is most comfortable and **supplemental oxygen** (>60%) corrects hypoxaemia. **Loop diuretics** (e.g. furosemide i.v.) initially relieve dyspnea by reducing LV preload (i.e. pulmonary venodilation). Subsequent diuresis lowers fluid load and cardiac filling pressures. **Nitrates** (i.v., sublingual) are also effective venodilators while simultaneously dilating coronary arteries in IHD. **Diamorphine** is a potent pulmonary venodilator and reduces Vo_2 by relieving anxiety. **Bronchodilators** (e.g. salbutamol) reverse bronchospasm but may precipitate arrhythmias. Continuous positive airways pressure (**CPAP**) reduces hypoxaemia and work of breathing and is often effective in HF (Chapter 16). **Arrhythmia** control is essential (Chapter 32).

Low-output left ventricular failure

When pulmonary oedema has been controlled, treatment aims to improve LV function, CO, DD and prognosis. **ACE inhibitors** reduce afterload, increase CO, reduce symptoms (e.g. fatigue) and prolong survival. They benefit most HF patients except when contraindicated (e.g. renal failure) or if side-effects occur (e.g. cough). Selective **beta-blockers** (e.g. bisoprolol) improve prognosis by reducing myocardial ischaemia and arrhythmias but may precipitate pulmonary oedema, heart block or bronchospasm. **Calcium channel blockers (CCBs)** alleviate DD by reducing hypertension and coronary vasospasm. However, tachycardia and impaired contractility limit use. **Digoxin** has inotropic effects and is useful in HF with AF. **Prophylactic anticoagulants** reduce thromboembolic events.

Right ventricular failure

Diuresis reduces peripheral oedema but is detrimental if high RV filling pressures are required to maintain CO. Afterload reduction with pulmonary vasodilators (e.g. CCBs) is usually limited by hypotension. **Oxygen therapy** relieves cor pulmonale (Chapter 41).

Cardiogenic shock

This may require **inotropic agents** or **intra-aortic balloon pumps** to maintain CO and BP (Chapter 7). **Phosphodiesterase inhibitors** (milrinone) stimulate cardiac contractility and peripheral vasodilation. Similarly, new **calcium sensitizers** (e.g. levosimendin) enhance contractility. Early **ventilatory support** improves survival (Chapters 16, 18).

Pearl of wisdom

Fatigue is the principal symptom in chronic heart failure and is alleviated by increasing cardiac output (e.g. afterload reduction, heart rate control) but not diuretics

35 Cardiac emergencies

Figure 35a Clinical features of hypertension-induced end organ damage

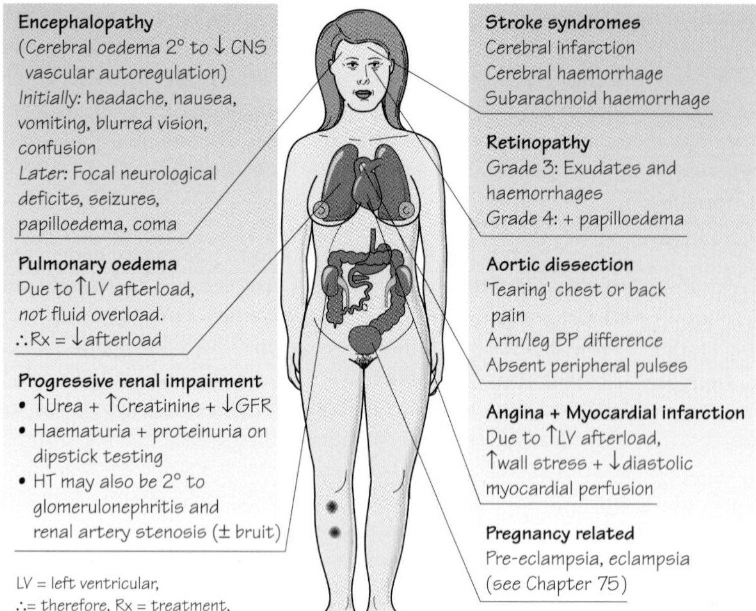

Encephalopathy
(Cerebral oedema 2° to ↓ CNS vascular autoregulation)
Initially: headache, nausea, vomiting, blurred vision, confusion
Later: Focal neurological deficits, seizures, papilloedema, coma

Pulmonary oedema
Due to ↑LV afterload, not fluid overload.
∴Rx = ↓afterload

Progressive renal impairment
• ↑Urea + ↑Creatinine + ↓GFR
• Haematuria + proteinuria on dipstick testing
• HT may also be 2° to glomerulonephritis and renal artery stenosis (± bruit)

LV = left ventricular,
∴= therefore, Rx = treatment,
GFR = glomerular filtration rate,
2° = secondary, ↓ = decreased, ↑ = increased
CNS = central nevous system

Stroke syndromes
Cerebral infarction
Cerebral haemorrhage
Subarachnoid haemorrhage

Retinopathy
Grade 3: Exudates and haemorrhages
Grade 4: + papilloedema

Aortic dissection
'Tearing' chest or back pain
Arm/leg BP difference
Absent peripheral pulses

Angina + Myocardial infarction
Due to ↑LV afterload,
↑wall stress + ↓diastolic myocardial perfusion

Pregnancy related
Pre-eclampsia, eclampsia
(see Chapter 75)

Figure 35b Organisms causing endocarditis

Organism	% Cases and notes
Streptococcus viridans	45-50%; the most usual cause; often related to poor dentition
Staphylococcus aureus	20-25%; most common cause of acute endocarditis; often associated with i.v. drug abuse
Staphylococcus epidermidis	Often follows valve replacement surgery
Streptococcus faecalis	~5%; common after abortion in women + genitourinary surgery in older men
Gram-negative organisms e.g. Haemophilus influenzae	Less common; occurs in drug addicts and following heart valve surgery
Other bacteria e.g. gonococcus, brucella, Coxiella burneti (Q fever), Chlamydia	Rare
Fungi	Rare: Immunosuppressed patients

Figure 35c Echocardiogram of mitral valve endocarditis

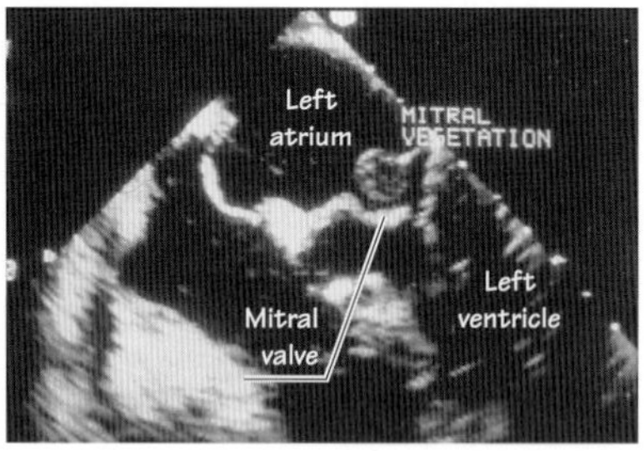

Left atrium
MITRAL VEGETATION
Mitral valve
Left ventricle

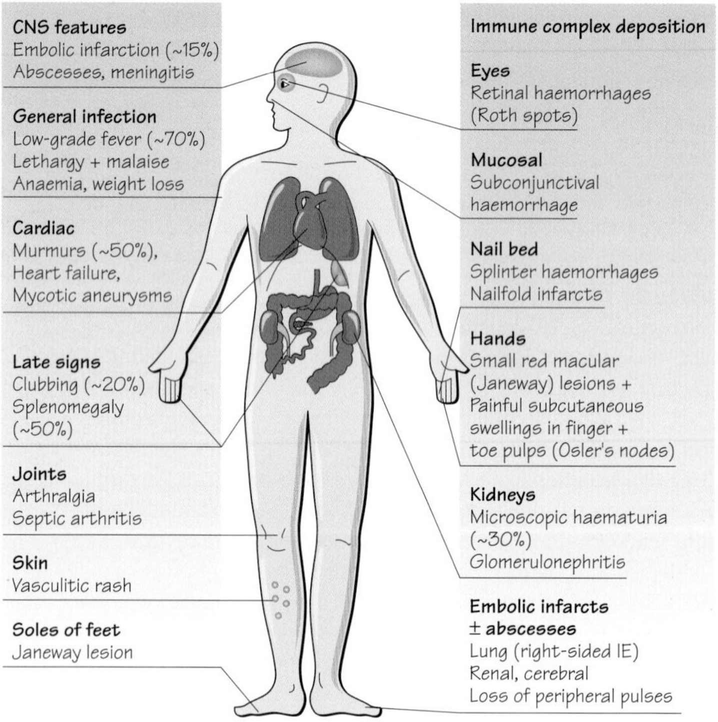

Figure 35e Needle pericardiocentesis (aspiration of percardial effusion)

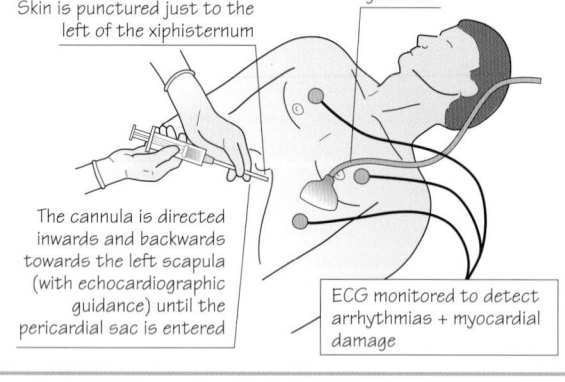

Skin is punctured just to the left of the xiphisternum

Echocardiographic guidance

The cannula is directed inwards and backwards towards the left scapula (with echocardiographic guidance) until the pericardial sac is entered

ECG monitored to detect arrhythmias + myocardial damage

Figure 35d Clinical features of Infective endocarditis (IE)

CNS features
Embolic infarction (~15%)
Abscesses, meningitis

General infection
Low-grade fever (~70%)
Lethargy + malaise
Anaemia, weight loss

Cardiac
Murmurs (~50%),
Heart failure,
Mycotic aneurysms

Late signs
Clubbing (~20%)
Splenomegaly (~50%)

Joints
Arthralgia
Septic arthritis

Skin
Vasculitic rash

Soles of feet
Janeway lesion

Immune complex deposition

Eyes
Retinal haemorrhages (Roth spots)

Mucosal
Subconjunctival haemorrhage

Nail bed
Splinter haemorrhages
Nailfold infarcts

Hands
Small red macular (Janeway) lesions +
Painful subcutaneous swellings in finger + toe pulps (Osler's nodes)

Kidneys
Microscopic haematuria (~30%)
Glomerulonephritis

Embolic infarcts ± abscesses
Lung (right-sided IE)
Renal, cerebral
Loss of peripheral pulses

Hypertensive emergencies

• *Definition*: severe hypertension (HT) is a systolic BP (SBP) >220–240 mmHg or a diastolic BP (DBP) >120–140 mmHg. In the past, hypertensive emergencies (HEs) were termed either 'accelerated' or 'malignant', the latter associated with more advanced retinopathy (±organ damage). Current HE classification is based on the presence of **life-threatening organ damage (LTOD)**, which determines the urgency for treatment. When

Critical Care Medicine at a Glance, Third Edition. Richard Leach. © 2014 John Wiley & Sons, Ltd. Published 2014 by John Wiley & Sons, Ltd.

LTOD is present (e.g. aortic dissection), reduce BP to safe levels (DBP ~100–110 mmHg) within <1–2 hours. However, rapid falls in BP can cause strokes, accelerated renal failure and myocardial ischaemia. Therefore, in the absence of LTOD, gradual reduction of BP over >6–72 hours is preferred.

- *Aetiology*: most HEs are due to inadequate or discontinued therapy for benign essential HT. However, in young (<30 years) or black patients, >50% have a secondary cause (e.g. renovascular disease, phaeochromocytoma, endocrine (Chapter 51), drug-induced [e.g. cocaine]). Pregnancy-related HT is discussed in Chapter 75. **Pathophysiology**: most organ damage is due to arteriolar necrotizing vasculitis and loss of vascular autoregulation.
- *Clinical features* of severe HT/HE are illustrated in Figure 35a. **Prognosis**: untreated severe HT with LTOD has a 1-year mortality >90%.

Management

- *Severe HT with LTOD* is a medical emergency requiring admission for monitoring. **Occasionally**, immediate BP reduction is required (e.g. dissecting aneurysm) using potent, titratable, vasodilator infusions. In these cases, arterial BP monitoring is mandatory. **Intravenous therapies** include: (a) **sodium nitroprusside,** a rapidly reversible, arteriovenous dilator, always administered by infusion pump to avoid hypotensive episodes. Prolonged use causes cyanide poisoning; (b) **glycerol trinitrate,** an arteriovenous dilator, is particularly useful if ischaemic heart disease (IHD) or pulmonary oedema co-exist; (c) **labetalol,** an $\alpha + \beta$-blocker, is valuable for hypertensive encephalopathy but may exacerbate asthma, heart failure and heart block; (d) **rarely used agents** include hydralazine and diazoxide, which are difficult to titrate. Angiotensin-converting enzyme (ACE) inhibitors can cause severe hypotension and are best avoided.
- *Severe HT without LTOD* rarely presents the same therapeutic crisis. When possible, **oral** regimes are used to lower DBP to ~100 mmHg over ~24–72 hours. Sublingual **nifedipine** has a rapid onset of action, short half-life and is titratable. Oral beta-blockers, ACE inhibitors and calcium antagonists are introduced as normal.

Infective endocarditis

Infection of heart valves or endocardium is usually **subacute** and causes a chronic illness when due to non-virulent organisms (e.g. *Streptococcus viridans*). However, it can be **acute** with a fulminant course when due to virulent organisms (e.g. *Staphylococcus*). Figure 35b lists organisms that cause infective endocarditis.

- *Aetiology*: it is most common in older people with degenerative aortic and mitral valve disease but it also affects those with prosthetic valves, or rheumatic or congenital heart disease. Abnormal valves are more susceptible to infection following dental or surgical procedures. Normal valves are occasionally infected by virulent organisms (e.g. staphylococcal valve infection with i.v. drug abuse).
- *Clinical features* are illustrated in Figure 35d. **Systemic embolization** causes splenic, lung, renal and cerebral infarcts (±abscesses). **Immune complex deposition** produces nail bed splinter haemorrhages, retinal haemorrhage (Roth spots), mucosal haemorrhage (e.g. subconjunctival) and painful nodules in finger pulps (Osler's nodes). Microscopic haematuria and splenomegaly are common.
- *Diagnosis* is initially clinical and suspected in any patient with fever, anaemia, raised ESR/CRP, microscopic haematuria, new heart murmurs, flu-like symptoms or weight loss. Repeatedly positive blood cultures (~50–80%) and echocardiography confirm the diagnosis. Transthoracic echocardiography (Figure 35c) detects

<50% of vegetations. Transoesophageal studies are more sensitive.

- *Management*: look for and treat underlying infection (e.g. dental abscesses). Start empiric broad-spectrum antibiotic therapy (e.g. benzylpenicillin/aminoglycoside) and adjust when microbiological results and antibiotic sensitivities are available. Treatment is usually for 3–6 weeks. Severely damaged native valves (±heart failure) and infected prosthetic valves often require surgical replacement.
- *Prognosis*: the high mortality (~15%) in developed contries is due to prosthetic valve infection. **Prophylactic antibiotics** are given to patients with valvular heart disease before dental or potentially septic procedures (e.g. cystoscopy)

Pericardial emergencies

Acute pericarditis

Acute pericarditis is due to infection (mostly viral), myocardial infarction (MI), uraemia, connective tissue disease, trauma, tuberculosis (TB) and neoplasia. An immunologically mediated febrile pleuropericarditis (Dressler's syndrome) can occur 2–6 weeks after MI (~2%).

- *Clinical features* include severe, positional (i.e. relief sitting forward), retrosternal chest pain and pericardial rub on auscultation.
- *Investigation*: ECG shows concave ST segment elevation in all leads. Cardiac enzymes may be elevated with myocarditis.
- *Management*: anti-inflammatory drugs (e.g. aspirin) relieve discomfort. Steroids are required occasionally (e.g. Dressler's syndrome).

Pericardial effusion

Pericardial effusion is due to infection (e.g. TB), uraemia, MI, aortic dissection, myxoedema, neoplasia and radiotherapy.

- *Clinical features*: cardiac tamponade occurs when pericardial fluid impairs ventricular filling, reducing cardiac output (CO). Breathlessness and pericarditic pain often precede acute cardiovascular collapse. Examination may reveal a raised jugular venous pressure (JVP) that increases on inspiration (Kussmaul's sign), hypotension with a paradoxical pulse (i.e. BP falls >15 mmHg during inspiration) and distant heart sounds.
- *Investigation*: ECG (reduced voltage), CXR (globular cardiomegaly) and echocardiography (pericardial fluid and tamponade-induced right ventricular diastolic collapse) are diagnostic.
- *Management*: echocardiography-directed, pericardial drainage is required for tamponade (Figure 35e).

Constrictive pericarditis

Progressive pericardial fibrotic constriction (e.g. TB) may cause tamponade. Surgical removal of the pericardium may be necessary.

Other cardiac emergencies

Acute valve lesions, type A ascending aorta dissection, trauma (Chapter 71), myocarditis and congenital heart disease may also present as cardiac emergencies.

Pearl of wisdom

Consider prophylactic antibiotics in patients with prosthetic heart valves or valvular disease before any procedure (e.g. catheterization)

36 Deep venous thrombosis and pulmonary embolism

Figure 36a Pulmonary angiograms (A,D) and V/Q scans (B,E = ventilation scans, C,F = perfusion scans) in a normal patient and a patient with a massive right-sided pulmonary embolism. The angiogram (D) shows complete occlusion of the right pulmonary artery. On the V/Q scan there is loss of right lung perfusion (F) but normal ventilation (E)

NORMAL   PULMONARY EMBOLISM

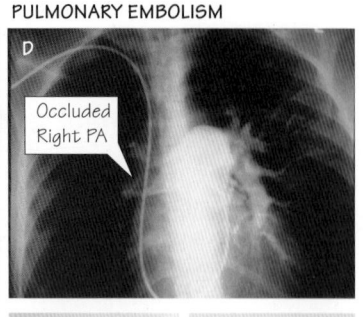

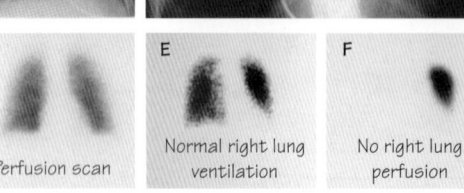

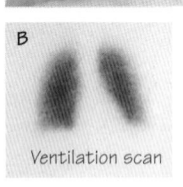
Ventilation scan

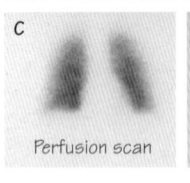
Perfusion scan

Normal right lung ventilation

No right lung perfusion

Figure 36b Contrast CT scan showing contrast in the heart and pulmonary arteries (PA). Both the right and left PA show irregular defects consistent with pulmonary emboli

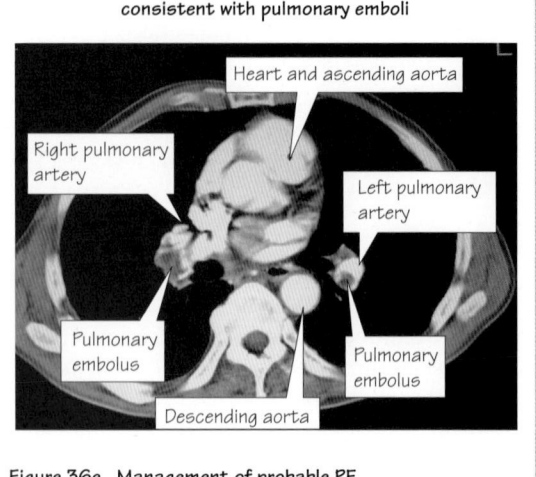

Figure 36c Risk factors for DVT and PE

• Recent Surgery (<12 wks)	Hip, knee, gynaecological procedures
• Trauma	Spinal trauma, limb fractures
• General factors	Age, obesity, smoking, oral contraceptive pill, immobility for >3 days in last 4 weeks, previous DVT/PE or family history, post-partum
• Underlying disease	Malignancy, sepsis, stroke, autoimmune disease
• Cardiovascular disease	Low flow states (e.g. heart failure)
	Vascular injury (e.g. atherosclerosis)
• Inherited disorders (less common)	Deficiencies (e.g. antithrombin III, protein C, protein S)
	Clotting disorders (e.g. Factor V Leiden, antiphospholipid syndrome)

Figure 36d DVT prophylaxis

Risk of DVT	Patient	Regime
Low (<1%)	<40 years old, minor surgery (<1 hr) Minimal immobility	Early ambulation Compression stockings
Moderate (5-10%)	>40 years old, surgery (>1 hr), cardiac, medical problems, CVA, hypercoaguability	Low dose heparin (UFH or LMWH)
High (>15%)	Complicated surgery, hip or knee surgery hip fracture, trauma	Full dose LMWH or warfarin

LMWH=low molecular weight heparin, UFH=unfractionated heparin, CVA=cerebrovascular accident

Figure 36e Management of probable PE

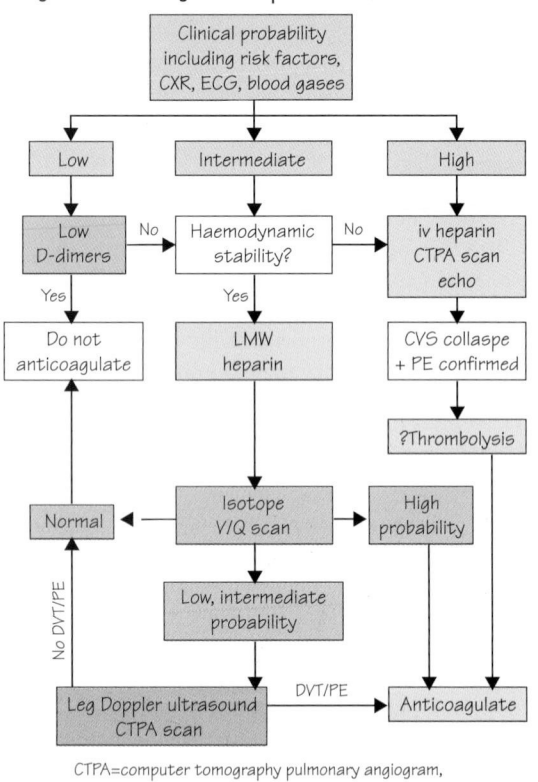

CTPA=computer tomography pulmonary angiogram, DVT=deep venous thrombosis, CVS=cardiovascular, PE=pulmonary embolism, V/Q=ventilation/perfusion

Venous stasis, hypercoagulability and vascular injury (Virchow's triad) predispose to deep venous thrombosis (DVT) of which pulmonary embolism (PE) is the most significant complication. Appropriate clinical suspicion and a systematic approach to investigation reduce frequently missed diagnoses. **Risk factors** for venous thromboembolism (VTE) are listed in Figure 36c. Up to 70% of high-risk patients without prophylaxis develop DVT (e.g. hip replacement surgery). **Epidemiology**: VTE affects $\sim$70/10^6 UK population/year, a third with PE and two-thirds with DVT alone.

Deep venous thrombosis

Most clinically significant PEs ($\sim$90%) arise from DVTs that originate in the calves and propagate above the knees. Clots confined to the calves ($\sim$65%) are of little importance, but half the 15–25% that extend into the femoral and iliac veins release PEs. Occasional axillary or subclavian DVTs are due to central lines or surgery and associated emboli are small. The risk of PE is greatest during early clot proliferation and decreases once thrombus has organized.

• **Clinical features** are non-specific including mild fever and calf swelling, tenderness, erythema and warmth. *Homan's sign* (calf pain on foot dorsiflexion) may dislodge thrombus and is best avoided. Clinical examination fails to detect >50% of DVT.

• **Diagnosis**: D-dimers are fibrin degradation products created when fibrin is lysed by plasmin. **D-dimers assays** are sensitive but not specific for DVT. They increase with infection, inflammation and malignancy. Thus, a negative D-dimer excludes but a raised assay cannot confirm VTE. A **Doppler ultrasound scan (USS)** is performed if the D-dimer is raised or clinical probability high, but it may fail to detect $\sim$30% of proximal DVTs. Venography is rarely necessary.

• **Prevention**: stop smoking and contraceptive pills, lose weight and treat infection or heart failure before elective surgery. Prophylaxis is essential after surgery and in high-risk patients, and depends on the level of risk (Figures 36c, 36d). It includes pneumatic compression devices, regular leg exercises and early mobilization. Unfractionated heparin (UFH) and low molecular weight heparin (LMWH) reduce post-operative DVTs by $\sim$50% and PEs by $\sim$65–75%.

• **Treatment**: LMWH is as effective as UFH for prevention of clot extension and PE in DVT. Subsequent oral anticoagulation with warfarin is required for $\geq$6 weeks.

Pulmonary embolism

PE occurs when thrombus, usually from an iliac or femoral DVT, passes through the venous system and right heart and occludes a pulmonary artery (PAr) with respiratory and circulatory consequences. Hypoxaemia is mainly due to ventilation/perfusion (V/Q) mismatch and increased ventilatory dead space necessitates increased ventilation to maintain a normal $P_a\text{CO}_2$. Reduced surfactant in affected areas causes atelectasis. Circulatory collapse occurs with >50% PAr obstruction. Pre-existing heart failure, rate of onset and degree of PAr obliteration determine clinical and cardiovascular effects. **Massive PE** due to large central PAr emboli may cause catastrophic circulatory collapse and hypoxaemia. **Multiple small PEs** with extensive segmental PAr occlusions cause breathlessness, hypoxia and right ventricular (RV) failure but may be well tolerated due to adaptive responses. A **single small PE** occluding a segmental PAr may cause dyspnoea, haemoptysis and pleuritic pain due to pulmonary infarction (<25% cases). Small emboli can be fatal with co-existing lung or heart disease.

Clinical presentation

PEs present with pleuritic pain and haemoptysis in $\sim$65%, isolated dyspnoea in $\sim$25% and circulatory collapse in $\sim$10% of cases.

Dyspnoea does not occur in $\sim$30% of confirmed cases. Non-specific features include anxiety, tachypnoea, tachycardia, cough, sweating and syncope. RV failure with hypotension and elevated jugular venous pressure (JVP) occurs in severe PE. **Chest radiograph (CXR)** findings are often unremarkable but include atelectasis and wedge infarcts. **Electrocardiograms (ECGs)** show non-specific ST segment changes and, rarely, after a large PE, RV strain with an $S_1Q_3T_3$ pattern, right axis deviation and right bundle branch block. **Arterial blood gas (ABG)** abnormalities include a widened A-a gradient, hypoxaemia and hypocapnia (despite increased dead space). PE should be considered in all hypoxaemic patients with a normal CXR.

Diagnosis

Figure 36e illustrates management of suspected PE.

• **Spiral CT scans** (Figure 36b): have replaced V/Q isotope scans as the investigation of choice. They are sensitive (70–95%; highest for proximal emboli) and specific ($\geq$90%) for PE and useful when parenchymal disease (e.g. chronic obstructive pulmonary disease [COPD]) limits V/Q scan interpretation.

• **Isotope V/Q scans** have significant limitations (Figure 36a). A negative perfusion scan effectively rules out PE and a 'high probability' scan (i.e. segmental perfusion defects with normal ventilation) has a >85% probability of PE. High clinical suspicion with a 'high probability' V/Q scan has a positive predictive value >95%. Unfortunately, most V/Q scans are indeterminate with a 15–50% likelihood of PE (i.e. not diagnostic), necessitating further imaging.

• **Doppler USS**: confirmation of lower limb DVT precludes the need for further investigation as treatment is required. Absence of DVT combined with a low probability V/Q scan permits withholding treatment whereas a negative USS with an intermediate probability V/Q scan (or cardiopulmonary disease) necessitates CT scanning.

• **Transthoracic and transoesophageal echocardiography** may reveal RV dysfunction and main PAr emboli (but not lobar/segmental emboli) respectively.

• **Pulmonary angiography**: a rarely used diagnostic standard.

Treatment

Therapy is similar to that for established DVT:

• **Anticoagulation** stops propagation of DVT and allows organization. Immediate therapy may prevent further life-threatening emboli in those at high risk. **Heparin (UFH or LMWH)** for 5–7 days followed by warfarin for 3–6 months is standard therapy. Monitor UFH and warfarin because subtherapeutic levels increase VTE risk. LMWH is more bioavailable and does not require monitoring. Patients with inherited or acquired hypercoagulability may require lifelong anticoagulation(Chapter 69). If contraindications prevent anticoagulation (e.g. haemorrhagic stroke) or recurrent PE occur while anticoagulated, insertion of an **inferior vena cava filter** may prevent further PE.

• **Thrombolytic therapy** hastens clot breakdown, corrects perfusion defects and alleviates RV dysfunction. Prognosis is not improved in patients without massive PE but bleeding complications increase, including a 0.3–1.5% risk of intra-cerebral haemorrhage. Consequently, thrombolysis is only recommended in life-threatening PE with compromised haemodynamics.

Pearl of wisdom

Consider pulmonary embolism (PE) in any hypoxaemic patient with a normal chest radiograph (CXR)

37 Chest imaging and bronchoscopy

Figure 37 Evaluation of the CXR includes all the following:

① Date: ② Name:

③ AP/PA: Is it AP (anteroposterior)
   or PA (posteroanterior)?
   (Heart size cannot be measured if AP)

④ Is it well positioned? The trachea should be midway between clavicles

⑤ Penetration: The disc spaces should be just visible through the cardiac shadows
   (underpenetrated = plethoric lungs
      overpenetrated = dark lungs)

⑥ Soft tissues and breast shadows
   (mastectomy in a female)

⑦ Right diaphragm 2 cm higher than left
   (raised when paralysed, flat in asthma/COPD)

⑧ Check ribs for fractures, metastases

⑨ Right heart border = right atrium

⑩ Hilium = bronchi, arteries and veins

⑪ Superior vena cava

⑫ Aortic arch

⑬ Left heart border = left ventricle

⑭ Pulmonary vessels

⑮ Trachea and main bronchi

⑯ Lung fields

(a)   Chest radiograph interpretation

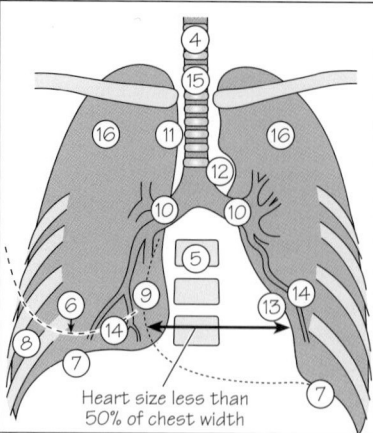

Heart size less than
50% of chest width

Normal chest X-ray

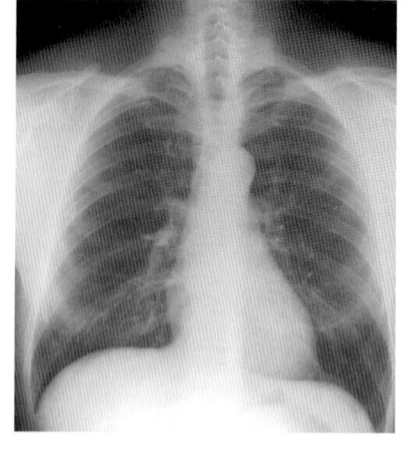

---

① Thoracic vertebral bodies

② Scapula

③ Pulmonary trunk and hilium

④ Descending aorta

⑤ Head of clavicle

⑥ Trachea

⑦ Arch of aorta

⑧ Ascending aorta

⑨ Anterior space (thymus)

⑩ Heart

⑪ Sternum

⑫ Diaphragm

(b)   Chest radiograph interpretation

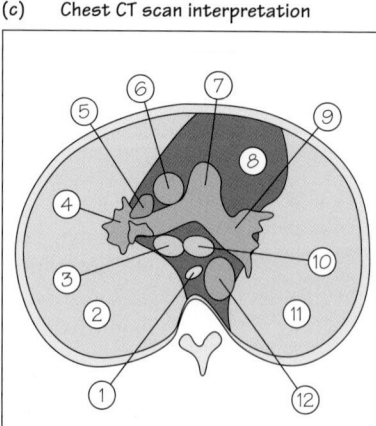

Normal lateral X-ray

L

---

① Oesophagus

② Right lung

③ Right main bronchus

④ Right pulmonary artery and branches

⑤ Superior vena cava

⑥ Ascending aorta

⑦ Pulmonary trunk

⑧ Mediastinum and heart

⑨ Left pulmonary artery and branches

⑩ Left main bronchus

⑪ Left lung

⑫ Descending aorta

(c)   Chest CT scan interpretation

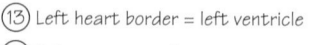

Normal, contrast enhanced, chest CT scan at the level of the pulmonary artery bifurcation

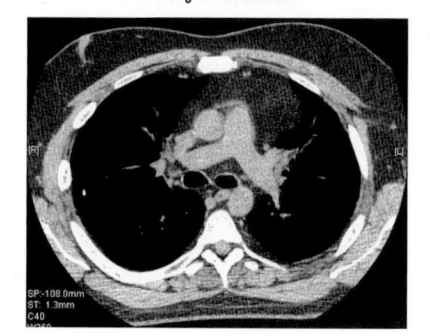

SP:-108.0mm
ST: 1.3mm
C40

Standard (two-dimensional) chest X-rays are the mainstay of thoracic imaging and detect, diagnose or follow morphological abnormalities in the chest. They account for over 50% of thoracic imaging procedures and are important in critical illness because the procedure can be performed by mobile X-ray units. Development of digital, three-dimensional computed tomography (CT) scans and physiological (e.g. ventilation/perfusion [V/Q] scans) imaging has further enhanced diagnostic capability but requires patient transfer to the radiology department, which can be hazardous and time consuming in critical illness. Magnetic resonance images (MRI) are less useful in chest disease. Specific radiographical abnormalities are discussed in individual chapters.

Posteroanterior (PA) chest radiographs (CXRs) should be performed upright in full inspiration although this is often difficult in the critically ill. Lateral films are occasionally helpful. Figures 37a and 37b illustrate the features and interpretation of the normal CXR. Portable anteroposterior (AP) films magnify the heart and mediastinum and limit assessment of lung parenchyma. A standard PA CXR allows two-dimensional visualization of both lungs, diaphragmatic position, the trachea, main carina, main stem bronchi, major and minor fissures and mediastinal structures including the great vessels (e.g. aorta) and heart. In respiratory disease, abnormal lung parenchymal infiltrates or consolidation, enlarged hilar and/or paratracheal lymph nodes, volume loss, enlarged pulmonary arteries or cardiac enlargement may be detected. In suspected pleural effusions, lateral decubitus films allow visualization of as little as 50 mL of fluid. Digital CXRs allow detailed views of the denser portions of the thorax and show finer detail of the lung parenchyma.

Computed tomography allows thin slice axial images and detailed examination of intrathoracic structures. It can detect small lesions and determine their relationship to other intrathoracic structures. New technology allows complete axial scanning of the thorax with a single breath-hold. Gross CT scan features are shown in Figure 37c and examples are shown in several chapters. Indications for CT scans are:

- *Thoracic and mediastinal tumours/masses*: to detect and assess operability and prognosis of tumours by determining size, presence of abnormal lymph nodes (e.g. mediastinal, axillary), location and relationship to other structures.
- *Lung parenchymal disease*: to detect and localize interstitial lung infiltrates, bronchiectasis, cavities, bulla and fluid collections.
- *Pleural disease*: to determine the cause of pleural effusions and assess asbestos-related plaques and pleural tumours (e.g. mesothelioma).
- *Pulmonary emboli (PE)*: administration of intravenous contrast allows imaging of the pulmonary blood vessels and detection of emboli (Chapter 36).

V/Q scans are usually performed in the evaluation of pulmonary embolism (Chapter 36). Gamma cameras visualize radiopharmaceuticals injected into venous blood (perfusion) or inhaled (ventilation). Thromboembolism classically causes a V/Q mismatch, with absence of perfusion in the presence of ventilation. Unfortunately, many PEs result in indeterminate V/Q scans with small mismatches or matched V/Q deficits, requiring additional studies to demonstrate thromboemboli. Contrast CT scans have largely superseded V/Q scans as the first-line investigation to detect PE. Quantitative V/Q scans are used before lung resection surgery, to assess regional and residual lung function.

Pulmonary angiography visualizes the vasculature following injection of contrast medium (Chapter 36). It may be required in patients with pulmonary hypertension, pulmonary vascular disease (e.g. vasculitis, arteriovenous malformations) and very occasionally to confirm PE. These studies are often preceded by echocardiography to visualize right ventricular function and estimate pulmonary artery pressure using Doppler imaging.

Positron emission tomography (PET) uses a fluorinated analogue of glucose (FDG) to produce lung images that highlight areas of increased glucose metabolism. Malignant cells have increased glucose uptake and appear as increased densities on PET images. Recent studies demonstrate that PET is useful in distinguishing between benign and malignant pulmonary nodules and in detecting small nodal metastases that are not seen on CT scans. For these indications, sensitivity and specificity was 80–97% with false-positives in infection or granulomatous inflammation. Whole body PET detects clinically inapparent distant metastases.

Bronchoscopy enables direct visualization of the fourth and fifth divisions of the endobronchial tree. Most bronchoscopies are performed as day cases under local anaesthetic in the sedated but awake patient, using a flexible fibreoptic instrument. It is a safe technique with a low complication rate. Saturation and heart rhythm should be monitored and supplemental oxygen administered during the procedure. Facilities for resuscitation should always be immediately available. In critical care units, flexible bronchoscopes can be passed through an endotracheal tube (ETT) or tracheostomy (>8 mm internal diameter [i.d.]). Attempts to pass an endoscope through an ETT with an i.d. <7.5 mm risks expensive 'surface degloving'. Always ensure adequate sedation before bronchoscopy. Thoracic surgeons use rigid bronchoscopes to obtain larger biopsies, to achieve better suctioning (e.g. haemoptysis) and to remove inhaled foreign bodies. Bronchoscopy is most often used to investigate CXR 'masses', visualize endobronchial tumours, assess operability and obtain biopsies, washings and brush samples for histological and cytological analysis. Bronchoscopy can also be used to diagnose parenchymal lung disease (e.g. transbronchial biopsy for histological examination) and to collect bronchoalveolar fluid (i.e. bronchoalveolar lavage) for diagnosis of infection (e.g. tuberculosis) in critically ill and immunocompromised patients (e.g. *Pneumocystis (carinii) jiroveci pneumonia*). Bronchoscopy also aids investigation of collapsed segments or lobes. Therapeutically, bronchoscopy is often used in ICU/HDU to aspirate sputum plugs, blood and secretions and to remove inhaled foreign bodies. It may also be used to place bronchial stents and treat endobronchial tumours (e.g. radiotherapy). Haemorrhage, pneumothorax and cardiac arrhythmia, although uncommon, are the main complications of fibreoptic bronchoscopy.

Pearl of wisdom
In critical illness, sudden hypoxaemia with lobar or segmental collapse on chest radiograph (CXR) is often due to a sputum plug

38 Community-acquired pneumonia

Figure 38a (i) Pneumonia affecting the right lower lobe

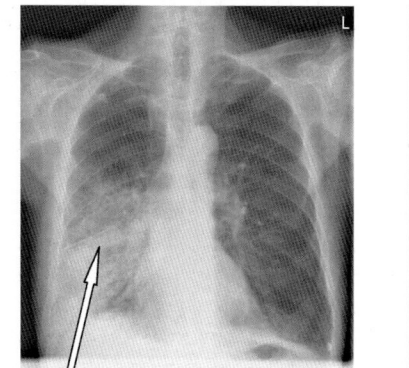

Consolidation right lower lobe

(ii) Pneumonia affecting lingula lobe

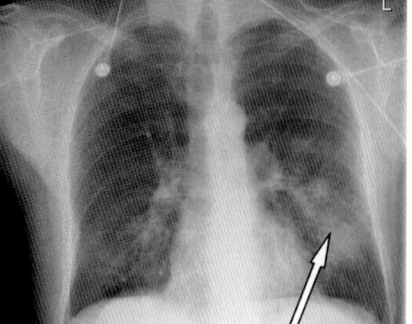

Consolidation lingula lobe

Figure 38b Risk factors for pneumonia

Age: >65, <5 years old
Chronic disease (e.g. renal, lung)
Diabetes mellitus
Immunosuppression: (e.g. drugs, HIV)
Alcohol dependency
Aspiration (e.g. epilepsy)
Recent viral illness (e.g. influenza)
Malnutrition
Mechanical ventilation
Postoperative (e.g. obesity, smoking)
Environmental (e.g. psitticosis)
Occupational (e.g. Q fever)
Travel abroad (e.g. paragonomiasis)
Air-conditioning (e.g. Legionella)

Figure 38c Micro-organisms and patological insults that cause pneumonia

Bacterial infections	Atypical infections	Fungal infection
Streptococcus pneumoniae	Mycoplasma pneumoniae	Aspergillus
Haemophilus influenzae	Legionella pneumophila	Histoplasmosis
Klebsiella pneumoniae	Coxiella burnetii	Candida
Pseudomonas aeruginosa	Chlamydia psittaci	Nocardia
Gram negative (E.coli)		

Viral infections	Protozoal infections	Other
Influenza	Pneumocystis carinii	Aspiration
Coxsackie	Toxoplasmosis	Lipoid pneumonia
Adenovirus	Amoebiasis	Bronchiectasis
Respiratory syncytial	Paragonomiasis	Cystic fibrosis
Cytomegalovirus		Radiation

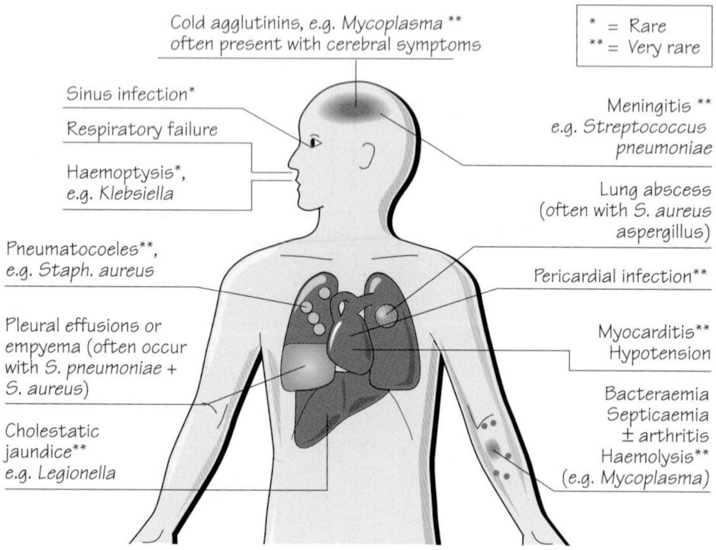

Figure 38e Management of CAP in patients admitted to hospital using the recently validated CURB-65 score

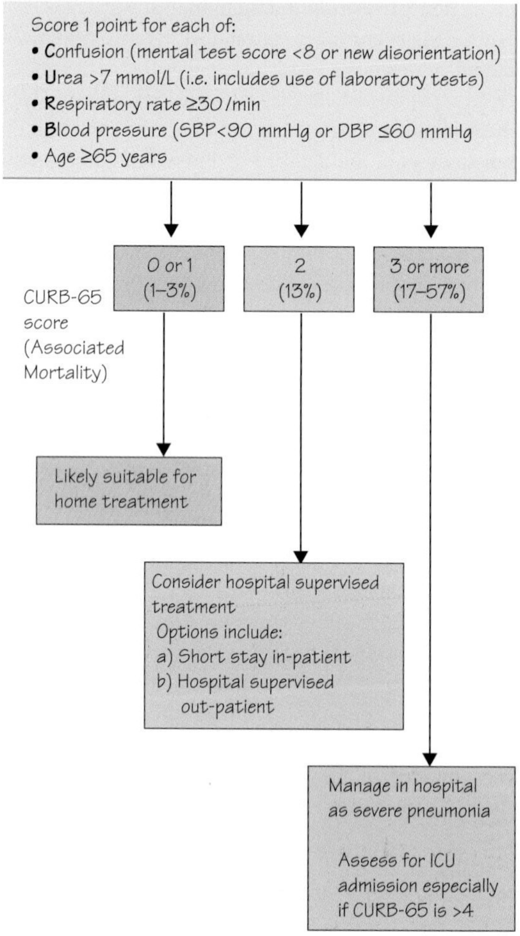

Score 1 point for each of:
• Confusion (mental test score <8 or new disorientation)
• Urea >7 mmol/L (i.e. includes use of laboratory tests)
• Respiratory rate ≥30/min
• Blood pressure (SBP<90 mmHg or DBP ≤60 mmHg)
• Age ≥65 years

CURB-65 score (Associated Mortality)

| 0 or 1 (1–3%) | 2 (13%) | 3 or more (17–57%) |

Likely suitable for home treatment

Consider hospital supervised treatment
Options include:
a) Short stay in-patient
b) Hospital supervised out-patient

Manage in hospital as severe pneumonia

Assess for ICU admission especially if CURB-65 is >4

Figure 38d Complications and infection specific features of pneumonia

* = Rare
** = Very rare

Cold agglutinins, e.g. Mycoplasma ** often present with cerebral symptoms

Sinus infection*

Respiratory failure

Haemoptysis*, e.g. Klebsiella

Pneumatocoeles**, e.g. Staph. aureus

Pleural effusions or empyema (often occur with S. pneumoniae + S. aureus)

Cholestatic jaundice** e.g. Legionella

Meningitis ** e.g. Streptococcus pneumoniae

Lung abscess (often with S. aureus aspergillus)

Pericardial infection**

Myocarditis** Hypotension

Bacteraemia Septicaemia ± arthritis Haemolysis** (e.g. Mycoplasma)

Definition

Pneumonia is an **acute lower respiratory tract (LRT) illness**, usually due to **infection**, associated with **fever, focal chest symptoms (±signs)** and **new shadowing on chest radiograph (CXR)** (Figure 38a). Figure 38c lists causes of pneumonia.

Classification

Microbiological classification of pneumonia is not practical because causative organisms may not be identified or diagnosis takes several days. Likewise **radiographic** appearance (e.g. lobar- [i.e. one lobe] or broncho-pneumonia [i.e. widespread, patchy

Critical Care Medicine at a Glance, Third Edition. Richard Leach. © 2014 John Wiley & Sons, Ltd. Published 2014 by John Wiley & Sons, Ltd.

involvement]) gives little information about cause. The following classification is widely accepted:

- **Community-acquired pneumonia (CAP)** describes LRT infections occurring before or within 48 hours of hospital admission in patients who have not been hospitalized for >14 days. The most frequently identified organism is *Streptococcus pneumoniae* (20–75%). 'Atypical' pathogens (e.g. *Mycoplasma pneumoniae*, *Chlamydia pneumoniae*, *Legionella* spp. [2–25%]) and viral infections (8–12%) are relatively common causes. *Haemophilus influenzae* and *Mycobacterium catarrhalis* occur in chronic obstructive pulmonary disease (COPD) exacerbations and staphylococcal infections may follow influenza. Alcoholic, diabetic, heart failure and nursing home patients are prone to staphylococcal, anaerobic and gram-negative organisms.
- **Hospital-acquired (nosocomial) pneumonia** (Chapter 39) describes LRT infections developing >2 days after hospital admission. Likely organisms are gram-negative bacilli (~65%) or staphylococci (~15%).
- **Aspiration/anaerobic pneumonia** follows aspiration of oropharyngeal contents due to impaired consciousness or laryngeal incompetence. Causative organisms include bacteroides and other anaerobes.
- **Opportunistic pneumonia** (Chapter 68) occurs in the immunosuppressed (e.g. chemotherapy, HIV) who are susceptible to viral, fungal, mycobacterial and unusual bacterial infections.
- **Recurrent pneumonia** is due to aerobic and anaerobic organisms in cystic fibrosis and bronchiectasis.

Epidemiology

- **Annual CAP incidence**: 5–11 cases per 1000 adult population; 15–45% require hospitalization of whom 5–10% are treated in intensive care. Incidence is highest in older people and infants. **Mortality** is 6–12% in hospitalized and 25–>50% in ICU patients. **Seasonal variation**: (e.g. mycoplasma in autumn, staphylococcus in spring) and annual cycles (e.g. 4-yearly mycoplasma epidemics) occur. Viral infections increase CAP in winter.

Risk factors

Factors increasing CAP risk are listed in Figure 38b. **Specific factors** include **age** (e.g. mycoplasma in young adults), **occupation** (e.g. brucellosis in abattoir workers, Q fever in sheep workers), **environment** (e.g. psittacosis with pet birds, ehrlichiosis due to tick bites) or **geographical** (e.g. coccidomycosis in southwest USA). Epidemics of *Coxiella burnetii* (Q fever) or *Legionella pneumophila* may be localized (e.g. Legionnaires' disease may involve a specific hotel due to air-conditioner contamination).

Diagnosis

The aims are to establish the **diagnosis**, identify **complications**, assess **severity** and determine **classification** to aid antibiotic choice.

Clinical features

These are not diagnostic without a CXR and cannot predict causative organisms (i.e. 'atypical' pathogens do not have characteristic presentations). **Symptoms** may be general (e.g. malaise, fever, myalgia) or chest specific (e.g. dyspnoea, pleurisy, cough, haemoptysis). **Signs** include cyanosis, tachycardia and tachypnoea, with focal dullness, crepitations, bronchial breathing and pleuritic rub on chest examination. In the young, older people and those with atypical pneumonias (e.g. mycoplasma) **non-respiratory features** (e.g. headache, confusion, diarrhoea) may predominate. **Complications** are shown in Figure 38d.

Investigations

Blood tests: white cell count (WCC) and C-reactive protein confirm infection; haemolysis and cold agglutinins occur in ~50% of mycoplasma infection; abnormal liver function tests suggest legionella or mycoplasma infection. **Blood gases** identify respiratory failure. **Microbiology**: no organism is isolated in ~33–50% of patients because of previous antibiotic therapy or poor specimen collection. Blood cultures, sputum, pleural fluid and bronchoalveolar lavage samples, with appropriate staining (e.g. Gram stain), culture and assessment of antibiotic sensitivity, determine the pathogen and effective therapy. **Serology** identifies mycoplasma infection but long processing times limit clinical value. Rapid antigen detection for legionella (e.g. urine) and pneumococcus (e.g. serum, pleural fluid) is more useful. **Radiology**: CXR (Figure 38a) and CT scans aid diagnosis, indicate severity and detect complications.

Severity assessment

Features associated with increased mortality and the need for high dependency unit (HDU) monitoring are: (a) **Clinical**: age > 60 years, respiratory rate > 30/min, diastolic blood pressure < 60 mmHg, new atrial fibrillation, confusion, multilobar involvement and co-existing illness. (b) **Laboratory**: urea > 7 mmol/L, albumin < 35 g/L, hypoxaemia Po_2 < 8 kPa, leucopenia (WCC < 4 × 10^9/L), leucocytosis (WCC > 20 × 10^9/L) and bacteraemia. **Severity scoring**: the CURB-65 score allocates points for **C**onfusion; **U**rea > 7 mmol/l; **R**espiratory rate > 30/min; low systolic (< 90 mmHg) or diastolic (< 60 mmHg) **B**lood pressure and age > **65** years, to stratify patients into mortality groups and appropriate management pathways (Figure 38c).

Management

- **Supportive measures** include oxygen to maintain P_ao_2 > 8 kPa (S_ao_2 < 90%) and intravenous fluid (±inotrope) resuscitation to ensure haemodynamic stability. **Ventilatory support**: consider non-invasive or mechanical ventilation in respiratory failure (Chapters 13, 16, 18). **Physiotherapy and bronchoscopy** aid sputum clearance.
- **Initial antibiotic therapy** represents the 'best guess', according to pneumonia classification and likely organisms, because microbiological results are not available for 12–72 hours. Therapy is adjusted when results and antibiotic sensitivities are available. The American and British Thoracic Societies (ATS, BTS) recommend the following initial antibiotic protocols for CAP:
  - **Non-hospitalized patients** are treated with oral amoxicillin (BTS) or a macrolide (e.g. clarithromycin) or doxycycline (ATS). Patients with severe symptoms or at risk of drug-resistant *S. pneumoniae* (e.g. recent antibiotics, co-morbidity) require a beta-lactam plus a macrolide or doxycycline; or an antipneumococcal fluoroquinolone (e.g. moxifloxacin) alone.
  - **Hospitalized patients**: initial therapy must cover both 'atypical' organisms and *S. pneumoniae*. An intravenous macrolide is combined with a beta-lactam or an antipneumococcal fluoroquinolone (ATS/BTS) or cefuroxime (BTS). If not severe, combined ampicillin and macrolide (oral) may be adequate. Cover staphylococcal infection after influenza and *H. influenzae* in COPD.

Pearl of wisdom

Risk of death in pneumonia increases 20-fold if two of the following are present: respiratory rate > 30/min, diastolic blood pressure (BP) < 60 mmHg or urea > 7 mmol/L

39 Hospital-acquired (nosocomial) pneumonia

Figure 39a (i) CXR (ii) CT scan from a patient with hospital-acquired pneumonia (HAP) showing consolidation, cavitation and abscess formation

(i)

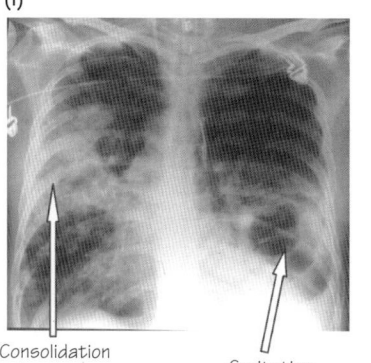

Consolidation

Cavitation

(ii)

Fluid filled abscess

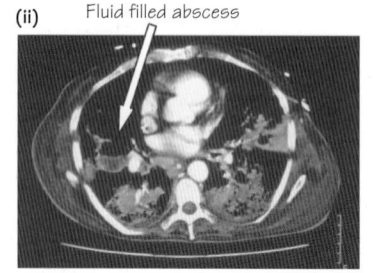

Figure 39b Risk factors and modifiable risk factors for HAP and VAP

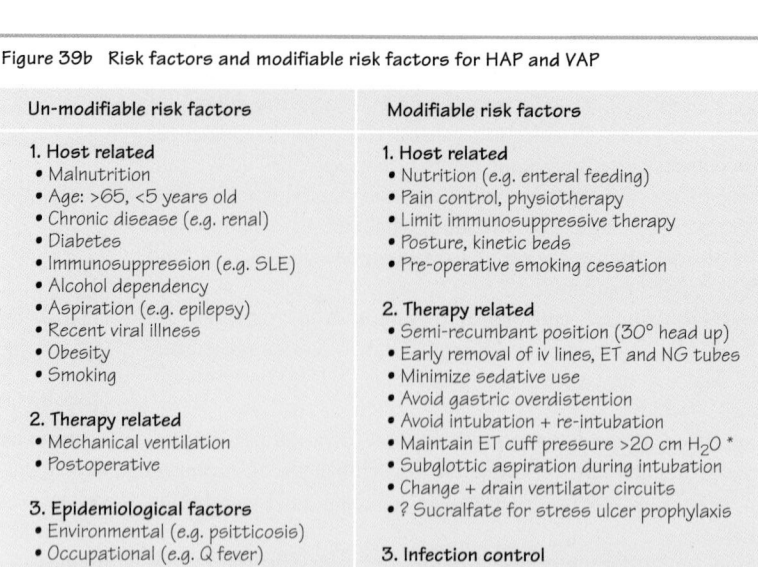

Un-modifiable risk factors	Modifiable risk factors
1. Host related • Malnutrition • Age: >65, <5 years old • Chronic disease (e.g. renal) • Diabetes • Immunosuppression (e.g. SLE) • Alcohol dependency • Aspiration (e.g. epilepsy) • Recent viral illness • Obesity • Smoking	**1. Host related** • Nutrition (e.g. enteral feeding) • Pain control, physiotherapy • Limit immunosuppressive therapy • Posture, kinetic beds • Pre-operative smoking cessation
2. Therapy related • Mechanical ventilation • Postoperative	**2. Therapy related** • Semi-recumbant position (30° head up) • Early removal of iv lines, ET and NG tubes • Minimize sedative use • Avoid gastric overdistention • Avoid intubation + re-intubation • Maintain ET cuff pressure >20 cm H_2O * • Subglottic aspiration during intubation • Change + drain ventilator circuits • ? Sucralfate for stress ulcer prophylaxis
3. Epidemiological factors • Environmental (e.g. psitticosis) • Occupational (e.g. Q fever) • Travel abroad (e.g. paragonomiasis) • Air-conditioning (e.g. Legionella)	**3. Infection control** • Hand washing, sterile technique • Patient isolation • Microbiological surveillance

Figure 39c Risk factors for multidrug-resistant pathogens causing hospital-acquired pneumonia

• Antimicrobial therapy in the previous 90 days
• Current hospitalization of >5 days
• High frequency of local antibiotic resistance
• Presence of risk factors for HCAP
  Hospitalization for >2 days in the previous 90 days
  Residence in a nursing home
  Home wound care or intravenous therapy
  Chronic dialysis within 30 days
  Family member with MDR pathogen
• Immunosuppressive disease and / or therapy

Figure 39d Pathogenesis of hospital-acquired pneumonia

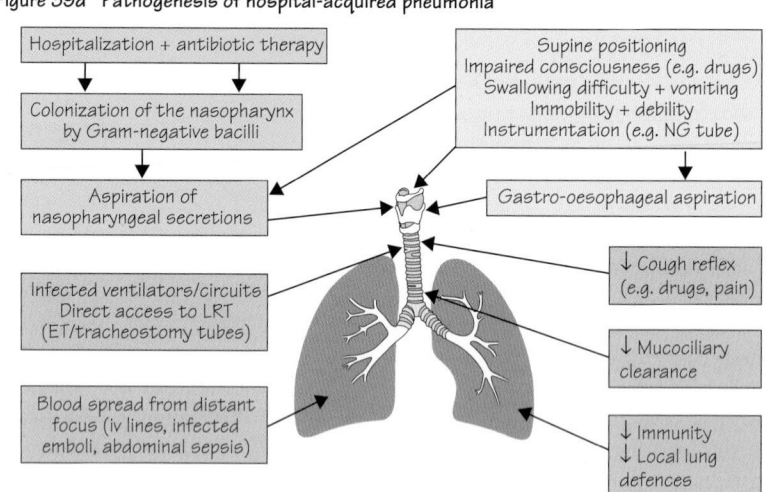

Hospitalization + antibiotic therapy

Colonization of the nasopharynx by Gram-negative bacilli

Aspiration of nasopharyngeal secretions

Infected ventilators/circuits Direct access to LRT (ET/tracheostomy tubes)

Blood spread from distant focus (iv lines, infected emboli, abdominal sepsis)

Supine positioning
Impaired consciousness (e.g. drugs)
Swallowing difficulty + vomiting
Immobility + debility
Instrumentation (e.g. NG tube)

Gastro-oesophageal aspiration

↓ Cough reflex (e.g. drugs, pain)

↓ Mucociliary clearance

↓ Immunity
↓ Local lung defences

Figure 39e Likely pathogens and empirical antibiotic treatment of hospital-acquired pneumonias

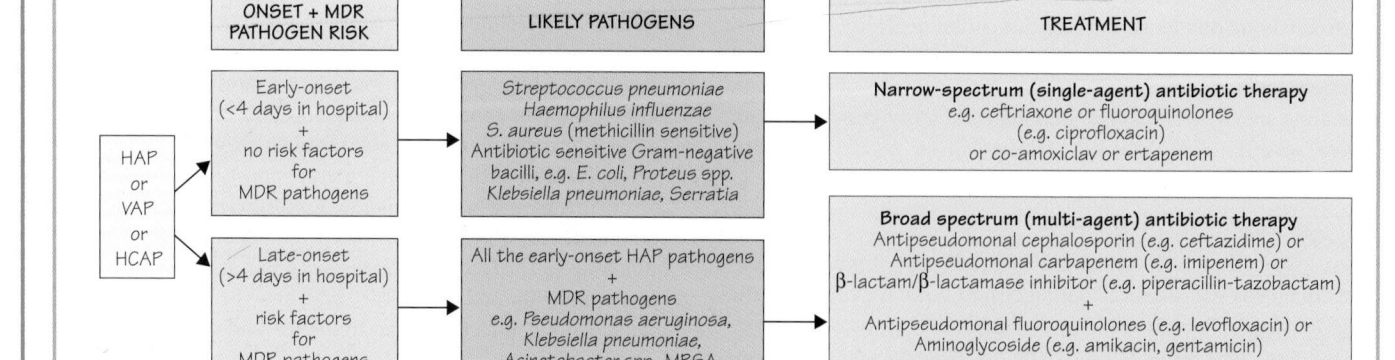

ONSET + MDR PATHOGEN RISK	LIKELY PATHOGENS	TREATMENT
HAP or VAP or HCAP → Early-onset (<4 days in hospital) + no risk factors for MDR pathogens	*Streptococcus pneumoniae Haemophilus influenzae S. aureus* (methicillin sensitive) Antibiotic sensitive Gram-negative bacilli, e.g. *E. coli, Proteus* spp. *Klebsiella pneumoniae, Serratia*	**Narrow-spectrum (single-agent) antibiotic therapy** e.g. ceftriaxone or fluoroquinolones (e.g. ciprofloxacin) or co-amoxiclav or ertapenem
Late-onset (>4 days in hospital) + risk factors for MDR pathogens	All the early-onset HAP pathogens + MDR pathogens e.g. *Pseudomonas aeruginosa, Klebsiella pneumoniae, Acinetobacter* spp., MRSA, *Legionella pneumophila*	**Broad spectrum (multi-agent) antibiotic therapy** Antipseudomonal cephalosporin (e.g. ceftazidime) or Antipseudomonal carbapenem (e.g. imipenem) or β-lactam/β-lactamase inhibitor (e.g. piperacillin-tazobactam) + Antipseudomonal fluoroquinolones (e.g. levofloxacin) or Aminoglycoside (e.g. amikacin, gentamicin) + Vancomycin or linezolid (if risk factors for MRSA)

Hospital-acquired (nosocomial) pneumonia (HAP) including **ventilator-associated pneumonia** (VAP) and **healthcare-associated pneumonia** (HCAP) affects 0.5–2% of hospital patients. It is a major cause of nosocomial infection (i.e. with wound and urinary tract infection). Pathogenesis, causative organisms and outcome differ from community-acquired pneumonia (CAP). Prevention, early antibiotic therapy and an awareness of the role of multidrug-resistant (MDR) pathogens improve outcome.

Definitions

HAP is pulmonary infection that develops >48 hours after hospital admission and which was not incubating at the time of admission. **VAP** is pneumonia >48–72 hours after endotracheal intubation. **HCAP** includes patients residing in nursing homes, receiving therapy (e.g. wound care, intravenous therapy) within 30 days or admitted to hospital for >2 days within 90 days of the current infection, or attending a hospital or haemodialysis clinic.

Epidemiology

Incidence varies between 5 and 10 episodes per 1000 discharges and is highest on surgical and intensive care unit (ICU) wards and in teaching hospitals. It lengthens hospital stay by between 3 and 14 days per patient. The risk of HAP increases 6- to 20-fold during mechanical ventilation (MV) and in ICU is responsible for 25% of infections and ~50% of prescribed antibiotics. VAP accounts for >80% of all HAP and occurs in 9–27% of intubated patients. **Risk factors** include CAP risk factors and those associated with HAP pathogenesis, some of which can be **prevented** (Figure 39b). **Mortality** is between 30% and 70%. **Early-onset HAP/VAP** (<4 days in hospital) is usually caused by antibiotic-sensitive bacteria and carries a better prognosis than **late-onset HAP/VAP** (>4 days in hospital), which is associated with MDR pathogens. In early onset HAP/VAP, prior antibiotic therapy or hospitalization predisposes to MDR pathogens and is treated as late-onset HAP/VAP. Bacteraemia, medical rather than surgical illness, VAP and late or ineffective antibiotic therapy increase mortality.

Pathogenesis

The oropharynx is colonized by enteric gram-negative bacteria in most hospital patients due to immobility, impaired consciousness, instrumentation (e.g. nasogastric tubes), poor hygiene or inhibition of gastric acid secretion. Subsequent aspiration of oral secretions (±gastric contents) causes HAP (Figure 39d).

Aetiology

Early or late onset and risk factors for infection with MDR organisms (Figure 39c) determine likely pathogens (Figure 39e). Aerobic gram-negative bacilli (e.g. *Klebsiella pneumoniae*, *Pseudomonas aeruginosa*, *Escherichia coli*) cause ~60–70% and *Staphylococcus aureus* ~10–15% of infections. *Streptococcus pneumoniae* and *Haemophilus influenza* may be isolated in early-onset HAP/VAP. In intensive care, >50% of *S. aureus* infections are methicillin-resistant (MRSA). *S. aureus* is more common in diabetics and ICU patients.

Diagnosis

This requires both **clinical** and **microbiological** assessment. Non-specific clinical features, concurrent illness (e.g. acute respiratory distress syndrome [ARDS]) and previous antibiotics, which limit microbiological evaluation, can make diagnosis difficult. **Clinical**: suspect HAP when new chest radiograph (CXR) infiltrates occur with features suggestive of infection (e.g. fever > 38°C, purulent sputum, leukocytosis, hypoxaemia). **Diagnostic tests**: confirm infection and establish the causative organism (±antibiotic sensitivity). They include blood tests and gases, serology, blood cultures, pleural fluid aspiration, sputum, endotracheal aspirates and bronchioalveolar lavage. CXR and CT scanning (Figure 39a) aid diagnosis and detect **complications** (e.g. cavitation, abscesses).

Management

Early diagnosis and treatment improve morbidity and mortality. Do not delay antibiotic therapy while awaiting microbiological results.

Supportive therapy

Supplemental **oxygen** maintains P_aO_2 >8 kPa (S_aO_2 <90%), **intravenous fluids** (±inotropes) preserve haemodynamic stability and **ventilatory support** (e.g. MV) corrects respiratory failure. **Physiotherapy** and **analgesia** aid sputum clearance post-operatively and in the immobilized patient. **Semi-recumbent** (i.e. 30° bed-head elevation) nursing of bed-bound patients reduces aspiration risk. Strict glycaemic control and attention to avoidable risk factors (Figure 39b) may improve outcome.

Antibiotic therapy

This is empirical while awaiting microbiological guidance. The key factor is whether the patient is at risk of MDR organisms. Figure 39e illustrates the American Thoracic Society guidelines for initial, empiric, intravenous antibiotic therapy. Local patterns of antibiotic resistance are used to modify these protocols.

• In **early-onset HAP/VAP** with no risk factors for MDR organisms, use **monotherapy** with a β-lactam/β-lactamase, third generation cephalosporin or fluoroquinolone antibiotic.

• In **late-onset HAP/VAP** or with risk factors for MDR pathogens (Figure 39c), start **combination therapy** (Figure 39e) with broad-spectrum antibiotics to cover MDR gram-negative bacilli and MRSA (e.g. vancomycin). Consider adjunctive therapy with inhaled aminoglycosides or polymyxin in patients not improving with systemic therapy.

A short course of therapy (e.g. 7 days) is appropriate if the clinical response is good. Resistant pathogens (e.g. *Pseudomonas aeruginosa*, *S. aureus*) may require 14–21 days' treatment. Focus therapy on causative organisms when culture data are available and withdraw unnecessary antibiotics. Sterile cultures (without new antibiotics for >72 hours) virtually rule out HAP.

Other pneumonias

• **Aspiration/anaerobic pneumonia**: anaerobic infection (e.g. *Bacteroides*) follows aspiration of oropharyngeal contents due to laryngeal incompetence or reduced consciousness (e.g. drugs). Lung abscesses are common. Antibiotic therapy should include anaerobic coverage (e.g. metronidazole).

• **Pneumonia during immunosuppression** (Chapter 68): HIV, transplant and chemotherapy patients are susceptible to viral (e.g. cytomegalovirus), fungal (e.g. *Aspergillus*) and mycobacterial infections, in addition to the normal range of organisms. HIV patients with CD4 counts <200/mm³, may also develop opportunistic infections such as *Pneumocystis (carinii)* jiroveci pneumonia (PCP) or toxoplasma. Severely immunocompromised patients require broad-spectrum antibiotic, anti-fungal and anti-viral regimes. PCP is treated with steroids and high-dose co-trimoxazole.

Pearl of wisdom

Multidrug-resistant (MDR) organisms are more likely to cause Hospital-acquired (nosocomial) pneumonia (HAP) if the patient has been in hospital for >4 days

40 Asthma

Figure 40a Factors increasing risk of death from asthma

Previous life-threatening asthma attack
(intubation, ICU admission)
Hospital/ER history
- ≥ 3 ER visits within past year
- 2 hospitalizations within past year
- Hospitalization/ER visit within past month

Medication history
- >2 inhalers/month of short-acting β2 agonist
- Current/recent use of systemic corticosteroids

Psychiatric/psychosocial problems
Low socioeconomic status and urban residence
Concurrent cardiovascular or lung disease
Illicit drug use

Figure 40b Triggers of an asthma attack

Upper respiratory infections
Inhalation of allergens
- Mould, pollen, animal dander, products of dust mites and cockroaches

Inhalation of irritants
- Tobacco smoke, strong odours, air pollution, occupational fumes

Environmental change
- Vacation, new home or workplace

Drugs (NSAIDs, β-blockers)
Food additives (sulfites)
Changes in weather
Exercise
Emotional upset
Hormonal factors
- Thyroid disease, menses, pregnancy

Figure 40c Measurement of pulsus paradoxus

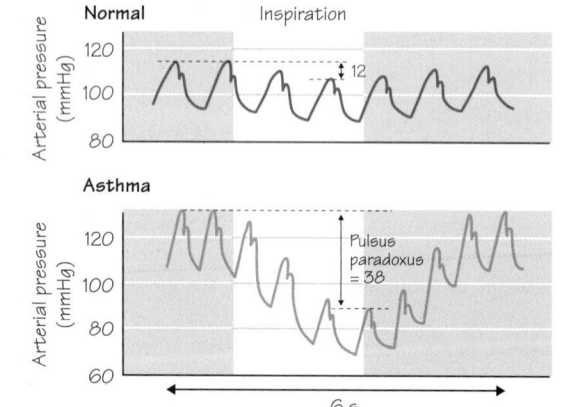

Slowly deflate a BP cuff and note the difference between the highest pressure at end inspiration and the rest of the respiratory cycle

Figure 40d Use of accessory muscles of respiration

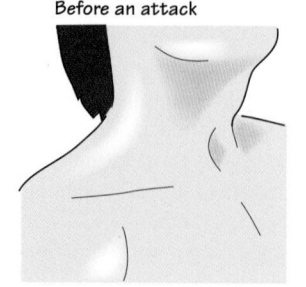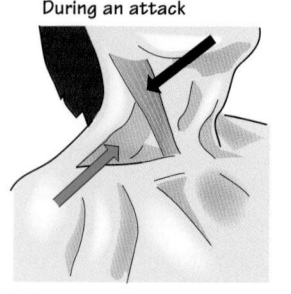

Note marked contraction of sternocleidomastoid (black arrow) and retraction of supraclavicular fossa (green arrow) during the attack

Figure 40e Spirometry in a normal subject and an asthmatic patient during an attack

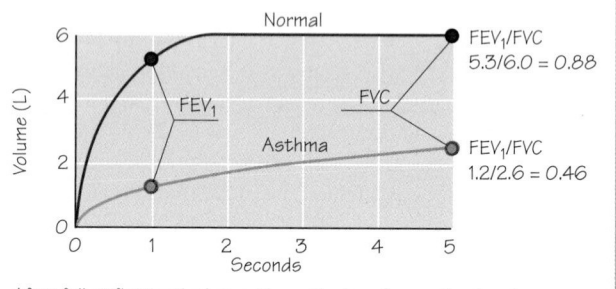

After fully inflating the lungs, the patient expires as hard as he can for as long as he can.
FEV_1 = forced expired volume in 1s. FVC = forced vital capacity,
Normally, FEV_1/FVC is >0.8

Figure 40f Measurement of (a) plateau pressure (P_{plat}) and (b) intrinsic (or auto) positive end-expiratory pressure ($PEEP_i$) in an asthmatic patient on positive pressure mechanical ventilation

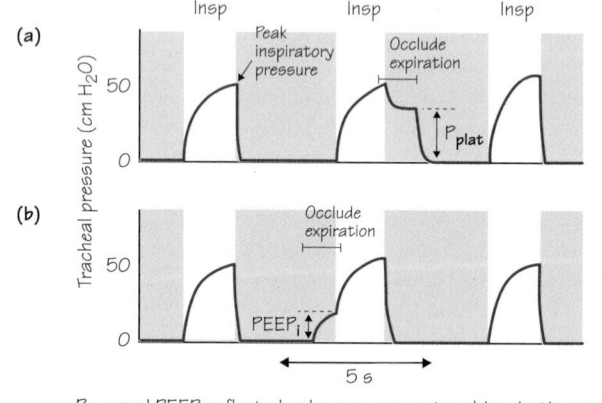

P_{plat} and $PEEP_i$ reflect alveolar pressures at end-inspiration and end-expiration, respectively, assuming the patient's muscles are relaxed

Critical Care Medicine at a Glance, Third Edition. Richard Leach. © 2014 John Wiley & Sons, Ltd. Published 2014 by John Wiley & Sons, Ltd.

Asthma is **reversible obstruction** of inflamed, hyperreactive airways manifested by recurrent episodes of wheezing, coughing and dyspnoea. It affects 5–10% of the population. **Prevalence** is increasing, particularly in children. Although **mortality is low** (2 deaths/year/100,000), it has increased for 20 years and is higher in black people. Factors increasing risk of death are shown in Figure 40a.

Pathogenesis

Airway inflammation, usually allergenic, is central to pathogenesis and derives from predominance of type 2, over type 1, T-helper lymphocytes due to genetic–environmental interactions in childhood. Characteristic airway changes include inflammatory cell accumulation, mediator release, epithelial denudation, submucosal oedema and fibrosis, goblet cell hyperplasia with mucous hypersecretion and hypertrophied hyperresponsive smooth muscle.

Pathophysiology Acute airway obstruction is triggered by many factors (Figure 40b). During an attack, the patient struggles to keep obstructed airways open by breathing at high lung volumes, using accessory muscles (Figure 40d). Work of breathing (WoB) increases because of high airways resistance, decreased lung compliance and reduced muscle efficiency. Heroic efforts sufficient to increase alveolar ventilation and lower P_aCO_2 despite increasing dead space fail to maintain airway patency, resulting in hypoxaemia due to regional hypoventilation (i.e. low ventilation/perfusion [V/Q] ratio). Hypoxic vasoconstriction and pulmonary capillary compression cause pulmonary hypertension, increased right ventricular (RV) afterload and right heart failure. Increased RV filling pressures may push the interventricular septum into the left ventricular (LV) cavity, decreasing LV end-diastolic volume. During inspiration, marked falls in pleural pressure impair LV emptying, reducing systolic volume and causing exaggerated reductions (≥ 15 mmHg) in systolic blood pressure (pulsus paradoxus [Figure 40c]). If the attack does not abate, respiratory muscles become exhausted, leading to respiratory arrest and death.

Clinical features

Onset of asthma is usually gradual but may be sudden. Episodic wheeze, cough and nocturnal waking with breathlessness are typical. The history may reveal a seasonal pattern, precipitating causes (Figure 40b) and risk factors for death (Figure 40a). **Physical examination** detects wheeze with prolonged expiration on chest auscultation and signs of hyperinflation (e.g. hyperresonance).

- **Severe asthma** is characterized by a peak expiratory flow rate (PEFR) < 50% of predicted, agitation, difficulty completing sentences, respiratory rate > 25/min, sweating, accessory muscle use and pulsus paradoxus (Figure 40c).
- **Life-threatening asthma** with respiratory failure (±impending arrest) is indicated by confusion, drowsiness, silent chest, PEFR < 33% predicted, paradoxical thoracoabdominal excursions (i.e. outward abdominal and inward sternal movement during inspiration), bradycardia, pulsus paradoxus and hypercapnia (±hypoxaemia).

Investigation

Initially **arterial blood gases** (ABGs) demonstrate hypoxaemia (or normoxia), hypocapnia and alkalosis. A rise in P_aCO_2 (i.e. PaCO2 >6 kPa) suggests impending respiratory failure. **Chest radiography** excludes other pathology (e.g. pneumothorax). **Electrocardiography** may show RV strain. **FEV₁** (Figure 40e) or **PEFR** assess severity and monitor therapy.

Initial management

- **Primary pharmacological therapy** is essential in all patients and includes inhaled short-acting β₂-**adrenergic agonists** (e.g. albuterol, salbutamol) and **intravenous (i.v.) corticosteroids**, which are given until sustained improvement is achieved. Systemic β₂-adrenergic agonists (e.g. salbutamol) have no advantage over inhaled therapy.
- **Secondary pharmacological therapy** is given if improvement does not occur within 6–24 hours, although evidence of benefit is limited. Inhaled **ipratropium bromide** reduces airways obstruction caused by cholinergic mechanisms. Although i.v. **magnesium sulphate** may improve severe asthma, avoid its use in renal failure or heart block. The role of i.v. **aminophylline** is controversial. It dilates airway and pulmonary vascular smooth muscle and increases respiratory muscle contractility by inhibiting phosphodiesterases; however, monitor serum levels closely to avoid serious toxic effects (e.g. seizures).
- **Respiratory therapy** establishes adequate oxygenation and relieves dyspnoea. Treat all patients with high-dose (~60%) **supplemental oxygen** (Chapter 14) to correct hypoxaemia. **Non-invasive positive pressure ventilation (PPV)** (Chapter 16) may alleviate fatigue and improve gas exchange. Using tight-fitting facemasks, modest levels of positive pressure are administered during expiration (~5 cmH₂O) and inspiration (10–15 cmH₂O) to reduce the effort required to initiate and sustain airflow into hyperinflated lungs, where end-expiratory alveolar pressure may exceed atmospheric pressure (intrinsic or auto-PEEP). *Risks* include worsened hyperinflation, agitation and aspiration. Occasionally, removing mucus plugs by **bronchoalveolar lavage** may relieve obstruction.

Management of deteriorating asthma

- **HDU/ICU admission** is required if severe asthma deteriorates during initial therapy, fails to improve after ≥6 hours' treatment or if respiratory arrest is imminent or complications (e.g. pneumothorax) occur.
- **Mechanical ventilation** (MV) is required in ventilatory failure, coma or cardiopulmonary arrest (Chapter 18). Deep **sedation** allows **controlled hypoventilation**, a strategy that reduces hyperinflation by increasing expiratory time. Resulting CO_2 retention, due to reduced ventilation, is termed '**permissive hypercapnia**' and associated respiratory acidosis (pH < 7.2) may require correction with sodium bicarbonate. Paralytic agents interact with corticosteroids to cause post-paralytic myopathy (Chapter 64) but cannot always be avoided. Volume-control ventilation is used in patients making little respiratory effort, or intermittent mandatory ventilation if respiratory effort is not reduced by sedation. In both modes, the rate (≤10/min) and volume of ventilator breaths (≤6 ml/kg) should be minimized. Inspiratory flow should be rapid (≥100 L/min) but the associated increase in peak inspiratory pressure (usually ≥50 cmH₂0) should not cause this strategy to be abandoned. Better indicators of lung volume are plateau pressure (P_{plat}) and the level of intrinsic or auto-PEEP (PEEP$_i$), measured as shown in Figure 40f to estimate alveolar pressure at end-inspiration and end-expiration, respectively. Safe levels are unknown, but P_{plat} < 30 and PEEP$_i$ < 10 cmH₂O are likely to reduce risks. Intubated patients who deteriorate may respond to a trial of general anaesthesia with halothane or isoflurane.

Pearl of wisdom
Wheeze is a poor indicator of asthma severity; beware the silent chest

41 Chronic obstructive pulmonary disease

Figure 41a   Risk factors for COPD

Smoking
Age >50 years old; prevalence ~5-10%
Male gender
Childhood chest infections
Airways hyperreactivity
• Asthma/atopy
Low socioeconomic status
α_1-Antitrypsin deficiency
Heavy metal exposure
• Cadmium
Atmospheric pollution

Figure 41c   Spirometry.

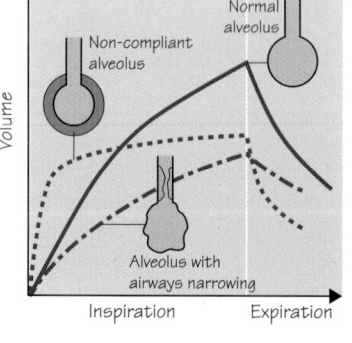

FEV$_1$/FVC ratio decreases in COPD

Normal ————	COPD ·········	COPD –·–·–·
FEV$_1$/FVC = >0.8	FEV$_1$/FVC = <0.8	Irreversible <15% increase in FEV$_1$ with bronchodilators

Figure 41b   Pathophysiology of chronic bronchitis and emphysema

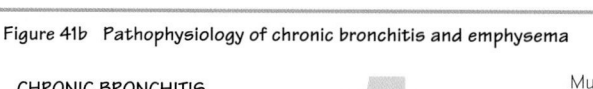

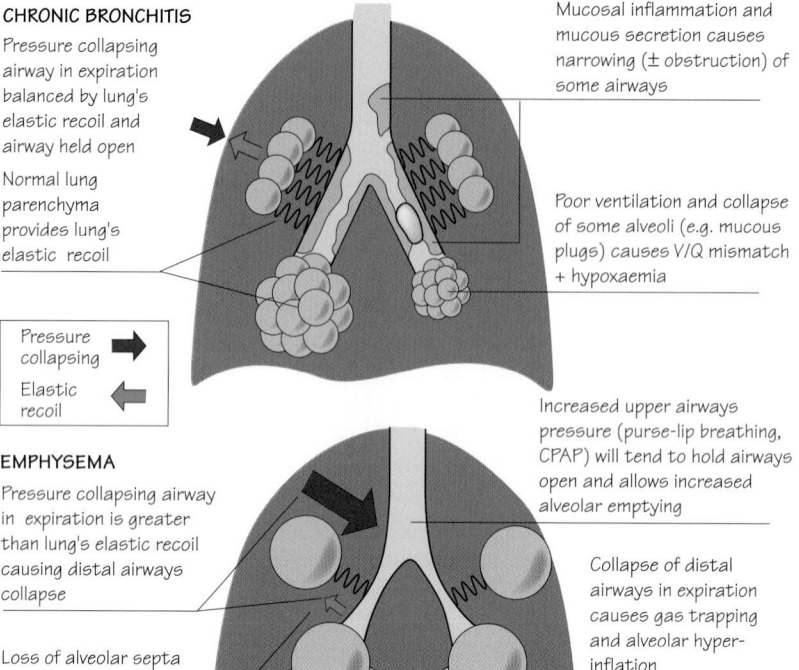

CHRONIC BRONCHITIS

Pressure collapsing airway in expiration balanced by lung's elastic recoil and airway held open

Normal lung parenchyma provides lung's elastic recoil

Pressure collapsing ➡
Elastic recoil ⬅

EMPHYSEMA

Pressure collapsing airway in expiration is greater than lung's elastic recoil causing distal airways collapse

Loss of alveolar septa and capillaries reduces the lung's elastic recoil. Large air spaces (bullae) develop

Mucosal inflammation and mucous secretion causes narrowing (± obstruction) of some airways

Poor ventilation and collapse of some alveoli (e.g. mucous plugs) causes V/Q mismatch + hypoxaemia

Increased upper airways pressure (purse-lip breathing, CPAP) will tend to hold airways open and allows increased alveolar emptying

Collapse of distal airways in expiration causes gas trapping and alveolar hyper-inflation

Figure 41d   Mechanical ventilation in COPD requires an adequate inspiratory time to ensure alveolar inflation (i); increased expiratory time to prevent gas trapping (ii); ± ventilator (extrinsic) PEEP to balance auto-PEEP and reduce gas trapping and work of breathing (iii)

(i) Adequate inspiratory time
A short inspiratory time results in incomplete inflation of alveoli with narrowed airways causing V/Q mismatching and hypoxaemia

Volume

Normal alveolus
Non-compliant alveolus
Alveolus with airways narrowing

Inspiration — Expiration

Time constant (TC) determines alveolar filling
Time constant = compliance × resistance
• Non-compliant alveoli have short TC
• Alveoli with narrowed airways have long TC

(ii) Increased expiratory time
A long expiratory time is required to prevent gas trapping because the rate of alveolar deflation is decreased due to:
1. Airways obstruction: which slows expiration. A short expiratory time causes incomplete alveolar emptying (gas trapping)

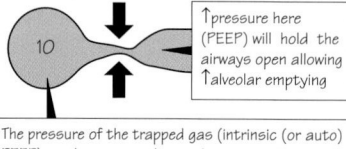

10 ← Reduced airflow ➡

2. Distal airways collapse: initially reduces airflow and then causes gas trapping (Fig b)

10

↑pressure here (PEEP) will hold the airways open allowing ↑alveolar emptying

The pressure of the trapped gas (intrinsic (or auto) PEEP) can be measured at end expiration by occluding the expiratory limb of the ventilator

A reduction in breath rate (8–10 /min) increases both inspiratory and expiratory times

(iii) Reduced work of breathing (WoB)
Hyperinflation increases WoB which can be reduced by bronchodilation, ↑expiratory time (i.e. ↓ breath rate) and ventilator (extrinsic) PEEP matched to auto-PEEP

No PEEP added

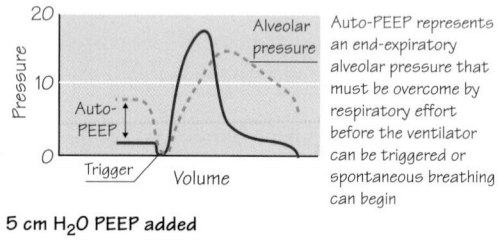

Auto-PEEP represents an end-expiratory alveolar pressure that must be overcome by respiratory effort before the ventilator can be triggered or spontaneous breathing can begin

5 cm H$_2$O PEEP added

PEEP similar to the auto-PEEP added downstream from the site of flow limitation does not significantly slow expiratory airflow but reduces the inspiratory work of breathing

Critical Care Medicine at a Glance, Third Edition. Richard Leach. © 2014 John Wiley & Sons, Ltd. Published 2014 by John Wiley & Sons, Ltd.

Chronic obstructive pulmonary disease (COPD) is characterized by irreversible, expiratory airflow obstruction, hyperinflation, mucous hypersecretion and increased work of breathing (WoB). Typically, smoking and other risk factors (Figure 41a) accelerate the normal age-related decline in expiratory airflow and cause chronic respiratory symptoms, disability and respiratory failure punctuated by intermittent acute exacerbations (AEs).

Pathophysiology

In COPD, emphysema and chronic bronchitis often co-exist but are different processes (Figure 41b):

- **Emphysema** destroys **alveolar septa and capillaries**, partly due to inadequate anti-protease defences. Smoking causes *centrilobular* emphysema with mainly upper lobes involvement, whereas α_1-antitrypsin deficiency causes *panacinar* emphysema, which affects lower lobes. Lung tissue loss results in bullae, reduced elastic recoil and impaired diffusion capacity. Airways obstruction follows distal airways collapse at end-expiration due to loss of 'elastic' radial traction from normal lung tissue (Figure 41b). Resulting hyperinflation enhances expiratory airflow but inspiratory muscles work at a mechanical disadvantage (i.e. increased WoB).
- **Chronic bronchitic** airways obstruction is due to **chronic mucosal inflammation**, mucous gland hypertrophy, **mucous hypersecretion** and **bronchospasm** (Figure 41b). Lung parenchyma is unaffected.

Diagnosis

Spirometry (Figure 41c) demonstrates airflow obstruction (**FEV$_1$/FVC ratio <0.7**), which is largely irreversible with bronchodilator or steroid therapy (i.e. <15% increase in FEV$_1$). In **emphysema**, resting arterial blood gases (ABGs) are usually normal because alveolar septa and capillaries are destroyed in proportion. Exercise desaturation and increased ventilation are due to reduced diffusion capacity. Lung function tests show impaired diffusion (D$_L$CO, KCO) and increased lung volumes (total lung capacity [TLC], functional residual capacity [FRC], residual volume). Chest radiography (CXR) reveals hyperinflation (e.g. flat diaphragm), narrow mediastinum, bullae and less vascular markings. In **bronchitis**, diffusion and lung volumes are normal but ventilation/perfusion (V/Q) mismatching may cause hypoxaemia. CXR shows more vascular markings but normal lung volumes.

Clinical features

The concept of emphysematous '**pink puffers**' and bronchitic '**blue bloaters**' is unreliable because most patients have elements of both. **Emphysematous patients** tend to be **thin, breathless** and **tachypnoeic**, with signs of hyperinflation (e.g. barrel chest, purse-lipped breathing, accessory muscle use). Chest auscultation reveals distant breath sounds and prolonged expiratory wheeze. **Chronic bronchitis** is defined as daily morning cough and mucus production for 3 months over 2 successive years. These patients are often less breathless despite potential **hypoxaemia** (±polycythaemia). Reduced respiratory drive leads to **CO$_2$ retention** with associated bounding pulse, vasodilation, confusion, headache, flapping tremor and papilloedema. Hypoxaemia-induced renal fluid retention (±right heart failure) causes **cor pulmonale** (i.e. hepatomegaly, ankle oedema, raised central venous pressure [CVP]). **Pulmonary hypertension** is a late feature due to hypoxic pulmonary vasoconstriction and/or extensive capillary loss.

Management

Established COPD is irreversible but **smoking cessation** reduces symptoms, AEs and disease progression. **Pharmacological therapy**: inhaled β-agonists (e.g. salbutamol) and anticholinergics (e.g. tiotropium bromide) alleviate symptoms and improve lung function, with additive effects when combined. Theophyllines improve exercise tolerance and ABGs but do not alter spirometry. Inhaled corticosteroids are recommended in severe COPD (FEV$_1$ <50% predicted; or >2 steroid requiring AEs/year). Long-term oral corticosteroids are avoided because they benefit <25% of patients and cause significant side-effects. Mucolytics help a few patients with excessive sputum production. **Pulmonary rehabilitation** strengthens respiratory muscles, increases exercise tolerance, improves quality of life and reduces hospitalizations but spirometry is unchanged. **Home oxygen therapy** for >15 hours/day improves survival in chronically hypoxaemic (P_ao$_2$ < 7.5 kPa) patients. **Prophylaxis**: pneumococcal and influenza vaccinations reduce AEs. **Surgery**: lung volume reduction or transplantation occasionally benefit carefully selected patients.

Prognosis: yearly mortality is ∼25% when FEV$_1$ is <0.8 L. This is increased by co-existing cor pulmonale, hypercapnia and weight loss.

Acute exacerbations

The cause is often unknown but infection, pulmonary embolism (PE), pneumothorax, ischaemic heart disease (IHD), arrhythmias, drugs and metabolic disturbances can precipitate AEs.

- **General management**: fluid balance can be difficult, especially in cor pulmonale. Thromboembolic prophylaxis is essential. Electrolyte correction and nutrition improve respiratory muscle strength. **Oxygen therapy (OT)** relieves life-threatening hypoxia and the small $P_a$co$_2$ increase that occurs in most cases is of no consequence. In a few patients with reduced hypoxic respiratory drive (±hypercapnia), OT causes hypoventilation and further CO$_2$ retention. However, on the steep part of the oxyhaemoglobin dissociation curve, small P_ao$_2$ increases do not cause much CO$_2$ retention but significantly increase arterial oxygen content. Monitor OT with serial ABGs to achieve a P_ao$_2$ > 8 kPa without a substantial rise in $P_a$co$_2$ (Chapters 13, 14). **Pharmacological therapy**: high-dose, aerosolized β-agonists and anticholinergic bronchodilators improve symptoms and gas exchange. Short courses of oral corticosteroids (i.e. 30 mg/day for 10 days) improve lung function and hasten recovery. Direct antibiotic therapy at likely organisms (e.g. *H. influenza*) and adjust according to microbiological results. **Respiratory therapy** aids sputum clearance (Chapter 19). Timely **non-invasive ventilation (NIV)**, as discussed in Chapter 16, may reverse early respiratory failure.

- **Mechanical ventilation (MV)** can be life-saving but may be associated with prolonged weaning (Chapters 18, 19) and complications (e.g. pneumothorax). Dynamic hyperinflation, raised intrathoracic pressure and patient-ventilator dyschrony are treated with bronchodilators, increased expiratory time, decreased minute ventilation and by setting ventilator positive end-expiratory pressure (PEEP) at auto-PEEP levels (Figure 41d). Do not over-ventilate patients with CO$_2$ retention to avoid metabolic alkalosis. In end-stage COPD, ventilatory support may be limited to NIV (Chapter 16).

Pearl of wisdom

Hypercapnoea occurs in 1 in 10 chronic obstructive pulmonary disease (COPD) patients, but do not deny potentially life-saving oxygen therapy (OT) to other COPD patients

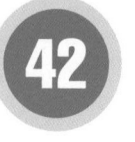 **Acute respiratory distress syndrome**

Figure 42a   Acute respiratory distress syndrome

Pathophysiology

Systemic inflammatory response (sepsis/trauma)

Direct alveolar damage (aspiration/pneumonia)

Endotoxin IL-1, IL-6, TNFα

White cell activation

White cell adhesion and migration

IL-1, IL-8 Increased permeability and consolidation

Decreased surfactant with alveolar collapse

H_2O

Alveolar flooding

Endothelial and alveolar cell damage

Loss of surfactant and increased permeability

Widespread alveolar and dependent consolidation

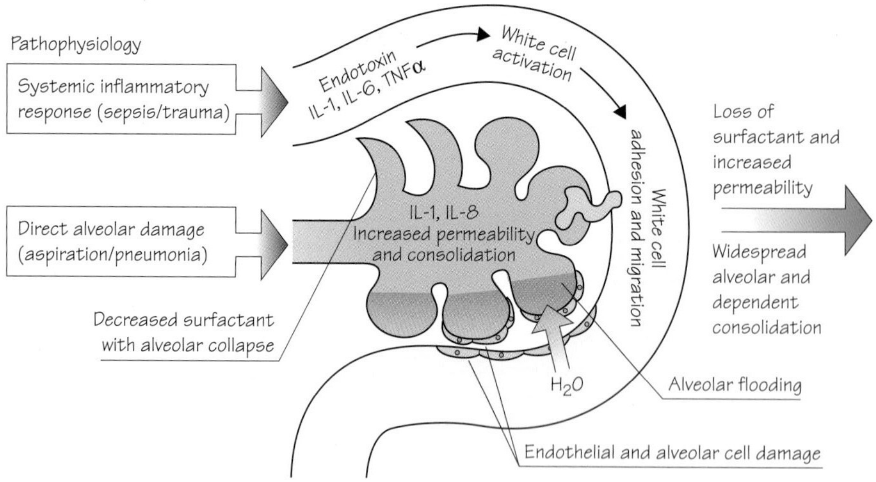

CXR of aspiration-induced ARDS

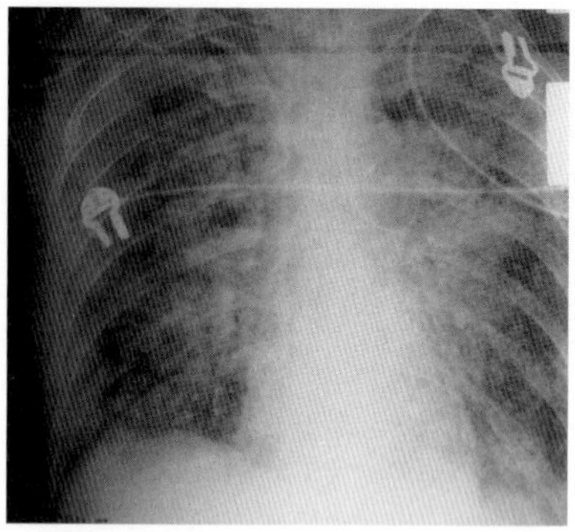

CT scan of ARDS

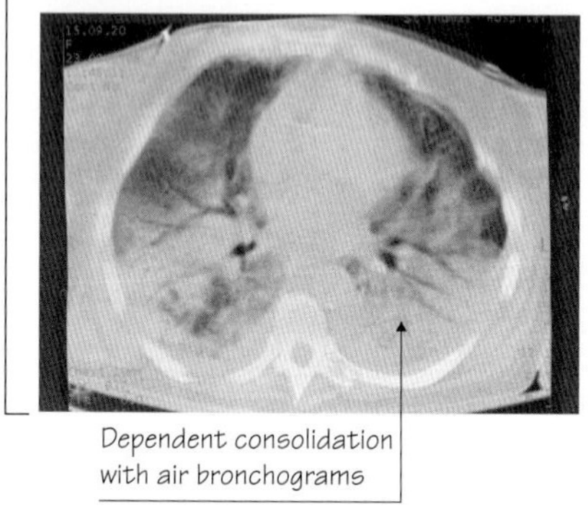

Dependent consolidation with air bronchograms

Figure 42b   Ventilator-induced lung damage

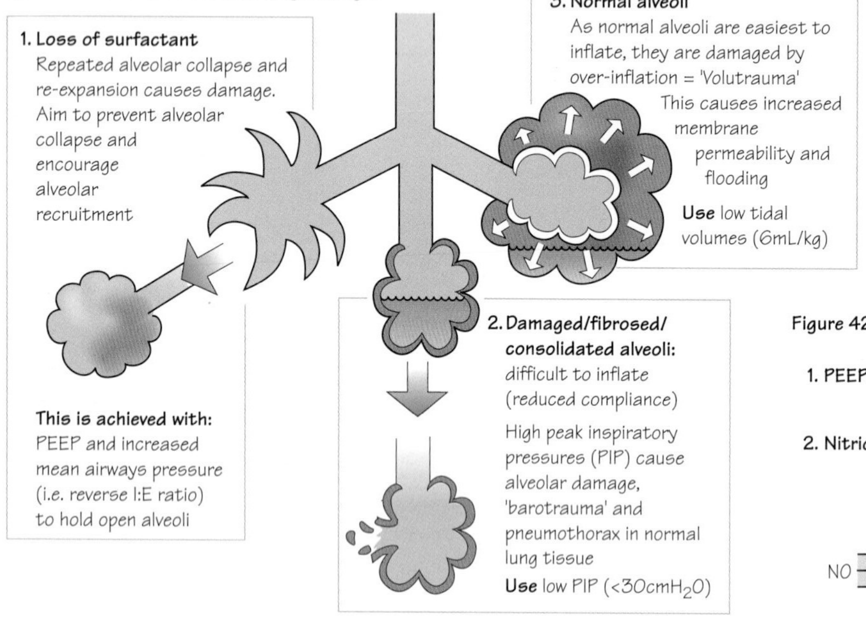

1. Loss of surfactant
Repeated alveolar collapse and re-expansion causes damage. Aim to prevent alveolar collapse and encourage alveolar recruitment

This is achieved with:
PEEP and increased mean airways pressure (i.e. reverse I:E ratio) to hold open alveoli

3. Normal alveoli
As normal alveoli are easiest to inflate, they are damaged by over-inflation = 'Volutrauma'
This causes increased membrane permeability and flooding
Use low tidal volumes (6mL/kg)

2. Damaged/fibrosed/consolidated alveoli:
difficult to inflate (reduced compliance)
High peak inspiratory pressures (PIP) cause alveolar damage, 'barotrauma' and pneumothorax in normal lung tissue
Use low PIP (<30cmH$_2$O)

Figure 42d   V/Q matching

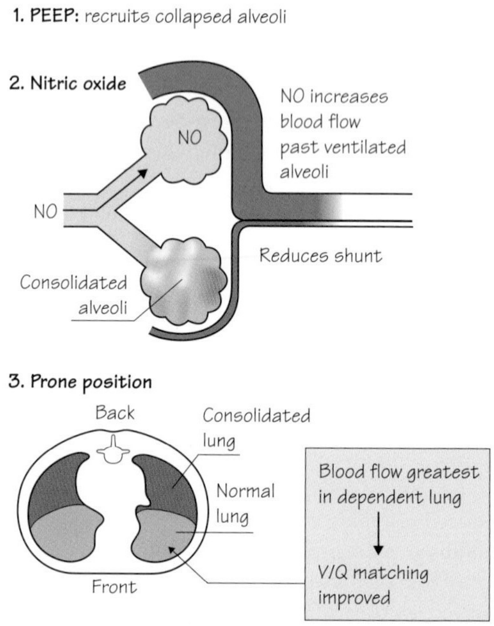

1. **PEEP:** recruits collapsed alveoli

2. **Nitric oxide**

NO

NO

Consolidated alveoli

NO increases blood flow past ventilated alveoli

Reduces shunt

3. **Prone position**

Back

Consolidated lung

Normal lung

Front

Blood flow greatest in dependent lung

V/Q matching improved

Figure 42c   Common causes of ARDS

Direct pulmonary	Indirect
Infective (pneumonia, tuberculosis)	Sepsis
Pulmonary trauma	Non-thoracic trauma
Near-drowning	Burns
Toxic gas inhalation	Haemorrhage, multiple transfusion
Smoke	Post arrest
NO_2, NH_3, Cl_2	Bowel infarction
Phosgene	Anaphylactic
Oxygen toxicity ($F_iO_2 > 0.8$)	Pancreatitis
Inhalation of gastric contents (pH < 2)	Uraemia, toxins, eclampsia
	Drugs (salicylates, barbiturates)

Acute respiratory distress syndrome (ARDS) is most simply defined as 'leaky lung syndrome' or 'low pressure (i.e. non-cardiogenic) pulmonary oedema'. It describes acute inflammatory lung injury, often in previously healthy lungs, mediated by a uniform pulmonary pathological process (Figure 42a) in response to a variety of direct (i.e. inhaled) or indirect (i.e. blood-borne) insults (Figure 42c). During the **acute inflammatory phase** of ARDS (Figure 42a), cytokine-activated neutrophils and monocytes adhere to alveolar epithelium or capillary endothelium, releasing inflammatory mediators and proteolytic enzymes. These damage the integrity of the alveolar–capillary membrane, increase permeability and cause alveolar oedema. Reduced surfactant production causes alveolar collapse and hyaline membrane formation. Progressive hypoxaemia and respiratory failure are due to ventilation/perfusion (V/Q) mismatch and loss of functioning alveoli. The later **healing, fibroproliferative phase** causes progressive pulmonary fibrosis and associated pulmonary hypertension.

Diagnosis

The internationally agreed 2012 Berlin definition of ARDS:
- **Acute onset** within 1 week of the insult
- **Bilateral diffuse opacities on the chest radiograph (CXR)**
- **Non-cardiac origin for pulmonary oedema** (nor fluid overload).
- **Oxygenation**: defines the severity of the ARDS. Mild ARDS is a P_aO_2/F_iO_2 (P/F) of 200–300 mmHg; moderate, a P/F of 100–200 mmHg and severe, a P/F of <100 mmHg (all with end-expiratory pressure (PEEP)/continuous positive airways pressure (CPAP) ≥5 cmH$_2$O). P/F is calculated as follows: if P_aO_2 is 80 mmHg on 80% inspired oxygen, $P_aO_2/F_iO_2 = 80/0.8 = 100$ mmHg. Mild ARDS equates to the previous definition of acute lung injury.

Epidemiology and prognosis

The incidence of ARDS is ~2–8 cases/100,000 population/year. Mortality is ~27% in mild, ~32% in moderate and ~45% in severe ARDS and is determined by the precipitating condition (trauma <35%, sepsis ~50%, aspiration pneumonia ~80%) and increased by age (>60 years old) and associated sepsis. The cause of death is multi-organ failure (MOF) and <20% die from hypoxaemia alone.

Clinical features

The **acute inflammatory phase** lasts 3–10 days and results in hypoxaemia and MOF. It presents with progressive breathlessness, tachypnoea, cyanosis, hypoxic confusion and lung crepitations. These features are not diagnostic and are frequently misinterpreted as heart failure. During the **healing, fibroproliferative phase**, lung scarring and pneumothoraces are common. Secondary chest and systemic infections occur in both phases.

Investigation and monitoring

Routine measurements include temperature, respiratory rate, S_aO_2 and urine output. Haemodynamic monitoring of central venous pressure (CVP), cardiac output (CO), lung water and occasionally left atrial pressure (e.g. PiCCO, PAC) ensures appropriate fluid balance and adequate tissue oxygen delivery (Chapter 3). Serial arterial blood gas (ABG) measurements and occasionally capnography (Chapter 3) monitor gas exchange. Regular microbiological samples (e.g. bronchial lavage) identify secondary infection early. **Radiology** (Figure 42a): serial CXRs detect progression of diffuse bilateral pulmonary infiltrates. Early CT scans often demonstrate dependent consolidation and later scans pneumothoraces, pneumatocoeles and fibrosis.

Management

Initially identify and treat the precipitating cause. In mild ARDS, oxygen therapy, diuretics and physiotherapy may preserve gas exchange. However, if respiratory failure progresses, non-invasive ventilation (NIV) (Chapter 16) with CPAP improves oxygenation and may avoid the need for mechanical ventilation (MV). In more severe disease, MV with high-inspired oxygen concentrations is necessary. Because of reduced lung compliance, high peak inspiratory pressures (PIPs) are required to achieve normal tidal volumes (T_v). These high pressures cause lung damage termed 'barotrauma' (e.g. pneumothorax). 'Volutrauma' describes damage to healthy alveoli due to over-distension (Figure 42b).

- **Mechanical Ventilation** must avoid oxygen toxicity (i.e. F_iO_2 < 80%), limit pressure-induced lung damage and volutrauma, optimize alveolar recruitment and oxygenation, and avoid circulatory compromise due to high intrathoracic pressures. A **'protective' lung ventilation strategy** of low T_v (6 ml/kg) and low PIP (<30 cmH$_2$O) prevents lung damage (Chapter 19) while high PEEP (>10 cmH$_2$O) and long inspiratory to expiratory (I:E) times (i.e. 2:1 instead of the normal 1:2) recruit collapsed alveoli. No ventilatory mode is proven to be superior, although pressure-controlled modes (Chapter 18) are often favoured. The CO_2 retention, termed 'permissive hypercapnia', resulting from low T_v strategies is usually tolerated with adequate sedation.
- **Conservative (i.e. 'dry') fluid management** limits alveolar oedema related to the increased alveolar permeability. Maintain adequate CO and organ perfusion at lower left atrial pressures (LAPs) using vaso-inotropic drugs rather than aggressive fluid filling. In the acute phase, diuretics reduce pulmonary oedema and may improve oxygenation.
- **General measures**: include good nursing care, physiotherapy, nutrition, sedation and infection control. Reduce metabolic demand by controlling fever, shivering and agitation (e.g. paracetamol, sedatives). No specific drug therapy (e.g. steroids, anti-inflammatory agents, surfactant) has been consistently beneficial in clinical ARDS trials. High-dose steroid therapy at 7–10 days, to reduce the development of pulmonary fibrosis, remains controversial.
- **Additional measures**: inhaled nitric oxide (NO) increases perfusion of ventilated alveoli by vasodilating surrounding vessels, improving V/Q matching and reducing shunt fraction (Figure 42d). Unfortunately, initial P_aO_2 improvements are not sustained. Mortality is subsequently increased due to formation and toxicity of potent oxygen radicals (e.g NO_2). **Prone positioning**: consolidation is usually dependent and blood flow is greatest in the dependent areas; improved V/Q matching can be achieved by turning the patient prone so that previously non-dependent, non-consolidated, ventilated lung becomes dependent and perfused (Figure 42d). **Bronchoscopy** improves ventilation and V/Q matching by removing sputum plugs and secretions. **Extracorporeal membrane oxygenation (ECMO)** techniques to oxygenate blood or remove CO_2 are effective in children and increasing evidence suggests benefit in adults. **Chest drainage**: pneumothorax and pneumatocoeles are common during the late fibroproliferative phase and may be difficult to detect on CXR. The importance of CT scanning to localize and guide drainage of these air 'locules' has only recently been appreciated.

Pearl of wisdom

Acute respiratory distress syndrome (ARDS) is a post-inflammatory, non-cardiogenic 'leaky lung' syndrome followed by a fibroproliferative healing phase

Pneumothorax and air leaks

Figure 43a Pneumothorax

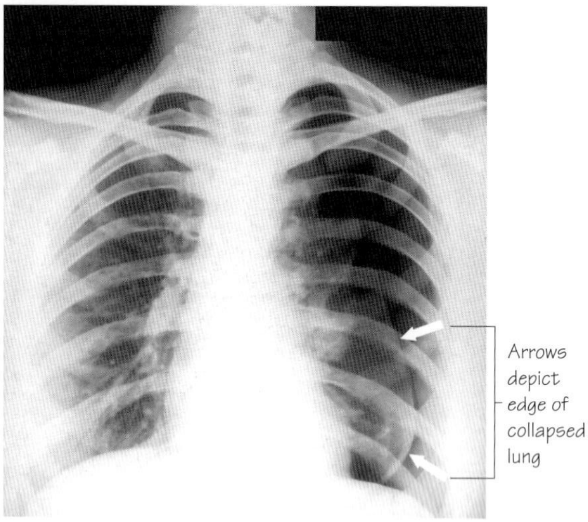

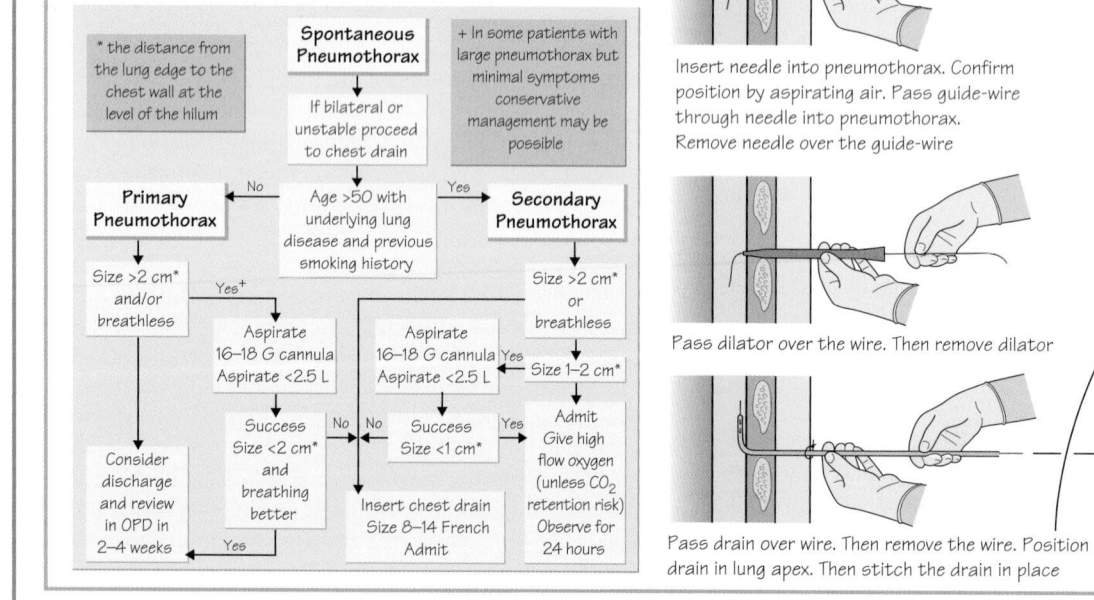

Arrows depict edge of collapsed lung

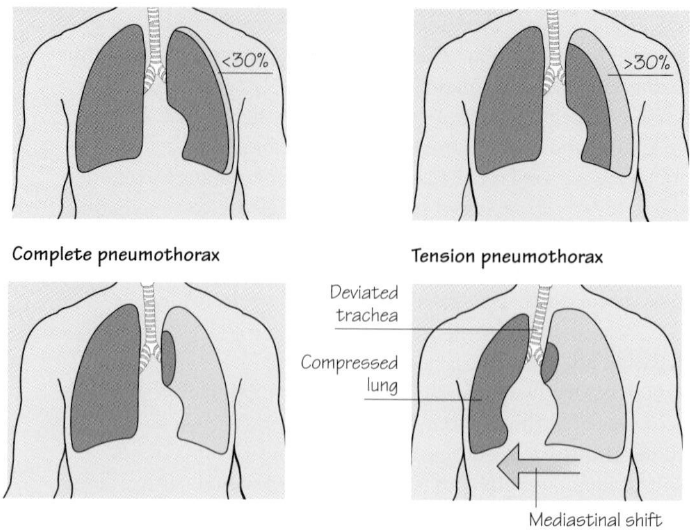

Small pneumothorax <30%

Moderate pneumothorax >30%

Complete pneumothorax

Tension pneumothorax
Deviated trachea
Compressed lung
Mediastinal shift

Figure 43b Pneumothorax management

Type of pneumothorax	Degree of collapse		
	Complete	Moderate	Small
Primary	Aspirate/ chest drain	Aspirate	Observe
Secondary	Chest drain	Chest drain	Chest drain
Traumatic/ Iatrogenic	Chest drain	Chest drain	Observe/ chest drain

Figure 43c Spontaneous pneumothorax management

* the distance from the lung edge to the chest wall at the level of the hilum

+ In some patients with large pneumothorax but minimal symptoms conservative management may be possible

Spontaneous Pneumothorax
→ If bilateral or unstable proceed to chest drain

Age >50 with underlying lung disease and previous smoking history
— No → Primary Pneumothorax
— Yes → Secondary Pneumothorax

Primary Pneumothorax
Size >2 cm* and/or breathless
Yes+ →
Aspirate 16–18 G cannula Aspirate <2.5 L
Success Size <2 cm* and breathing better
Consider discharge and review in OPD in 2–4 weeks

Secondary Pneumothorax
Size >2 cm* or breathless
Size 1–2 cm*
Aspirate 16–18 G cannula Aspirate <2.5 L
Yes →
Success Size <1 cm*
Admit Give high flow oxygen (unless CO$_2$ retention risk) Observe for 24 hours

Insert chest drain Size 8–14 French Admit

Figure 43d Seldinger technique for insertion of a chest drain

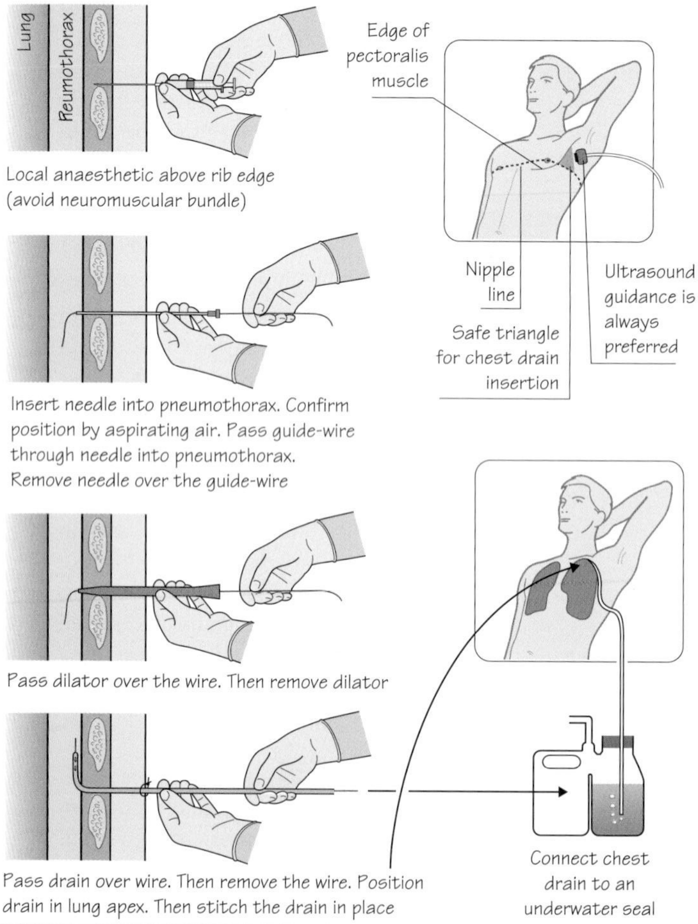

Lung
Pneumothorax

Local anaesthetic above rib edge (avoid neuromuscular bundle)

Insert needle into pneumothorax. Confirm position by aspirating air. Pass guide-wire through needle into pneumothorax. Remove needle over the guide-wire

Pass dilator over the wire. Then remove dilator

Pass drain over wire. Then remove the wire. Position drain in lung apex. Then stitch the drain in place

Edge of pectoralis muscle

Nipple line

Safe triangle for chest drain insertion

Ultrasound guidance is always preferred

Connect chest drain to an underwater seal

Pneumothorax (i.e. a collection of air between the visceral and parietal pleura causing a real rather than potential pleural space) and air leaks are common in critical illnesses. Recognition and early drainage can be life-saving. Predisposing and precipitating factors include necrotizing lung disease, chest trauma, ventilator-associated lung injury and cardiothoracic surgery.

Pneumothorax classification

1 Primary spontaneous pneumothorax (PSP) is the most common type of pneumothorax. It is due to rupture of apical subpleural air-cysts ('blebs') and is rarely associated with significant physiological disturbance. PSP usually affects tall, 20–40-year-old men (M:F 5:1) without underlying lung disease. Prevalence is $8/10^5$/year, rising to $200/10^5$/year in subjects >1.9 m in height. Likelihood of recurrence is >60% following a second PSP and pleurodesis is recommended to fuse the visceral and parietal pleura using either medical (e.g. pleural insertion of talc) or surgical (e.g. abrasion of the pleural lining) techniques.

2 Secondary pneumothorax (SP) is often associated with respiratory diseases that damage lung architecture (e.g. chronic obstructive pulmonary disease [COPD], fibrotic lung disease, pneumonia), and occasionally rare or inherited disorders (e.g. Marfan's, cystic fibrosis). The incidence of SP increases with age and the severity of the underlying lung disease. These patients usually require hospital admission because even a small SP in a patient with reduced respiratory reserve may have more serious implications than a large PSP. Mechanically ventilated (MV) patients with lung disease are at particular risk of SP because of associated high pressures ('barotrauma') and alveolar over-distension ('volutrauma'). 'Protective' ventilation strategies using low-pressure, limited-volume ventilation reduces this risk (Chapters 18, 19, 42).

3 Traumatic (iatrogenic) pneumothorax (TP) follows blunt (e.g. road traffic accidents) or penetrating (e.g. stab wounds) chest trauma (Chapter 73). Therapeutic procedures (e.g. line insertion, chest surgery) often cause iatrogenic pneumothorax.

A **tension pneumothorax** may complicate PSP or SP but is most common in MV patients and following TP. It occurs when air accumulates in the pleural cavity faster than it can be removed. Increased intrathoracic pressure causes mediastinal shift, lung compression, impaired venous return and shock due to reduced cardiac output (CO). It is a medical emergency and fatal if not rapidly relieved by drainage. Detection is a clinical diagnosis; awaiting chest radiography (CXR) confirmation may be life-threatening. Immediate drainage with a 14G needle in the second intercostal space in the midclavicular line is essential. A characteristic 'hiss' of escaping gas confirms the diagnosis. A chest drain is then inserted.

Clinical assessment: pneumothorax is graded and treated according to Figures 43a and 43b. Sudden breathlessness and/or sharp pleuritic pain suggest a pneumothorax. Most PSPs are small (<30%), and cause few symptoms other than pain. Clinical signs can be surprisingly difficult to detect, but in large pneumothoraces reduced air entry and hyper-resonant percussion over one hemithorax are characteristic and may be associated with tachypnoea and cyanosis. Cardiorespiratory compromise can develop rapidly in a tension pneumothorax or in MV patients and requires immediate drainage. **Monitoring** reveals tachycardia, hypotension and desaturation. **Blood gases** identify respiratory failure. **CXR** confirms the diagnosis (Figure 43a). **CT scans** detect localized pneumothoraces following trauma or MV.

Management: immediate supportive therapy includes supplemental oxygen and analgesia. Figure 43c illustrates spontaneous pneumothorax management, which depends on cause (i.e. PSP, SP), size and symptoms.

- Drain tension pneumothoraces immediately. Small PSPs (Figure 43c) are simply observed and spontaneous reabsorption confirmed on outpatient CXR. Large, symptomatic PSP (>2 cm between lung edge and chest wall at hilar level) are initially aspirated, under ultrasound (US) guidance, through a 16–18G needle using a 50-ml syringe connected to a three-way tap and underwater seal. Successful aspiration is confirmed by lung re-expansion on repeat CXR. Occasionally chest drainage is required if aspiration fails or in large PSP with respiratory failure.

- In general, SP and TP **always** require hospital admission and most need chest drain insertion (Figure 43b). The 'Seldinger' technique (i.e. chest drain inserted over a guide wire) is popular but complications have been reported (e.g. lung trauma). Recent recommendations advise daytime insertion under mandatory US guidance (Figure 43d). In difficult cases, chest drains can be inserted using relatively safe 'blunt dissection' techniques. Multiple chest drains may be needed in patients with loculated pneumothoraces. During MV, high airways pressures and positive end-expiratory pressure (PEEP) encourage persistent leaks. 'Protective' ventilation and the lowest airway pressures compatible with adequate gas exchange should be used (Chapter 19).

- Persistent drain leakage suggests development of a bronchopleural fistula (BPF). High-flow drain suction with pressures of 5–30 cmH$_2$O opposes visceral and parietal pleura encouraging spontaneous pleurodesis but early surgical advice is essential. Video-assisted thoracoscopy is as effective as thoracotomy at correcting BPF but causes less respiratory dysfunction.

- Remove chest drains when CXR confirms lung expansion and there has been no air leakage through the drain for >24 hours. Drains should not be clamped before removal. After adequate analgesia, the drain is pulled out during inspiration and the drain site secured with 'purse string' sutures.

Air leaks

Pneumomediastinum describes air in the mediastinal–pleural reflection, outlining the heart and great vessels on CXR. Air may also dissect along perivascular sheaths into the neck causing **subcutaneous emphysema (SE)** or around the heart with **pneumopericardium**, which may cause tamponade. Air leaks follow ventilator-induced barotrauma or traumatic damage to the trachea (e.g. tracheostomy), bronchus and oesophagus (Chapter 73). SE causes localized (e.g. neck) or grotesque facial and body swelling. It has a characteristic crackling sensation on palpation. The voice may have a nasal quality and auscultation over the precordium may reveal a 'crunch' with each heart beat (Homan's sign). Management includes good drainage of pneumothorax and 'protective' ventilation strategies (Chapters 18, 19). Failure to resolve should prompt investigation (e.g. bronchoscopy) to detect unrecognized air leaks and issues decreasing chest drain efficiency.

Pearl of wisdom

Tension pneumothorax is a clinical, life-threatening diagnosis requiring immediate drainage; do not await a chest radiograph (CXR)

44 Respiratory emergencies

Figure 44a Patient positioning during massive haemoptysis

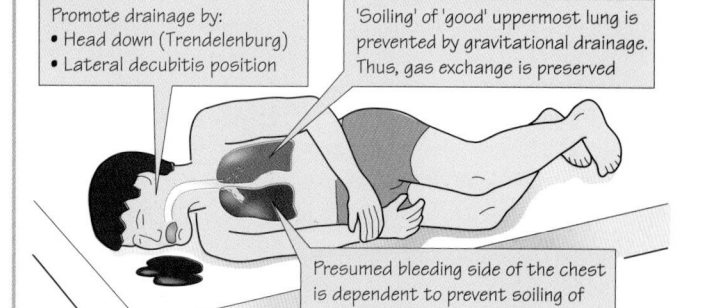

Promote drainage by:
• Head down (Trendelenburg)
• Lateral decubitis position

'Soiling' of 'good' uppermost lung is prevented by gravitational drainage. Thus, gas exchange is preserved

Presumed bleeding side of the chest is dependent to prevent soiling of unaffected lung

Figure 44b The Heimlich manoeuvre for expulsion of an aspirated foreign body. Follow steps 1–3

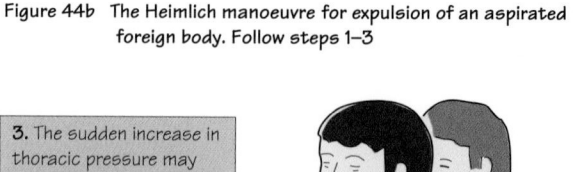
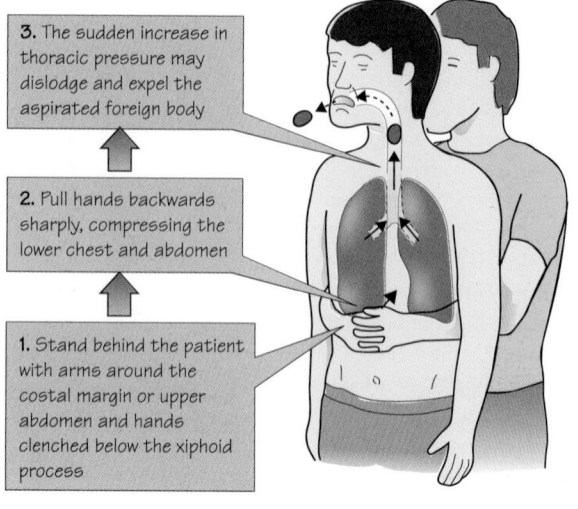

3. The sudden increase in thoracic pressure may dislodge and expel the aspirated foreign body

2. Pull hands backwards sharply, compressing the lower chest and abdomen

1. Stand behind the patient with arms around the costal margin or upper abdomen and hands clenched below the xiphoid process

Figure 44c Causes of massive haemoptysis

Infective (~80%)	Malignant (~20%)	Other
Tuberculosis	Lung cancer	• Pulmonary infarction
Pneumonia	Metastatic cancer	• Adenoma
Lung abscess	Lymphoma	• Trauma
Bronchiectasis		• Alveolar haemorrhage
Aspergillus		• Vasculitis

Figure 44d Bronchial angiogram showing a localized area of bleeding

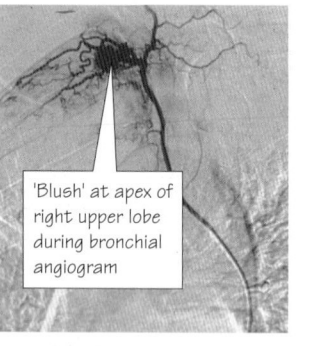

'Blush' at apex of right upper lobe during bronchial angiogram

Figure 44e CXR of aspiration pneumonia occuring 6hrs after gastric aspiration

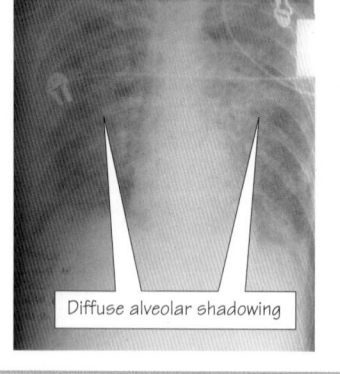

Diffuse alveolar shadowing

Figure 44f Diseases that may present as respiratory emergencies. Also see neuromuscular, endocrine and neurological chapters 47–52, 54, 60–67

Cause	Comments
CNS depression Coma (e.g. metabolic) CVA Sedation, self-poisoning	Perioperative sedation (e.g. benzodiazepines), self-poisoning (e.g. opiates) and strokes are associated with respiratory failure due to: • high risk of aspiration • loss of respiratory drive
Neurological diseases Myasthenia gravis Guillain-Barre syndrome Restrictive wall defects (e.g. kyphoscoliosis) Myopathies Motor neurone disease	Require close monitoring as sudden respiratory failure may occur. Other problems include: • progressive respiratory muscle weakness • inadequate cough • atelectasis due to loss of mobility • laryngeal incompetence with aspiration
Infections Poliomyelitis Tetanus Diphtheria Botulism Tuberculosis (TB)	• Respiratory failure may develop within hours of polio infection. Bulbar lesions cause aspiration and pneumonia • A toxin-mediated disease due to *Clostridium tetani* causing muscle rigidity, severe spasms, respiratory failure, bulbar lesions + CVS instability • Respiratory failure is due to laryngeal obstruction by characteristic pharyngeal membrane or toxin-mediated polyneuritis • Potent neurotoxins produced by *Clostridium botulinum* inhibit presynaptic acetylcholine release causing respiratory failure • Acute respiratory failure occurs with massive haemoptysis or sudden rupture of pus into the bronchial tree with acute miliary TB
Endocrine disorders • Thyroid • Adrenal • Pituitary	Endocrine disorders can be complicated by respiratory failure due to CNS depression, muscle weakness or electrolyte imbalance

CNS=central nervous system, CVA=cerebrovascular accident, CVS=cardiovascular system

Massive haemoptysis

Definition: expectoration of >600 ml of blood in 24 hours.
Causes: infection causes ~80% of cases (Figure 44c).
Prognosis: death is usually due to asphyxia, not blood loss, and is related to pathology, lung function and rate of bleeding (i.e. 600 ml in <4 hours or >16 hours, causes 70% or 5% mortality, respectively).
Clinical evaluation: haematemesis and nose bleeds must be distinguished from haemoptysis. Food particles suggest haematemesis; purulent secretions, bronchiectasis or lung abscesses; chest radiograph (CXR), apical cavities, tuberculosis (TB) or mycetoma; and

Critical Care Medicine at a Glance, Third Edition. Richard Leach. © 2014 John Wiley & Sons, Ltd. Published 2014 by John Wiley & Sons, Ltd.

haematuria, alveolar haemorrhage syndromes. Localization of the bleeding site may be difficult because blood aspiration results in diffuse clinical (e.g. crepitations) and CXR features. **Investigations** include serology, blood gases, clotting profile, CXR and sputum microbiology (e.g. acid fast bacilli).

Management involves:

1 Airways protection: assess bleeding severity and prevent asphyxia (e.g. clear secretion, oxygen therapy [OT]). **Promote airways drainage** by placing the patient slightly head down in the lateral decubitus position (Figure 44a). This prevents alveolar 'soiling' of the 'good' lung. Suppress cough (e.g. codeine) and withhold physiotherapy to reduce bleeding. Consider mechanical ventilation (MV) if haemoptysis causes respiratory failure. The unaffected lung can be independently ventilated by placing the endotracheal tube (ETT) in the corresponding main bronchus or by using a double lumen tube until bleeding is controlled.

2 Determine the site and cause of bleeding: early fibreoptic bronchoscopy allows examination of upper lobes and subsegmental bronchi, which account for ~80% of bleeding sites. Rigid bronchoscopy facilitates suctioning in severe haemorrhage but limits inspection. CT scans identify structural abnormalities (e.g. tumours) and bronchial arteriography, pulmonary angiography or nuclear scans detect active bleeding (Figure 44d).

3 Control of bleeding: immediate measures include bronchoscopic iced-saline (±epinephrine) lavages, topical fibrin or tamponade of affected bronchi using balloon catheters.

- **Bronchial artery embolization** is initially successful in >70% of cases, especially in those with dilated bronchial arteries (e.g. bronchiectasis). However, re-bleeding occurs in >50% within 3 months. Serious complications (e.g. paraplegia) follow anterior spinal artery thrombosis (~5%).
- **Surgical therapy** has the best outcomes but only medical management is possible in diffuse or end-stage disease (e.g. cancer, FEV$_1$ <40% predicted).

4 General measures: include fluid replacement, antibiotics and bronchodilators.

Aspiration syndromes

High-risk groups for aspiration include those with depressed conscious level (e.g. drug overdose), laryngeal incompetence (e.g. bulbar syndromes) and the critically ill. The clinical scenario depends on the type and volume of aspiration; peri-anaesthetic aspiration of large volumes of gastric contents rapidly progresses to acute respiratory distress syndrome (ARDS), whereas repeated microaspiration (e.g. bulbar palsy) causes pneumonia. A high index of suspicion is required because aspiration is not always witnessed.

- **Solid particulate matter** (e.g. peanuts, coins, teeth): can be aspirated. Partially masticated food is most common giving rise to the *'café-coronary'* syndrome. **Partial obstruction** causes stridor, cough, wheeze, atelectasis and recurrent pneumonia. **Complete obstruction** prevents breathing and speech, followed by cyanosis, coma and death. If a sharp blow to the back of the chest fails to dislodge the particle, the Heimlich manoeuvre is attempted (Figure 44b). If this fails, perform an emergency cricothyroidectomy by inserting a large bore needle or sharp implement through the cricothyroid membrane (Chapter 19). Urgent bronchoscopy follows to remove the obstruction.

- **Fluid aspiration**: gastric contents (pH < 2) are most frequently aspirated. Large volumes rapidly cause respiratory failure, pulmo-

nary oedema and ARDS. Right lower lobe involvement is common (~60%) because the right main bronchus is the most direct path of aspiration. CXR shows infiltrates in ~90% of cases (Figure 44e). **Prevention is essential** (i.e. nasogastric [NG] tube, pre-operative fasting) because treatment is largely supportive including airways clearance, OT, bronchodilators, antibiotics, continuous positive airways pressure [CPAP] or MV. Neither steroid therapy nor bronchoscopy is beneficial. Preventing pneumonia due to microaspiration (e.g. post-cerebrovascular accident [CVA]) is difficult and includes the use of thickened feeds, upright posture and NG feeding.

- **Near-drowning** is a common cause of accidental death. It is often associated with alcohol consumption or a primary medical event (e.g. myocardial infarction [MI]). Although more frequent in rivers, lakes or sea, deaths may occur at home in small volumes of water (e.g. bath). **Freshwater aspiration** inhibits pulmonary surfactant causing atelectasis, pulmonary shunt and hypoxaemia. Rapid lung absorption of hypotonic freshwater causes initial hypervolaemia, haemolysis and hyperkalaemia. Hypertonic **seawater aspiration** pulls fluid into alveoli causing hypovolaemia, shunting and hypoxaemia. Profound hypothermia (<30°C) is common in near-drowning and predisposes to resistant arrhythmias particularly during rough handling or cardiopulmonary resuscitation (CPR). Always rewarm patients before terminating CPR (Chapter 6). Do not perform the Heimlich manoeuvre because gravitational drainage of aspirated water is just as effective, without risking arrhythmias. Treatment is largely supportive. Overnight observation is recommended because late (>12 hours) pulmonary oedema can occur. The degree of hypoxic brain damage determines outcome (Chapter 72) and mortality is similar in fresh or seawater.

Upper airways obstruction

Causes include aspirated particulate matter, inhaled toxic gases and burns (Chapter 76), trauma (Chapter 73), anaphylaxis, laryngeal oedema, laryngospasm and large airway stenoses. Obstruction by the tongue should be excluded and prevented with a pharyngeal airway (Chapter 15). Extubation can be associated with laryngospasm due to oedema or irritation during ETT removal. **Treatment**: severe respiratory distress requires immediate intubation. In less critical situations, nebulized epinephrine (±salbutamol) with intravenous steroids may reduce oedema and spasm sufficiently to avoid intubation. Helium and oxygen mixtures may improve gas flow through obstructed airways.

Other respiratory emergencies

There is an extensive list of infective, neuromuscular and endocrine diseases that predispose to respiratory emergencies (Figure 44f). Although rare in countries with advanced public health programmes, poliomyelitis, tetanus, diphtheria and TB remain common causes of respiratory emergencies in the developing world.

Pearl of wisdom

In near-drowning, extended cardiopulmonary resuscitation (CPR) and rewarming are justified despite prolonged, hypothermic immersion, because high-quality survival can occur, especially in the very young

45 Acute kidney injury: pathophysiology and clinical aspects

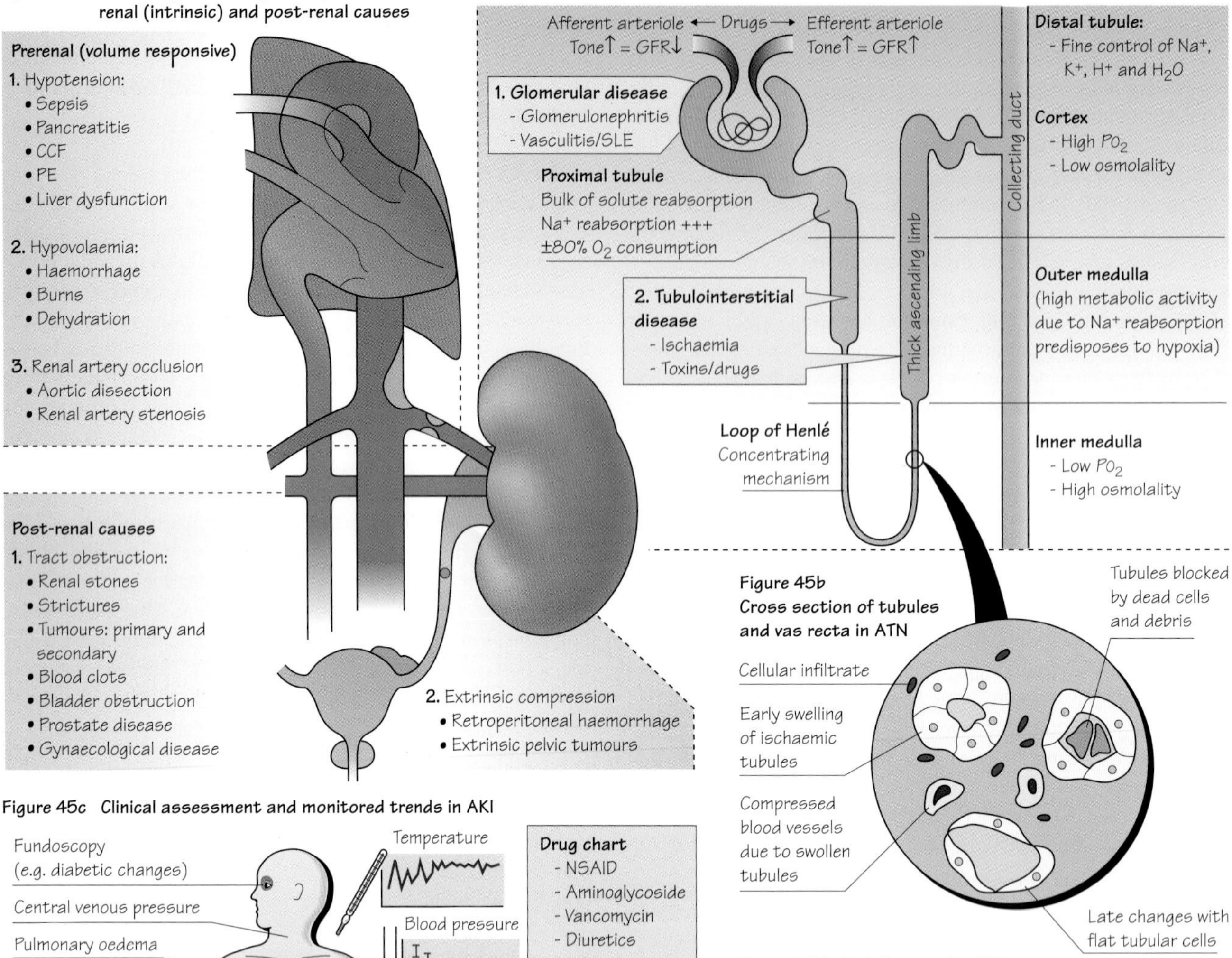

Figure 45a Prerenal (volume responsive), renal (intrinsic) and post-renal causes

Prerenal (volume responsive)

1. Hypotension:
   - Sepsis
   - Pancreatitis
   - CCF
   - PE
   - Liver dysfunction

2. Hypovolaemia:
   - Haemorrhage
   - Burns
   - Dehydration

3. Renal artery occlusion
   - Aortic dissection
   - Renal artery stenosis

Post-renal causes

1. Tract obstruction:
   - Renal stones
   - Strictures
   - Tumours: primary and secondary
   - Blood clots
   - Bladder obstruction
   - Prostate disease
   - Gynaecological disease

2. Extrinsic compression
   - Retroperitoneal haemorrhage
   - Extrinsic pelvic tumours

Renal (intrinsic) causes

Afferent arteriole ← Drugs → Efferent arteriole
Tone↑ = GFR↓   Tone↑ = GFR↑

1. Glomerular disease
- Glomerulonephritis
- Vasculitis/SLE

Proximal tubule
Bulk of solute reabsorption
Na^+ reabsorption +++
±80% O_2 consumption

2. Tubulointerstitial disease
- Ischaemia
- Toxins/drugs

Loop of Henlé
Concentrating mechanism

Thick ascending limb

Collecting duct

Distal tubule:
- Fine control of Na^+, K^+, H^+ and H_2O

Cortex
- High PO_2
- Low osmolality

Outer medulla
(high metabolic activity due to Na^+ reabsorption predisposes to hypoxia)

Inner medulla
- Low PO_2
- High osmolality

Figure 45b
Cross section of tubules and vas recta in ATN

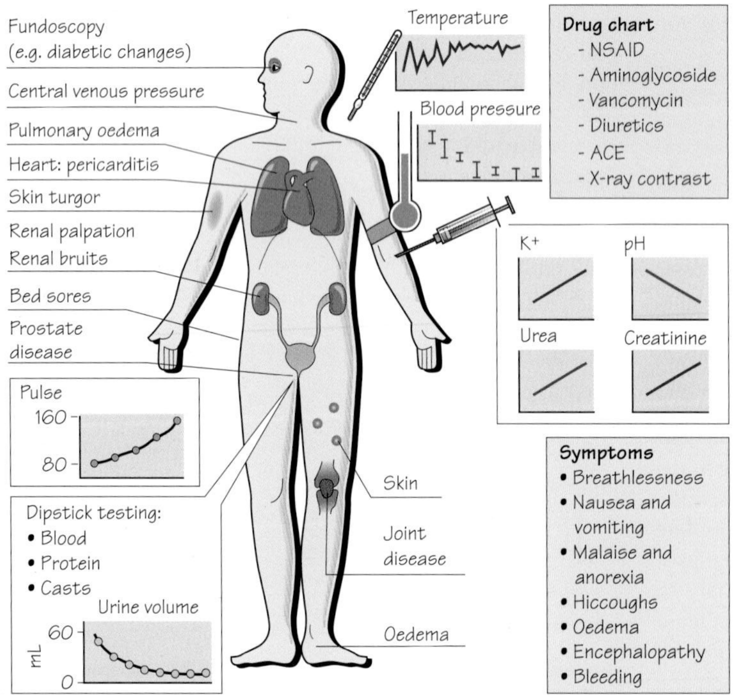

- Cellular infiltrate
- Early swelling of ischaemic tubules
- Compressed blood vessels due to swollen tubules
- Tubules blocked by dead cells and debris
- Late changes with flat tubular cells

Figure 45c Clinical assessment and monitored trends in AKI

- Fundoscopy (e.g. diabetic changes)
- Central venous pressure
- Pulmonary oedema
- Heart: pericarditis
- Skin turgor
- Renal palpation
- Renal bruits
- Bed sores
- Prostate disease

Temperature

Blood pressure

Drug chart
- NSAID
- Aminoglycoside
- Vancomycin
- Diuretics
- ACE
- X-ray contrast

K^+ pH

Urea   Creatinine

Pulse
160
80

Dipstick testing:
- Blood
- Protein
- Casts

Urine volume
60
mL
0

- Skin
- Joint disease
- Oedema

Symptoms
- Breathlessness
- Nausea and vomiting
- Malaise and anorexia
- Hiccoughs
- Oedema
- Encephalopathy
- Bleeding

Figure 45d Risk factors for AKI

Previous renal dysfunction	Diuretic use and abuse
More common in older people	Drugs (e.g. NSAID)
Pre-existing cardiac failure	X-ray contrast media
Hypovolaemia	Sepsis
Hypertension	Rhabdomyolysis
Peripheral vascular disease	Hypercalcaemia
Diabetes mellitus	

Figure 45e Prerenal (volume responsive) versus renal (intrinsic) oliguria

	Normal	Prerenal	Renal
Urine osmolality (mOsm/kg)	400–500	>500	<400
Urinary sodium (mmol)	10–20	<20	>40
Urine: plasma creatinine ratio	20–40	>40	<20

NB: Concurrent drug therapy (i.e. diuretics) and pre-existing chronic kidney disease make interpretation difficult

Definition

Acute kidney injury (AKI) is an abrupt reduction in kidney function defined as an increase in serum creatinine (SCr) of $\geq 26.4\,\mu mol/L$ within 48 hours; or an increase in SCr of 1.5-fold above baseline that has occurred within 7 days; or a reduction in urine output (UO; $<0.5\,ml/kg/h$ for $>6\,h$). AKI severity (Appendix 2) is classified as:

- **Stage I**: SCr increase $\geq 26.4\,\mu mol/L$ (0.3 mg/dl) **or** SCr 1.5–1.9 times baseline **or** UO $<0.5\,ml/kg/h$ for >6–12 hours.
- **Stage II**: SCr increase of 2.0–2.9 times baseline; **or** UO $<0.5\,ml/kg/h$ for >12 hours.
- **Stage III**: SCr increase $\geq 352\,\mu mol/L$ (4.0 mg/dl) **or** SCr >3.0 times baseline **or** UO $<0.3\,ml/kg/h$ for >24 hours **or** anuria for 12 hours.

Classification and causes (Figure 45a)

1 Pre-renal (volume responsive) AKI ($\sim55\%$): inadequate renal perfusion (e.g. hypotension, hypovolaemia, vascular occlusion) causes ischaemia and acute tubular necrosis (ATN).

2 Renal (intrinsic) AKI ($\sim30\%$): causes include:

- **Glomerular**: glomerulonephritis, vasculitis (e.g. Goodpasture's syndrome).
- **ATN and tubulointerstitial disease (TID)** are due to ischaemia, toxicity (e.g. drugs, heavy metals, contrast media) and the release of free haemoglobin (i.e. during haemolysis [e.g. haemolytic–uraemic syndrome]) or myoglobin (i.e. in rhabdomyolysis [e.g. trauma]). AKI also follows tubular precipitation of calcium in acute hypercalcaemia or 'light chains' in myeloma.
- **Drugs and toxins**: non-steroidal anti-inflammatory drugs (NSAIDs) cause renal arteriolar vasoconstriction by inhibiting normal prostaglandin-induced vasodilation. In hypovolaemic patients, this seriously reduces renal blood flow (RBF) and glomerular filtration rate (GFR). NSAIDs also precipitate AKI in chronic kidney disease (CKD) and those using diuretics (e.g. cirrhosis). Radiocontrasts, tacrolimus and amphotericin cause vasoconstriction, whereas aminoglycosides and cephalosporins are direct tubular toxins. ACE inhibitors block the angiotensin-mediated efferent arteriolar vasodilation that maintains GFR. Many drugs may cause TID (e.g. antibiotics, diuretics).

3 Post-renal AKI ($\sim15\%$): due to urinary tract obstruction. Resulting back pressure inhibits GFR and causes ischaemia. AKI only occurs if both kidneys are obstructed.

Pathophysiology

Renal ischaemia contributes to most cases of AKI due to failure of complex vascular control mechanisms. Blood pressure (BP) is a poor indicator of renal hypoperfusion because local autoregulatory feedback mechanisms act to maintain GFR and the renal renin–angiotensin mechanism raises BP despite hypovolaemia. The juxta-medullary region (i.e. proximal tubule, thick ascending limb of the loop of Henlé) is most susceptible to ischaemia because: (a) active sodium absorption in this region accounts for 80% of renal oxygen consumption, and (b) most RBF ($\sim30\%$ cardiac output [CO]) is directed to the cortex, while medullary blood flow is limited to maintain the concentration gradient of osmolality. Reduced RBF ($\pm$toxicity) causes ATN and tubular cell death in this region due to this combined high oxygen demand and poor blood supply. Subsequent tubular blockage reduces GFR and swelling further compromises medullary perfusion (Figure 45b).

Clinical features

There are two characteristic clinical presentations:

- **Critical illness AKI**: Most AKIs occur in critically ill patients (ICU incidence ~20–50%) and after surgery, trauma or burns as part of the multiple organ dysfunction syndrome. Although renal ischaemia (i.e. hypotension) is the main cause, aetiology is often multifactorial (i.e. sepsis, drugs). Typically presentation is with oliguria and a rising SCr/urea ($\pm$metabolic acidosis, hyperkalaemia). In severe AKI, mortality is high ($>50\%$) but $>65\%$ of survivors recover renal function and discontinue renal replacement therapy (RRT).
- **Medical AKI**: 'Single organ' AKI, due to specific renal disease (e.g. glomerulonephritis), is less common. It usually presents as a failure to excrete nitrogenous waste rather than oliguria. Although mortality is low ($<10\%$), it can progress to CKD requiring RRT.

Clinical assessment (Figure 45c)

The history identifies factors that predispose to AKI (Figure 45d). Recent throat or skin infections and haematuria suggest glomerulonephritis. Haemoptysis is associated with vasculitis (e.g. Goodpasture's syndrome). Renal colic or male prostatism (e.g. frequency, poor stream) indicates post-renal obstruction. The past medical history may suggest possible associations (e.g. malignancy and hypercalcaemia) and sites of chronic infection (e.g. endocarditis).

Examination

Assess fluid status (e.g. hypovolaemia), cardiovascular function (e.g. tissue hypoperfusion) and exclude renal bruits. Fundoscopy identifies diabetic or hypertensive changes. Sites of sepsis and features of multisystem disease (e.g. arthritis) must be sought. Cardiac auscultation may reveal uraemic pericarditis or valve disease. Examine upper airways for signs of Wegener's granulomatosis and the chest for pulmonary oedema. Abdominal examination may detect polycystic kidneys, pelvic disease and bladder or prostatic enlargement.

- **Monitor** trends in: (a) **vital signs**: pulse, BP, central venous pressure (CVP), UO and weight; (b) **biochemical parameters**: urea, SCr, K^+, Ca^{2+} and pH. Creatine kinase detects rhabdomyolysis.

- **Investigations** include **haematology** to assess anaemia and haemolysis, **and reagent strip urinalysis** to detect blood, protein, glucose and ketones. Haematuria occurs in renal and post-renal disease; haemoglobin indicates haemolysis; proteinuria suggests glomerulonephritis, CKD or myeloma; and myoglobin suggests rhabdomyolysis. **Urine biochemistry** is not performed routinely but may differentiate between pre-renal and renal failure (Figure 45e). **Urine microscopy**: red cell casts confirm glomerulonephritis, granular casts occur in ATN and urinary eosinophils suggest interstitial nephritis. **Microbiology** identifies infection (e.g. urine, sepsis). **Immunology**: antinuclear antibodies are high in systemic lupus erythematosus (SLE). Antiglomerular basement membrane antibody indicates Goodpasture's syndrome and antineutrophil cytoplasmic antibodies (ANCA) suggest vasculitis (e.g. Wegener's). Low complement levels occur in SLE and post-infective glomerulonephritis. **Radiology**: early ultrasonography (<24 hours) determines kidney size and excludes renal tract obstruction. Small kidneys indicate CKD. Radioisotope studies and angiography evaluate perfusion. **Histology**: renal biopsy may be required to establish the cause.

Pearl of wisdom

The blood pressure (BP) is not always a good sign of renal perfusion status

46 Acute kidney injury: management and renal replacement therapy

Figure 46a   Acute renal failure

Absolute indications for RRT

1. Fluid (± salt) overload
2. Uncontrolled hyperkalaemia
3. Uraemic pericarditis
4. Metabolic acidosis (pH < 7.2)
5. Raised creatinine (no specific value but usually >700 μmol/L in AKI)
6. Encephalopathy

Figure 46b   Intermittent dialysis

Acute complications
- Headache
- Dialysis disequilibrium
- Air embolism
- Hypotension
- Arrhythmia (Hypokalaemia)
- Muscle cramps
- Line related complications

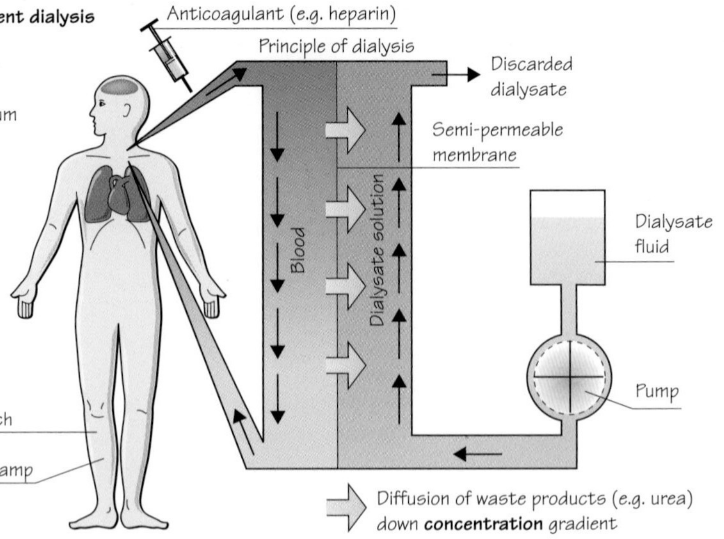

Anticoagulant (e.g. heparin)

Principle of dialysis

Discarded dialysate

Semi-permeable membrane

Dialysate fluid

Blood

Dialysate solution

Pump

Itch

Cramp

Diffusion of waste products (e.g. urea) down **concentration** gradient

Temporary access

Usually large-bore double lumen tube

Subclavian vein

Pearl of wisdom

Continuous haemofiltration is better tolerated in AKI patients with cardiovascular instability

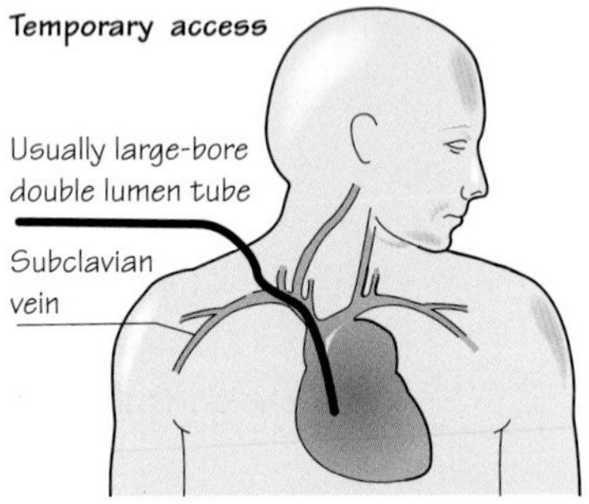

Real time ultrasound guidance should be used for all body and most femoral line placements

Figure 46c   Continuous haemofiltration

Advantages
- Slow and continuous
- Avoids rapid solute changes
- Suitable for haemodynamically unstable patients

Access
Double lumen central venous catheter

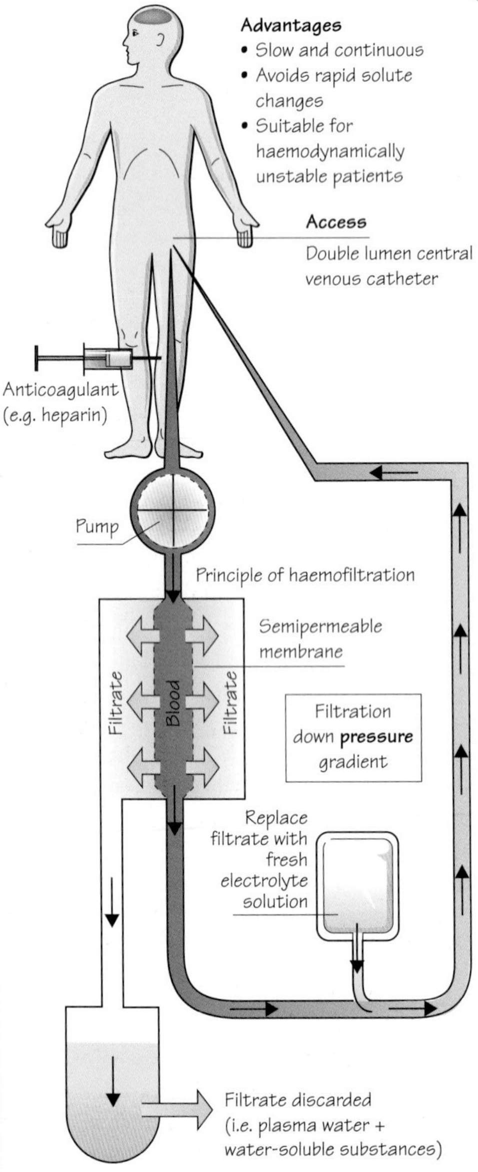

Anticoagulant (e.g. heparin)

Pump

Principle of haemofiltration

Semipermeable membrane

Filtrate

Blood

Filtrate

Filtration down **pressure** gradient

Replace filtrate with fresh electrolyte solution

Filtrate discarded (i.e. plasma water + water-soluble substances)

Figure 46d   Acute peritoneal dialysis

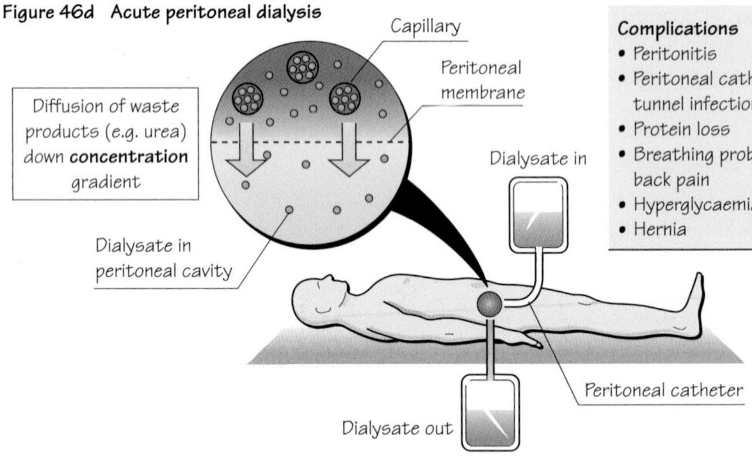

Capillary

Peritoneal membrane

Diffusion of waste products (e.g. urea) down **concentration** gradient

Dialysate in

Dialysate in peritoneal cavity

Peritoneal catheter

Dialysate out

Complications
- Peritonitis
- Peritoneal catheter tunnel infection
- Protein loss
- Breathing problems back pain
- Hyperglycaemia
- Hernia

Figure 46e   Treatment of hyperkalaemia

(K$^+$ >6.5mmol, with tented t-waves (± flat p waves or ↑p-r interval) or widened QRS complex, risks VF/VT)

1. Insulin (10U) in 50 mls of 50% glucose iv – Insulin encourages K$^+$ uptake into cells
2. Calcium gluconate (10%) 10 mls iv over 2 mins – Provides cardioprotection, K$^+$ not altered
3. Calcium resonium 30 g po/pr – Binds K$^+$ in gut
4. Nebulised salbutamol (2.5 mg) – Moves K$^+$ into cells
5. Dialysis/haemofiltration

K+ = potassium ion; iv = intravenous; po = per oral; pr = per rectum

Prevention and management

Acute kidney injury (AKI) is avoidable in 30% of cases. Simple preventative measures include early volume repletion, avoidance of nephrotoxins and timely recognition of renal dysfunction. Early AKI management includes:

1 Identification and treatment of the cause, including pre-renal, renal and post-renal pathology (e.g. steroids for vasculitis).

2 Fluid management: regular assessment of fluid and electrolyte balance is essential (Chapters 9, 10, 11). Monitor fluid intake, urine output (UO) and daily weight. A central venous catheter may be required to measure CVP. Volume replacement should match daily (e.g. urine) and insensible losses, with an additional 0.5 L/°C of fever. Inadequate perfusion and renal ischaemia (e.g. hypovolaemia, hypotension) cause most AKI and *must be corrected immediately*. If oliguria or renal dysfunction (i.e. rising urea, serum creatinine [SCr]) develop, consider:

- **Fluid challenges** ($\sim$0.5 L crystalloid over 15–30 min) – particularly if examination ($\pm$urinalysis) suggests a pre-renal cause. The aim is to raise CVP, blood pressure (BP), glomerular filtration rate (GFR) and UO. Further fluid challenges are guided by clinical assessment. In established AKI, oliguria may persist and further fluid challenges risk pulmonary oedema.
- **Diuretics**: although boluses or infusions of loop diuretics (e.g. furosemide) are sometimes recommended for their putative tubuloprotective effects (i.e. inhibition of sodium absorption reduces energy consumption and may alleviate ischaemia), there is no evidence that they prevent or treat AKI. In fact, they may cause harm (e.g. nephro-/ototoxicity) or potentiate drug toxicity (e.g. aminoglycosides) in hypovolaemic patients. However, they do induce diuresis in patients with fluid overload. In rhabdomyolysis, osmotic diuresis with mannitol will not prevent AKI but fluid resuscitation, high urinary flows and cautious urine alkalinization (pH > 6.5) with sodium bicarbonate (1.2%) solutions is recommended. **Low-dose 'renal' dopamine** has no role in AKI management despite its diuretic effects and may be harmful (e.g. arrhythmias).
- **Inotropes** (e.g. epinephrine) maintain GFR by increasing cardiac output (CO) and mean arterial pressure (MAP) (i.e. >70 mmHg) if fluid resuscitation is unsuccessful.

3 Oxygenation: optimize gas exchange (Chapter 14).

4 Sepsis must be identified and treated (e.g. antibiotics $\pm$ surgery).

5 Monitor biochemistry and drug levels: correct electrolyte imbalance/acidosis and adjust prescriptions.

6 Renal protection during imaging includes prophylactic fluid therapy (0.9% saline, 1 ml/kg/h for 12 hours pre- and post-procedure), iso-osmolar contrast media and stop specific drugs (e.g. angiotensin-converting enzyme [ACE] inhibitors, metformin) temporarily. Prophylactic *N*-acetylcysteine may be protective.

Established acute kidney injury

Once AKI is established, treatment is supportive. Management aims to: (a) prevent fluid overload; (b) maintain electrolyte and acid–base balance; and (c) limit accumulation of toxic metabolic waste by nutritional control and renal replacement therapy (RRT). In >65% of patients with acute tubular necrosis (ATN), renal function recovers after $\sim$2–60 days, heralded by a diuretic phase. AKI due to other causes (e.g. glomerulonephritis) may progress to chronic kidney disease (CKD) and long-term RRT.

General management

- **Fluid balance**: during anuric or oliguric periods, fluid replacement should match insensible loss ($\sim$0.5–1 L/day). If fluid overload causes pulmonary oedema (Chapter 34), it is treated with oxygen and pulmonary vasodilators (e.g. nitrates) while awaiting RRT to remove fluid. Diuretics, continuous positive airways pressure (CPAP) and venesection may help. Correct fluid and electrolyte losses during the diuretic phase of ATN recovery.

- **Electrolytes** are monitored daily and Na$^+$ and K$^+$ intake restricted. Calcium exchange resins, insulin with dextrose or RRT may be required to treat hyperkalaemia (Figure 46e). During AKI, SCr rises by $\sim$80–100 μmol/L/day but this depends on muscle mass, metabolic rate and tissue damage. The rate of rise of urea is more variable. Uraemic complications (e.g. pericarditis, seizures) develop at >50 mmol/L.

- **Nutritional support** improves outcome and early referral to a dietician is recommended. AKI patients are given 20–35 kcal/kg/day and up to 1.7 g amino acids/kg/day if hypercatabolic and on RRT. Vitamin supplements may be required.

- **Metabolic acidosis**: ideally RRT commences before respiratory distress or myocardial instability occur.

- **Uraemic bleeding** is usually due to platelet dysfunction. DDAVP (i.v.) may restore platelet function but clotting factors are ineffective.

- **General factors**: modify drug doses, control hypertension and prevent infection. Remove urinary catheters in anuric patients.

Renal replacement therapy

Absolute indications for RRT are listed in Figure 46a. Three main types of RRT are used in AKI. Continuous methods are better tolerated in haemodynamically unstable patients.

- **Intermittent dialysis** (Figure 46b): blood flows on one side, and a solution of crystalloids (dialysis fluid) is pumped in the opposite direction along the other side of a semipermeable membrane. Small molecules and toxic waste diffuse across the membrane according to imposed concentration gradients. Dialysis fluid composition aims to normalize plasma; small molecules like urea (60 Da) and creatinine (113 Da) are efficiently removed but larger molecules less so. Poor clearance of phosphate ions causes hyperphosphataemia. Dialysis corrects biochemical abnormalities and rapidly removes excess extracellular fluid ($\sim$2–4 hours). Hypokalaemia or hypovolaemia can occur, and may precipitate life-threatening hypotension or cardiac arrhythmias in unstable patients.

- **Continuous haemofiltration** (Figure 46c): plasma water and water soluble substances (<50 kDa) pass across a highly permeable membrane by convective flow (e.g. glomerular filtration). Unlike dialysis, urea, creatinine and phosphate are cleared at similar rates. Hypophosphataemia may occur if phosphate is not supplemented. Molecules like heparin are also efficiently cleared. The filtrate is discarded and replaced by a physiological solution. Low flow rates make haemofiltration less efficient at removing uraemic toxins but continuous use allows removal of any amount of fluid or nitrogenous waste. Ease of use in haemodynamically unstable patients is an advantage.

- **Acute peritoneal dialysis** (Figure 46d) uses hypertonic dialysate to draw fluid and solutes across the peritoneum after insertion of a peritoneal catheter. The dialysate (1–3 L) 'dwells' in the abdominal cavity for $\sim$4 hours before drainage. Abdominal pathology, infection risks and interference with ventilation limit use.

Pearl of wisdom

Acute kidney injury (AKI) is preventable in 30% of cases by early recognition, good fluid management and avoidance of nephrotoxic drugs

47 Electrolyte disturbances: sodium and potassium

Figure 47a Plasma osmolality and ADH release

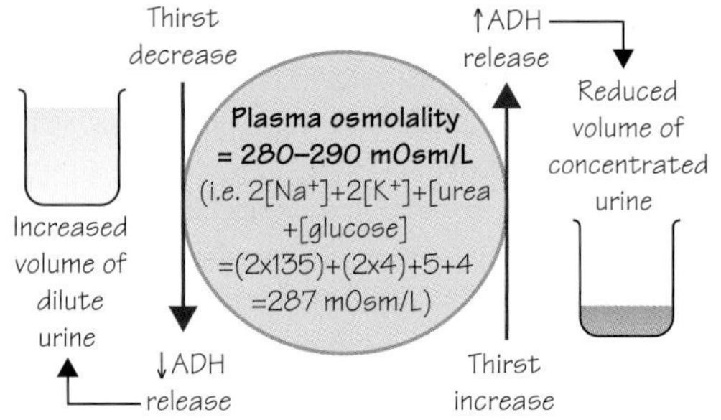

Thirst decrease

↑ADH release → Reduced volume of concentrated urine

Plasma osmolality = 280–290 mOsm/L
(i.e. 2[Na$^+$]+2[K$^+$]+[urea +[glucose]
=(2x135)+(2x4)+5+4
=287 mOsm/L)

Increased volume of dilute urine

↓ADH release

Thirst increase

Pearl of wisdom
Serum [Na$^+$] disorders are usually due to changes in water balance. Cause is determined from clinical volume status and urinary Na$^+$ (Figs 47b and 47f)

Figure 47c Hyponatraemia: clinical features

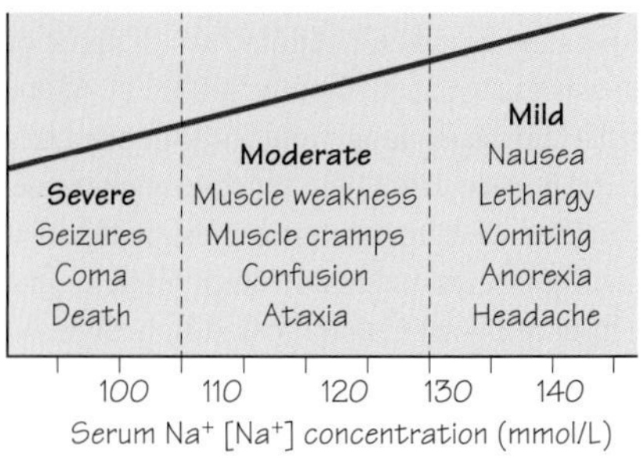

Severe	Moderate	Mild
Seizures	Muscle weakness	Nausea
Coma	Muscle cramps	Lethargy
Death	Confusion	Vomiting
	Ataxia	Anorexia
		Headache

Serum Na$^+$ [Na$^+$] concentration (mmol/L)
100 110 120 130 140

Figure 47b Clinical assessment and treatment of hyponatraemia

True hyponatraemia
Serum [Na$^+$] <130 mmol/L and osmolality <275 mosm/L

Measure serum [Na$^+$] and urine osmolality

Assess clinical volume status (TBW + TBNa$^+$):
- Hypovolaemia (TBW↓, TBNa$^+$↓↓)
- Euvolaemia (TBW↑, TBNa$^+$ normal)
- Hypervolaemia (TBW↑↑, TBNa$^+$↑)

Measure urine [Na$^+$]:
- >20 mmol/L / <20 mmol/L (Hypovolaemia)
- >20 mmol/L / <20 mmol/L (Euvolaemia)
- >20 mmol/L / <20 mmol/L (Hypervolaemia)

Underlying problem:
- Renal loss: Diuretics, Adrenal insufficiency, Na$^+$-losing nephropathy, Ketonuria
- Extra-renal loss: D and/or V, Intestinal obstruction, Fistulae, Sweating, Burns 'third spacing'
- Hypothyroidism, Adrenal insufficiency, SIADH, Drugs (e.g. carbamazepine)
- Water intoxication, Psychogenic polydipsia
- Renal failure
- Heart failure, liver failure/cirrhosis, Nephrotic syndrome, Excessive use of normal saline in acute illness or post-operatively

Treatment:
- Isotonic saline
- Water restriction
- Water restriction + diuretics

TBW = total body water, TBNa+ = total body sodium, D and/or V = diarrhoea or vomiting
SIADH = serum inappropriate antidiuretic hormone

Figure 47f Clinical assessment and treatment of hypernatraemia

Hypernatraemia serum [Na$^+$] >145 mmol/L

Measure serum [Na$^+$]

Assess clinical volume status (TBW + TBNa$^+$):
- Hypovolaemia (TBW↓, TBNa$^+$↓↓)
- Euvolaemia (TBW↓, TBNa$^+$ normal)
- Hypervolaemia (TBW↑, TBNa$^+$↑↑↑)

Measure urine [Na$^+$]:
- >20 mmol/L / <20 mmol/L (Hypovolaemia)
- Variable / Variable (Euvolaemia)
- >20 mmol/L / <20 mmol/L (Hypervolaemia)

Underlying problem:
- Renal loss: Diuretics, Na$^+$-losing nephropathy, Osmotic diuresis; Addison's disease
- Extra-renal loss: D and/or V, Sweating/burns, Respiratory loss
- Renal water loss
- Extra-renal water loss: Insensible loss in sweat + breath, impaired thirst (hypothalamic disease)
  - ↓ADH Central DI
  - ↑ADH Nephrogenic DI
- Iatrogenic, Hypertonic saline or tube feeding, Excessive salt ingestion
- Excess mineralocorticoid activity

Treatment:
- Isotonic saline and water or hypotonic saline
- Water administration and specific therapies
- Water replacement + diuretics

TBW = total body water, TBNa$^+$ = total body sodium, ADH = antidiuretic hormone,
DI = diabetes insipidus, D and/or V = diarrhoea and/or vomiting

Figure 47d SIADH diagnostic criteria

1. Decreased serum osmolality (<270 mOsm/kg H$_2$O)
2. Inappropriately concentrated urine (>100 mOsm/kg H$_2$O)
3. Elevated urinary Na$^+$
4. Euvolaemia
5. No other cause
   - No adrenal, pituitary, thyroid disease
   - No renal insufficiency
   - No diuretic use

Figure 47e Common causes of SIADH

Infection
- Pneumonia, meningitis, COPD

Neoplastic causes
- Lung cancer (most common), prostate
- GI tract, haematological, brain

Drugs
- Carbamazepine (↑ADH release)
- Cyclophosphamide (↑ADH action)

CNS causes
- Stroke, neoplasia, infection

Idiopathic

Post-operative pain

Figure 47g Causes of hypokalaemia (+ = common)

1. **Reduced intake**
   - Poor nutrition (e.g. fasting, anorexia nervosa)
2. **Increased output**
   Gastrointestinal loss$^+$
   - Vomiting, diarrhoea, fistulae,
   - Laxatives, long ileal loop, rectal villous adenoma
   Drugs loss$^+$
   - Diuretics, high dose penicillin
   Renal loss
   - Metabolic acidosis, metabolic alkalosis,
   - Mineralocorticoid excesses (e.g. steroid therapy, ectopic ACTH, Cushing's syndrome)
   - Primary hyperaldosteronism (Conn's syndrome) due to adrenal adenoma/carcinoma
   - Secondary hyperaldosteronism (e.g. hypertension, vomiting, heart failure, renal artery stenosis)
   - Hypercalcaemia, magnesium deficiency
   Renal tubular syndrome loss
   - Renal tubular acidosis, Bartter's or Fanconi syndrome
3. **Hypokalaemia with K$^+$ deficiency**
   - Intravenous insulin, β-sympathomimetic drugs, respiratory alkalosis, familial periodic paralysis, myeloproliferation

Figure 47h ECG changes with serum K$^+$ concentration

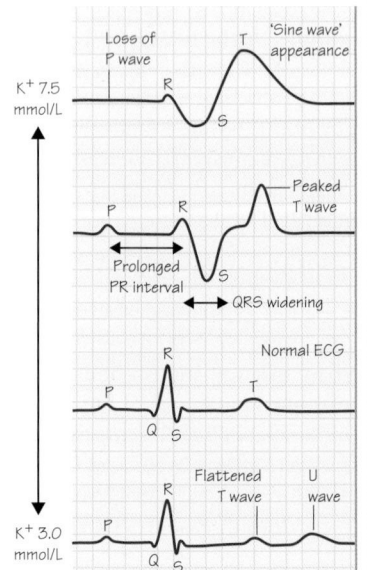

K$^+$ 7.5 mmol/L — Loss of P wave — 'Sine wave' appearance

Peaked T wave — Prolonged PR interval — QRS widening

Normal ECG

K$^+$ 3.0 mmol/L — Flattened T wave — U wave

Critical Care Medicine at a Glance, Third Edition. Richard Leach. © 2014 John Wiley & Sons, Ltd. Published 2014 by John Wiley & Sons, Ltd.

Hyponatraemia

Definition: a serum sodium (Na^+) concentration ($[Na^+]$) < 130 mmol/L. It affects 5–15% of hospital and >30% of elderly patients. Most hyponatraemia (Figures 47a, 47b) is closely linked to fluid balance with excess water relative to Na^+ in extracellular fluid (ECF). Cause and treatment are determined from volume status and urinary Na^+ (> or< 20 mmol/L; Figure 47b). Total body water (TBW) and Na^+ ($TBNa^+$) may be:

- **Increased (hypervolaemia)** (marked ↑TBW; moderate ↑$TBNa^+$) with peripheral oedema (i.e. ↑ECF). Figure 47b illustrates causes.
- **Normal (euvolaemia)** (modest ↑TBW; normal $TBNa^+$) with a slight ECF increase. Excessive use of 5% dextrose (or low Na^+) fluids is the most common cause.
- **Decreased (hypovolaemia)** (normal or ↓TBW; markedly ↓$TBNa^+$) associated with dehydration (↓ECF). Causes are **extra-renal** or **renal** (Figure 47b).

Clinical presentation depends on speed of onset, age and sex.
- **Acute onset hyponatraemia** (i.e. hours) reduces ECF osmolality causing water to move into cells. This intracellular oedema disrupts function, especially in the brain. Rapid correction is required to prevent confusion, coma and injury.
- **Chronic onset hyponatraemia** (i.e. days) allows cells to compensate (i.e. pump Na^+/other ions into ECF) preventing intracellular oedema. Consequently, moderate hyponatraemia ($[Na^+]$ 120–125 mmol/L) may be asymptomatic. Rapid correction of chronic hyponatraemia reverses the osmotic gradient and intracellular water moves into the ECF. This causes cell dehydration and central pontine demyelinolysis (brainstem neurone demyelination) with encephalopathy, quadriplegia and cranial nerve palsies.
- **Females** are more susceptible because oestrogen inhibits Na^+/K^+ ATPase pumps. Thus, sex hormone treatments (e.g. prostatic cancer) may cause hyponatraemia.

Clinical features (Figure 47c) of a $[Na^+]$ < 125 mmol/L include lethargy, agitation, confusion, muscle cramps, anorexia, nausea, altered tendon reflexes and, occasionally, raised intracranial pressure (ICP) with papilloedema, fits, respiratory depression (±Cheynes–Stokes breathing) and hypothermia.

Management: treat the cause (e.g. stop diuretics).
- **Acute-onset hyponatraemia** is corrected relatively rapidly. In acute hypovolaemic hyponatraemia, give intravenous (i.v.) normal (0.9%) saline and increase $[Na^+]$ by ~1 mmol/L/hr until $[Na^+]$ > 125 mmol/L. Measure $[Na^+]$ and $[K^+]$ frequently. Consider i.v. mannitol (100 ml 20%) for raised ICP.
- **Chronic hyponatraemia** is corrected slowly to prevent CPD (e.g. raise $[Na^+]$ by <0.5 mmol/L/hr).
- **Euvolaemic hyponatraemia** may not need treatment if asymptomatic. Restrict fluid intake if symptomatic.
- **Hypervolaemic hyponatraemia** is treated by restricting water intake (±diuretic therapy).

Syndrome of inappropriate antidiuretic hormone (SIADH) occurs when antidiuretic hormone (ADH) is raised (e.g. ectopic tumour release) despite a low plasma osmolality. Figures 47d and 47e list diagnostic criteria and causes. Treat the cause and restrict fluid. Demeclocycline, which inhibits renal ADH actions (i.e. tubular water reabsorption), may be needed.

Hypernatraemia

Definition: a $[Na^+]$ > 145 mmol/L, usually due to water deficiency. Common causes are impaired water intake (e.g. older people, infants) and hyperosmolar diabetic coma. Thirst is the main symptom but if $[Na^+]$ is >155 mmol/L, lethargy, irritability, fits, coma and death may occur. Figure 47f illustrates the assessment, causes and therapies for hypernatraemia.

Management: treat the cause and correct $[Na^+]$ cautiously (i.e. <0.5 mmol/L/hr) to prevent CPD. Monitor fluid balance and electrolytes closely. Hypovolaemic patients need 0.9% saline until haemodynamically stable and then 5% dextrose to correct $[Na^+]$. Hypervolaemia may require diuretics to remove excess Na^+/water.

Hypokalaemia

Definition: a serum potassium (K^+) concentration ($[K^+]$) < 3.5 mmol/L (normal 3.5–5.5 mmol/L). Average K^+ intake is ~40–70 mmol/day and total body K^+ (TBK^+) is ~3500 mmol, with ~95% intracellular ($[K^+]$ ~155 mmol/L). Thus, a 200 mmol TBK^+ loss only lowers serum $[K^+]$ by ~0.5 mmol/L. In acidosis, intracellular K^+ is displaced by hydrogen ions (H^+) causing hyperkalamia and renal K^+ loss. Rapid correction of acidosis (e.g. during diabetic ketoacidosis) moves K^+ intracellularly and can cause sudden serum hypokalaemia. **Causes** are listed in Figure 47g and include diuretic therapy, acute illness and gastrointestinal loss. Hypokalaemia also follows intracellular K^+ movement during acute illness and after insulin or salbutamol (i.e. β-receptor) therapy.

Clinical features include lethargy, intestinal ileus, metabolic alkalosis (i.e. renal H^+ loss), electrocardiogram (ECG) changes (Figure 47h), tachyarrhythmia and cardiac arrest. Profound weakness (i.e. paralysis, respiratory failure) occurs in severe hypokalaemia (i.e. $[K^+]$ < 2.2 mmol/L), Prolonged hypokalaemia can cause irreversible distal tubule damage and impairs concentrating ability (i.e. causes polyuria). Mild hypokalaemia is usually asymptomatic.

Management: treat the cause. If $[K^+]$ is <3 mmol/L, especially in those at risk of arrhythmias, give i.v. potassium chloride at a maximum rate of 20 mmol/hr. Give i.v. fluids with high K^+ concentrations (>20 mmol/L) centrally to avoid peripheral vein damage. Consider oral replacement (80–120 mg daily) if $[K^+]$ > 3–3.5 mmol/L unless the patient is 'nil-by-mouth' or vomiting.

Hyperkalaemia

Renal impairment is the main cause of hyperkalaemia (i.e. impaired K^+ excretion) and exacerbates other causes including mineralocorticoid deficiency (e.g. Addison's disease), K^+ retaining diuretics (e.g. amiloride), spironolactone and angiotensin-converting enzyme inhibitors. Potassium release also follows cell destruction (e.g. rhabdomyolysis). Hyperkalaemia is often asymptomatic but may cause muscle weakness. Figure 47h illustrates ECG changes.

Management: severe hyperkalaemia (i.e. $[K^+]$ > 6.9 mmol/L or ECG changes) is an emergency. Immediately lower $[K^+]$ with i.v. glucose and insulin (50 mls 50% glucose and 10U short-acting insulin), which moves K^+ intracellularly or use i.v. calcium gluconate (10 mls of 10% over 2 min) to stabilize the myocardium. Oral K^+ binding resin, calcium resonium, lowers $[K^+]$ in the short term but dialysis may be required for ongoing renal failure. In mild hyperkalaemia (i.e. $[K^+]$ < 6 mmol/L), reduce oral intake and stop K^+-retaining drugs.

48 Electrolyte disturbances: calcium

Figure 48a Hypocalcaemia

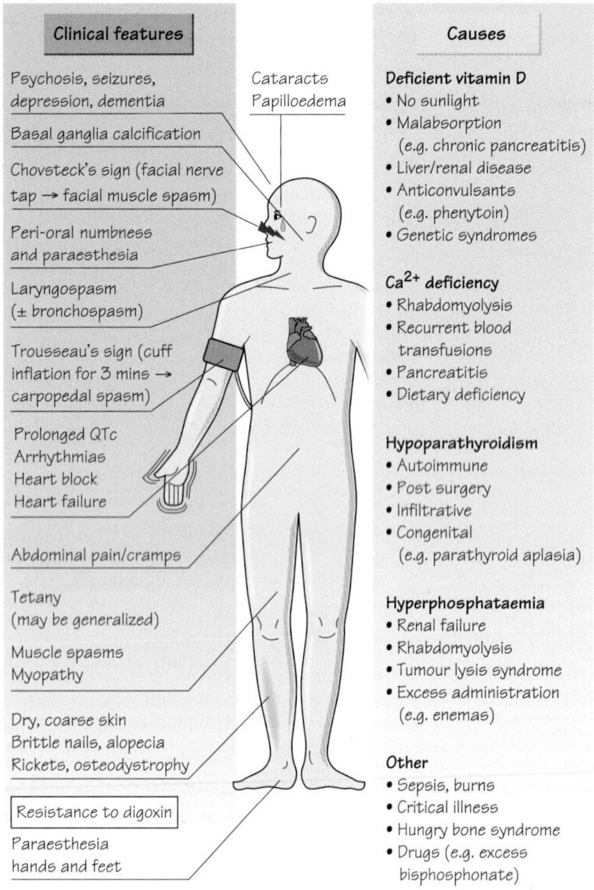

Clinical features

Psychosis, seizures, depression, dementia

Basal ganglia calcification

Chovsteck's sign (facial nerve tap → facial muscle spasm)

Peri-oral numbness and paraesthesia

Laryngospasm (± bronchospasm)

Trousseau's sign (cuff inflation for 3 mins → carpopedal spasm)

Prolonged QTc
Arrhythmias
Heart block
Heart failure

Abdominal pain/cramps

Tetany (may be generalized)

Muscle spasms
Myopathy

Dry, coarse skin
Brittle nails, alopecia
Rickets, osteodystrophy

Resistance to digoxin

Paraesthesia hands and feet

Cataracts
Papilloedema

Causes

Deficient vitamin D
• No sunlight
• Malabsorption (e.g. chronic pancreatitis)
• Liver/renal disease
• Anticonvulsants (e.g. phenytoin)
• Genetic syndromes

Ca^{2+} deficiency
• Rhabdomyolysis
• Recurrent blood transfusions
• Pancreatitis
• Dietary deficiency

Hypoparathyroidism
• Autoimmune
• Post surgery
• Infiltrative
• Congenital (e.g. parathyroid aplasia)

Hyperphosphataemia
• Renal failure
• Rhabdomyolysis
• Tumour lysis syndrome
• Excess administration (e.g. enemas)

Other
• Sepsis, burns
• Critical illness
• Hungry bone syndrome
• Drugs (e.g. excess bisphosphonate)

Figure 48b Hypercalcaemia

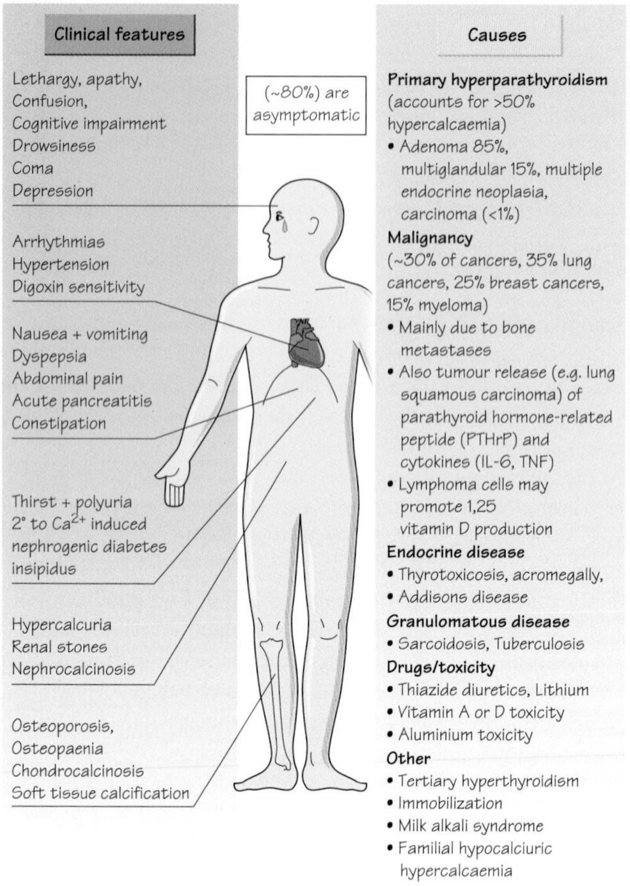

Clinical features

Lethargy, apathy,
Confusion,
Cognitive impairment
Drowsiness
Coma
Depression

Arrhythmias
Hypertension
Digoxin sensitivity

Nausea + vomiting
Dyspepsia
Abdominal pain
Acute pancreatitis
Constipation

Thirst + polyuria
2° to Ca^{2+} induced nephrogenic diabetes insipidus

Hypercalcuria
Renal stones
Nephrocalcinosis

Osteoporosis,
Osteopaenia
Chondrocalcinosis
Soft tissue calcification

(~80%) are asymptomatic

Causes

Primary hyperparathyroidism (accounts for >50% hypercalcaemia)
• Adenoma 85%, multiglandular 15%, multiple endocrine neoplasia, carcinoma (<1%)

Malignancy (~30% of cancers, 35% lung cancers, 25% breast cancers, 15% myeloma)
• Mainly due to bone metastases
• Also tumour release (e.g. lung squamous carcinoma) of parathyroid hormone-related peptide (PTHrP) and cytokines (IL-6, TNF)
• Lymphoma cells may promote 1,25 vitamin D production

Endocrine disease
• Thyrotoxicosis, acromegaly,
• Addisons disease

Granulomatous disease
• Sarcoidosis, Tuberculosis

Drugs/toxicity
• Thiazide diuretics, Lithium
• Vitamin A or D toxicity
• Aluminium toxicity

Other
• Tertiary hyperthyroidism
• Immobilization
• Milk alkali syndrome
• Familial hypocalciuric hypercalcaemia

Pearl of wisdom
Primary hyperparathyroidism is the most common cause of hypercalcaemia. About 80% of cases are due to a single parathyroid adenoma

Calcium

Calcium (Ca^{2+}) is the most abundant mineral in the body. About 98% is stored in bone. Plasma Ca^{2+} (2.25–2.65 mmol/L) is bound to albumin (±other proteins; ~40%), anions (e.g. bicarbonate; ~10%) or is in the free, ionized, physiologically active form (~50%). It is important for muscle contraction (±relaxation), skeletal and dental structure, clotting, cell membrane integrity, nerve transmission and regulation of cell signalling, hormone secretion and enzyme activity.

Calcium homeostasis

The gastrointestinal (GI) tract, bone and kidneys are key organs, and with parathyroid hormone (PTH) and 1,25-(OH)$_2$ vitamin D (1,25 vitamin D), maintain plasma calcium concentration ([Ca^{2+}])

in a narrow range (i.e. <2% variability). PTH secretion depends on serum magnesium concentration ([Mg^{2+}]); hypomagnesaemia inhibits PTH release even in severe hypocalcaemia.
• The GI tract normally absorbs ~40% (~10 mmol) of daily dietary Ca^{2+} intake but can increase this as required. Ca^{2+} uptake is active or passive. Following binding to calbindin, active transport is by Na$^+$/Ca^{2+}-ATPase and Na$^+$/Ca^{2+} exchangers, saturatable processes regulated by 1,25 vitamin D. Passive absorption is down a concentration gradient between the gut lumen and serosal surfaces. Absorption is inhibited by drugs (e.g. theophyllines), citrates and phytates.
• In the kidney, the proximal convoluted tubule (PCT) reabsorbs ~65% of filtered Ca^{2+}, a process closely linked to sodium and water balance, whereas PTH regulates reabsorption by the Loop

of Henle (~25%) and distal convoluted tubule (DCT; ~10%). PTH also stimulates renal production of 1,25 vitamin D, which increases intestinal Ca^{2+} and phosphate (PO^{4-}) absorption.

- Bone metabolism is regulated by PTH and 1,25 vitamin D. Normally bone formation and resorption are in balance with no net movement of Ca^{2+}. Osteoclastic activity (i.e. bone resorption) is increased by 1,25 vitamin D deficiency or hyperparathyroidism (hyperPTH).

Hypocalcaemia

Definition: a serum Ca^{2+} concentration ($[Ca^{2+}]$) < 1.75 mmol/L defines severe hypocalcaemia.

Clinical features (Figure 48a) depend on the rate of fall and severity of the hypocalcaemia and are worse when hypomagnesaemia and/or alkalosis co-exist. Patients are often relatively asymptomatic but can present with life-threatening features.

- *Acute hypocalcaemia* causes perioral paraesthesia, muscle and abdominal cramps, tetany in muscles supplied by long nerves, seizures, Trousseau's and Chvostek's signs (Figure 48a).
- *Chronic hypocalcaemia* also causes depression, irritability, dementia, movement disorders, papilloedema, prolonged QT interval, syncope (±occasional heart failure or angina), dry/brittle skin, alopecia, rickets, cataracts and basal ganglia calcification. It may be associated with alkalosis, hypokalaemia and hypomagnesaemia.

Causes (Figure 48a):
- *25-(OH)₂ vitamin D deficiency*: due to poor intake (e.g. older people, vegetarians), lack of sunlight, anticonvulsants (e.g. phenytoin), malabsorption (e.g. Crohn's disease, chronic pancreatitis) or loss of vitamin D binding proteins in nephrotic syndrome. *1,25-(OH)₂ vitamin D deficiency* is most commonly associated with renal disease with a glomerular filtration rate (GFR) < 30 mls/min (see later). Inherited disorders (e.g. vitamin D-dependent rickets type I and II due to 1-α-hydroxylase deficiency and end-organ resistance to 1,25 vitamin D respectively) are rare causes.
- *Acute or chronic kidney disease (CKD)* impair renal vitamin D hydroxylation (i.e. formation of 1,25 vitamin D) and promote PO^{4-} retention, which depresses $[Ca^{2+}]$. Secondary hyperPTH follows with osteoclast activation and characteristic bone and X-ray findings in the hands, skull (i.e. pepper-pot) and spine (i.e. rugger jersey). Treatment is with vitamin D and PO^{4-} binders. If untreated, parathyroid hyperplasia with autonomous PTH production causes tertiary hyperPTH and hypercalcaemia.
- *Hyperphospataemia*: due to CKD, rhabdomyolysis, tumour lysis syndrome or excess PO^{4-} absorption.
- *Hypoparathyroidism*: post-parathyroid/thyroid surgery, infiltrative disorders, congenital and pseudohyperparathyroidism. *Idiopathic autoimmune hypoparathyroidism* is rare and associated with vitiligo, parathyroid antibodies and other autoimmune conditions.
- *Other*: severe magnesium deficiency, drugs (e.g. bisphosphonates), acute pancreatitis, sepsis, burns.

Treatment should correct the cause and depends on severity, symptoms and rate of onset.
- *Acute symptomatic hypocalcaemia* ($[Ca^{2+}]$ < 1.75 mmol/L) is initially treated with a 10 ml i.v. bolus of 10% calcium gluconate

with electrocardiogram (ECG) monitoring. This can be followed by an infusion (i.e. 20 mls over 6 hrs) and then oral Ca^{2+} and vitamin D supplements. Treat co-existing hypomagnesaemia, hyperphosphataemia and hypokalaemia cautiously, especially in CKD.
- *Chronic hypocalcaemia* in CKD is treated with vitamin D metabolites (e.g. alphacalcidol) and oral Ca^{2+} supplements to prevent osteomalacia and vascular mineralization due to secondary hyperPTH.

Hypercalcaemia

Definition: a $[Ca^{2+}]$ > 2.6 mmol/L. It may be mild (2.6–3 mmol/L), moderate (3–3.5 mmol/L) or severe (>3.5 mmol/L). The key factors in diagnosis are PTH level, clinical picture and biochemical tests. Hypercalcaemia affects 5–50/10 000 population.

Causes (Figure 48b):
- *Primary hyperPTH* (85% adenoma; 15% multiglandular; rarely multiple endocrine neoplasia): is the most common cause (>50%) but over half are asymptomatic and only require observation. Female to male ratio is 2:1 and >90% of cases are >50 years old. PTH is raised. Definitive treatment involves surgical resection of adenomas. Treat associated transient post-operative hypocalcaemia with Ca^{2+} and vitamin D supplements.
- *Malignancy*: ~30% of cancers are associated with hypercalcaemia, usually due to bony metastases but also due to tumour release of PTH-related peptides (PTHrH) or cytokines. PTH levels are low.
- *Sarcoidosis and other granulomatous disease* cause steroid-sensitive hypercalcaemia.
- *Other causes* include drugs (e.g. thiazide diuretics), Vitamin A or D toxicity, tertiary hyperPTH in chronic renal failure (CRF), endocrine disease (e.g. thyrotoxicosis, acromegaly), familial hypocalciuric hypercalcaemia, milk alkali syndrome, aluminium toxicity and immobility.

Clinical features (Figure 48b) depend on $[Ca^{2+}]$ and rapidity of onset. Most cases are asymptomatic. Mild and moderate cases experience lethargy, depression, nausea, abdominal discomfort, constipation, thirst and polyuria. Acute, severe hypercalcaemia causes confusion, drowsiness and coma. Arrhythmias, hypertension and acute pancreatitis also occur. Chronic hypercalcaemia is associated with renal stone and bone disease.

Management: treatment decisions depend on symptoms, hypercalcaemia severity (>3 mmol/L), rate of onset, chronicity and the underlying cause, which should be corrected when possible.
- *Acute, symptomatic hypercalcaemia* (i.e. Ca^{2+} > 3.5 mmol/L) is a medical emergency. Initially rehydrate with normal (0.9%) saline (4 L over 24 h). Give loop diuretics when adequately hydrated (this reduces $[Ca^{2+}]$ by ~0.5 mmol/L). Bisphosphonates (i.v.) are effective in most cases (e.g. pamidronate 30–90 mg over 2–4 h) but use with care in CRF. Give steroids in haematological malignancies (e.g. myeloma) and granulomatous disorders. Calcitonin is only briefly effective due to tachyphylaxsis but may help in Paget's disease.
- *Chronic hypercalcaemia*: ensure adequate hydration and avoid thiazide diuretics. Use non-Ca^{2+} based phosphate binders in CRF and treat tertiary hyperPTH (i.e parathyroidectomy or cincalcet [to reduce PTH]).

49 Electrolyte disturbances: magnesium and phosphate

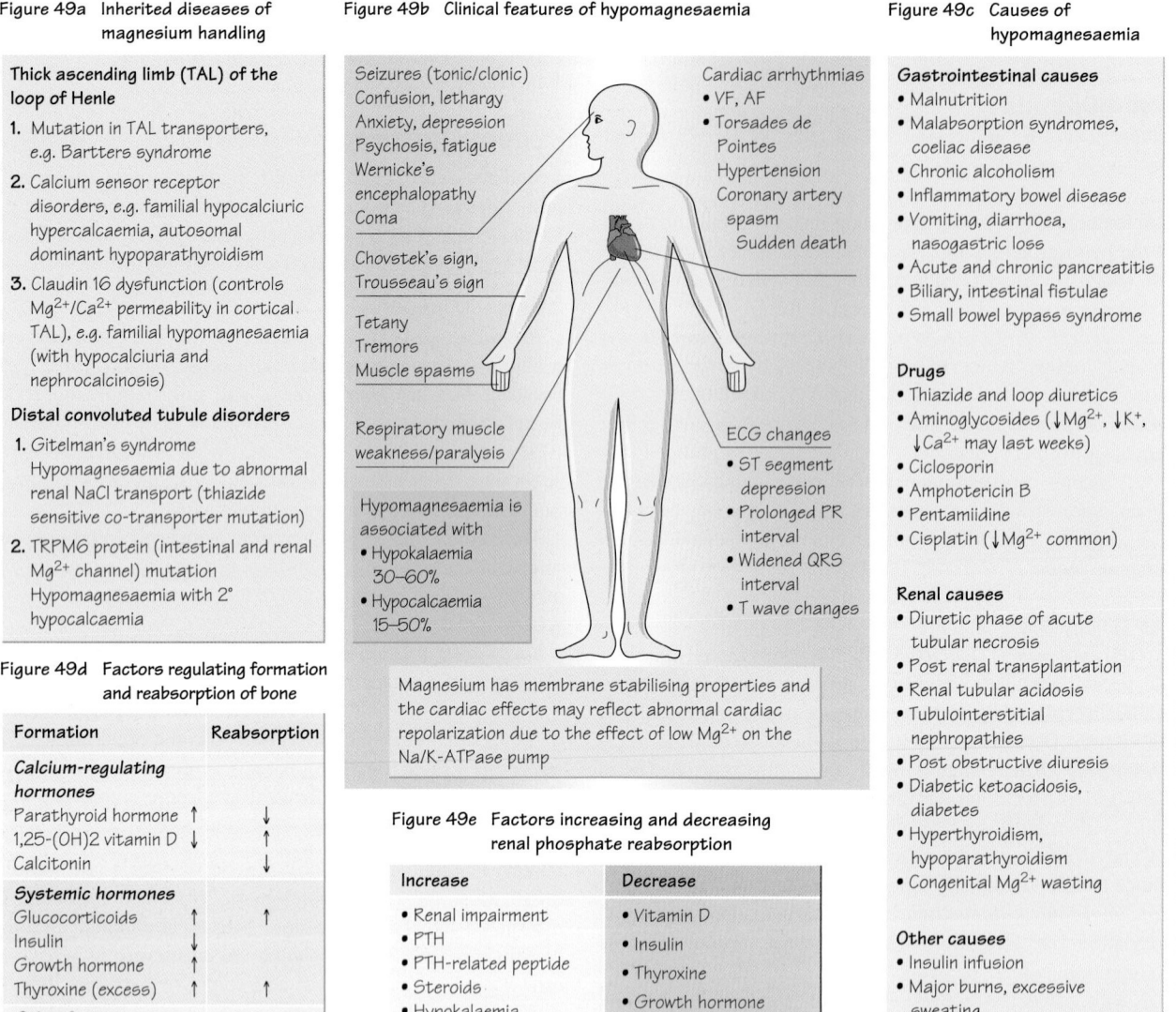

Figure 49a Inherited diseases of magnesium handling

Thick ascending limb (TAL) of the loop of Henle

1. Mutation in TAL transporters, e.g. Bartters syndrome
2. Calcium sensor receptor disorders, e.g. familial hypocalciuric hypercalcaemia, autosomal dominant hypoparathyroidism
3. Claudin 16 dysfunction (controls Mg^{2+}/Ca^{2+} permeability in cortical TAL), e.g. familial hypomagnesaemia (with hypocalciuria and nephrocalcinosis)

Distal convoluted tubule disorders

1. Gitelman's syndrome Hypomagnesaemia due to abnormal renal NaCl transport (thiazide sensitive co-transporter mutation)
2. TRPM6 protein (intestinal and renal Mg^{2+} channel) mutation Hypomagnesaemia with 2° hypocalcaemia

Figure 49b Clinical features of hypomagnesaemia

Seizures (tonic/clonic)
Confusion, lethargy
Anxiety, depression
Psychosis, fatigue
Wernicke's encephalopathy
Coma

Chovstek's sign, Trousseau's sign

Tetany
Tremors
Muscle spasms

Respiratory muscle weakness/paralysis

Hypomagnesaemia is associated with
• Hypokalaemia 30–60%
• Hypocalcaemia 15–50%

Cardiac arrhythmias
• VF, AF
• Torsades de Pointes
Hypertension
Coronary artery spasm
   Sudden death

ECG changes
• ST segment depression
• Prolonged PR interval
• Widened QRS interval
• T wave changes

Magnesium has membrane stabilising properties and the cardiac effects may reflect abnormal cardiac repolarization due to the effect of low Mg^{2+} on the Na/K-ATPase pump

Figure 49c Causes of hypomagnesaemia

Gastrointestinal causes
• Malnutrition
• Malabsorption syndromes, coeliac disease
• Chronic alcoholism
• Inflammatory bowel disease
• Vomiting, diarrhoea, nasogastric loss
• Acute and chronic pancreatitis
• Biliary, intestinal fistulae
• Small bowel bypass syndrome

Drugs
• Thiazide and loop diuretics
• Aminoglycosides ($\downarrow Mg^{2+}$, $\downarrow K^+$, $\downarrow Ca^{2+}$ may last weeks)
• Ciclosporin
• Amphotericin B
• Pentamiidine
• Cisplatin ($\downarrow Mg^{2+}$ common)

Renal causes
• Diuretic phase of acute tubular necrosis
• Post renal transplantation
• Renal tubular acidosis
• Tubulointerstitial nephropathies
• Post obstructive diuresis
• Diabetic ketoacidosis, diabetes
• Hyperthyroidism, hypoparathyroidism
• Congenital Mg^{2+} wasting

Other causes
• Insulin infusion
• Major burns, excessive sweating
• Hungry bone syndrome after parathyroidectomy
• Inappropriate ADH secretion

Figure 49d Factors regulating formation and reabsorption of bone

Formation		Reabsorption
Calcium-regulating hormones		
Parathyroid hormone	↑	↓
1,25-(OH)2 vitamin D	↓	↑
Calcitonin		↓
Systemic hormones		
Glucocorticoids	↑	↑
Insulin	↓	
Growth hormone	↑	
Thyroxine (excess)	↑	↑
Other factors		
Interleukin-1	↑	
Interleukin-6		↓
PTHrP	↑	↑

Figure 49e Factors increasing and decreasing renal phosphate reabsorption

Increase	Decrease
• Renal impairment	• Vitamin D
• PTH	• Insulin
• PTH-related peptide	• Thyroxine
• Steroids	• Growth hormone
• Hypokalaemia	• Low phosphate intake
• Volume expansion	• High calcium intake
• Chronic hypocalcaemia	

Pearl of wisdom

Mortality is increased fourfold in severe hypomagnesaemia (serum Mg^{2+} <0.3 mmol/L)

Magnesium

Magnesium (Mg^{2+}), the second most abundant intracellular cation, is stored in muscle, bone and soft tissues with <1% in extracellular fluid (ECF). Serum Mg^{2+} concentration ($[Mg^{2+}]$) is 0.7–1 mmol/L, with ~50% in the physiologically active, ionized form and ~50% bound to albumin or serum anions (e.g. phosphate). 'Total' $[Mg^{2+}]$ must be corrected for serum albumin.

Mg^{2+}, Ca^{2+} and phosphate homeostasis are closely linked. Mg^{2+} modulates functions dependent on intracellular Ca^{2+} (e.g. muscle contraction, insulin release) and is an essential co-factor in many clotting, neuromuscular and enzyme systems. The kidneys reab-

sorb ~95% of filtered Mg^{2+}, mainly in the ascending limb of the loop of Henle, but is inhibited by loop diuretics, osmotic diuresis, hypercalcaemia or saline infusions. Renal and diarrhoeal diseases cause significant Mg^{2+} loss. Figure 49a lists inherited disorders of Mg^{2+} handling.

Hypomagnesaemia

Definition: a $[Mg^{2+}]$ < 0.7 mmol/L. However, total body Mg^{2+} stores may be depleted by >20% despite a normal $[Mg^{2+}]$. Hypomagnesaemia occurs in chronic illness, elderly people (~30%), alcoholics (~30%), post-operatively, and those with refractory hypokalaemia or hypocalcaemia. It is severe ($[Mg^{2+}]$ <

0.5 mmol/L) in ~10% of hospital and ~65% of critically ill patients. Figure 49c lists causes.

Clinical features (Figure 49b): hypomagnesaemia is usually asymptomatic but can cause cardiac, muscular or neurological dysfunction. Many cases are associated with hypokalaemia (~60%) and/or hypocalaemia (~15–50%). A $[Mg^{2+}]$ of 0.5–0.7 mmol/L causes neuromuscular irritability and tremors; a $[Mg^{2+}] <$ 0.5 mmol/L can cause fits, tetany, arrhythmias and sudden death. Electrocardiogram (ECG) changes mimic hypokalaemia (i.e. prolonged PR interval, QRS complex widening, ST depression). Mg^{2+} has membrane-stabilizing properties and some arrhythmias only respond to Mg^{2+} replacement (e.g. Torsade de Pointes). Low $[Mg^{2+}]$ also causes hypertension, angina, muscle weakness, confusion, vertical nystagmus, Wernicke's encephalopathy and coma.

Treatment depends on cause and symptom severity. Use oral Mg^{2+} ~10–30 mmol/day if asymptomatic. Seizures, tetany and ventricular arrhythmias are treated with 4–8 mmol Mg^{2+} intravenously (i.v.) over 10–30 min, followed by an Mg^{2+} infusion (12–90 mmol) over 24 hours to maintain $[Mg^{2+}] > 0.5$ mmol/L. Monitor cardiac function. In renal failure, reduce infusions by ~50%. Severe deficiencies may need up to 160 mmol Mg^{2+} over ~5 days. Treat low $[K^+]$ and $[Ca^{2+}]$ as necessary. Amiloride reduces diuretic-induced and renal Mg^{2+} loss due to nephrotoxicity (e.g. cisplatin).

Hypermagnesaemia

Definition: a $[Mg^{2+}] > 1.0$ mmol/L is uncommon because the kidneys can excrete >95% of filtered Mg^{2+} if necessary. Consequently, hypermagnesaemia is common in renal impairment (glomerular filtration rate [GFR] <30 mls/min), particularly if Mg^{2+} intake is raised (e.g. laxatives, enemas, antacids). Hypermagnesiaemia also occurs in hypothyroidism, Addison's disease, rhabdomyolysis, lithium therapy and familial hypocalciuric hypercalcaemia.

Clinical features: a $[Mg^{2+}] < 2.0$ mmol/L is usually asymptomatic. Higher levels cause cardiovascular, metabolic and neuromuscular toxicity. Lethargy, nausea, vomiting and flushing occur at 2.0–2.9 mmol/L; bradycardia, hypotension, ECG changes (e.g. prolonged PR/QT intervals, widened QRS) and tendon reflex suppression between 2.0–5.0 mmol/L and coma, apnoea, ventricular arrhythmias, cardiac arrest and paralysis at >5 mmol/L. Parasympathetic inhibition (e.g. ileus, urinary retention, heart block), hyperkalaemia and mild hypocalcaemia also occur.

Treatment: avoid further Mg^{2+} administration (e.g. laxatives). Treat cardiovascular or respiratory toxicity with calcium gluconate (i.e. 10 mls of 10% solution i.v. over 10 min) to antagonize the effects of hypermagnesaemia. Normal saline increases renal Mg^{2+} excretion. Low Mg^{2+} dialysate reduces $[Mg^{2+}]$ by up to 50% in 4 hours during renal dialysis. Monitor $[K^+]$.

Phosphate

Phosphate (PO^{4-}), the most abundant intracellular anion, is mainly in bone and teeth as hydroxyapatite (~80%) and viscera and skeletal muscle (~20%). Phosphate is vital for adenosine triphosphate (ATP) production, oxyhaemoglobin binding, bone mineralization, buffering, signalling pathways, and in phospholipids, nucleoproteins and lipid membranes. Normal serum phosphate concentration ($[PO^{4-}]$) is 0.8–1.4 mmol/L.

Phosphorus is ubiquitous in food and ~40 mmol is absorbed daily by sodium phosphate (NaPi) co-transporters in the upper intestine. Absorption is increased by vitamin D, low serum PO^{4-} and raised parathyroid hormone (PTH). The kidneys control PO^{4-} homeostasis. Proximal tubule NaPi co-transporters reabsorb 80–95% of filtered PO^{4-}. Figure 49e illustrates factors altering renal PO^{4-} reabsorption. Figure 49d illustrates causes of bone formation and resorption.

Hypophosphataemia

A $[PO^{4-}] < 0.3$ mmol/L is considered severe. Patients at risk of low $[PO^{4-}]$ include those with malnutrition, sepsis, trauma, diabetic ketoacidosis and alcohol dependency.

Causes include vitamin D deficiency, raised PTH (or parathyroid-related peptide [PTHrP] release from tumours), volume expansion, diuretics, steroid excess, malabsorption, vomiting, PO^{4-} binding antacids, renal problems (e.g. failure, Fanconi syndrome) and genetic defects (e.g. autosomal dominant hypophosphataemic rickets). Internal redistribution, rather than deficiency, causes hypophosphataemia in treated diabetic ketoacidosis, respiratory alkalosis, acute leukaemia or refeeding syndrome.

Clinical features are due to impaired tissue oxygen delivery (increased affinity of haemoglobin for oxygen) and reduced ATP. Musculoskeletal effects include weakness, proximal myopathy, diaphragmatic weakness and osteomalacia (±bone pain). Acute onset may cause rhabdomyolysis, especially in malnourished or alcoholic patients, reduced cardiac contractility and impaired platelet function. Neurological features include paraesthesia, confusion, metabolic encephalopathy, polyneuropathy (e.g. like Guillain–Barré syndrome), seizures and coma. Renal consequences include glycosuria, hypercalcuria (increased bone turnover), Mg^{2+} excretion and hyperchloraemic metabolic acidosis.

Treatment depends on cause. In severe or symptomatic hypophosphataemia treatment aims to improve respiratory muscle strength and DO_2 (e.g. in critical illness). Give sodium phosphate infusions (10–20 mmol over 1–2 hours: max dose 60 mmol/24 h). Monitor $[Ca^{2+}]$, $[K^+]$ and $[Mg^{2+}]$ to avoid calcium precipitation, hypocalcaemia, arrhythmias and renal impairment. Consider oral supplements (~30 mmol/day) when ($[PO^{4-}]) > 0.6$ mmol/L.

Refeeding syndrome occurs 3–4 days after restarting feed in the malnourished. Initially $[PO^{4-}]$ is normal despite significant PO^{4-} depletion. Increased insulin secretion stimulates cellular uptake of PO^{4-}, K^+ and Mg^{2+} and may cause severe hypophosphataemia. Patients at risk include those with no food intake for >10 days, weight loss >15% and a body mass index (BMI) < 18 kg/m^2. In those at risk, start nutrition (oral or i.v.) at 5–10/kcal/kg/day and gradually increase over 7 days. Symptoms may develop at $[PO^{4-}]$ < 0.5 mmol/L, requiring i.v. phosphate therapy.

Hyperphosphataemia

Hyperphosphataemia is common in chronic kidney disease (CKD) and almost universal when GFR is <30 ml/min. Other causes include rhabdomyolysis, tumour lysis, hypoparathyroidism, acromegaly, thyrotoxicosis, steroid deficiency, excess intake (e.g. PO^{4-} absorption in enemas) and metabolic or respiratory acidosis.

Clinical features: symptoms are limited to those of hypocalcaemia. Elevation of $[Ca^{2+}] \times [PO^{4-}]$ product causes hypertension and ectopic calcification in blood vessels, myocardium and heart valves. Calcium deposition in subcutaneous and joint tissue causes painful necrosis. Asymptomatic corneal calcification and conjunctivitis also occur. Secondary hyperparathyroidism follows persistent hyperphosphataemia.

Treatment depends on severity and onset. ***Acute, severe hyperphosphataemia*** may be life-threatening when associated with hypocalcaemia. If renal function is intact, 0.9% saline infusion increases phosphate excretion. Consider haemodialysis in renal impairment or symptomatic hypocalaemia. ***Chronic hyperphosphataemia*** occurs in CKD. Restrict dietary PO^{4-} and Ca^{2+} intake. Maintain the $[Ca^{2+}] \times [PO^{4-}]$ product at <4.2 mmol²/L². Oral PO^{4-} binders prevent absorption and choice depends on the Ca^{2+} requirements. Measure PTH every 3 months in stage 5 CKD and keep PTH levels <2–4 times normal.

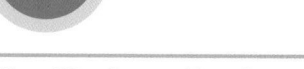

50 Diabetic emergencies

Figure 50a   Causes of hypoglycaemia

1. Usually related to diabetic therapy
Inadequate food intake, excessive exercise, accidental or deliberate overdose, prolonged drug effect (e.g. long-acting oral hypoglycaemics; chlorpropamide), poor clearance in renal failure (e.g. insulin)

2. General causes
Starvation, rebound hypoglycaemia after a large meal, alcohol, renal and liver disease, systemic diseases (e.g. sepsis, infection, hypothermia), endocrine disease (e.g. hypopituitarism, adrenal failure), poisoning or drug therapy (e.g. salicylate) and rare insulin secreting tumours (e.g. insulinomas) or insulin-like growth factor II producing tumours (e.g. pleural fibromas)

Figure 50b   Clinical features of hypoglycaemia

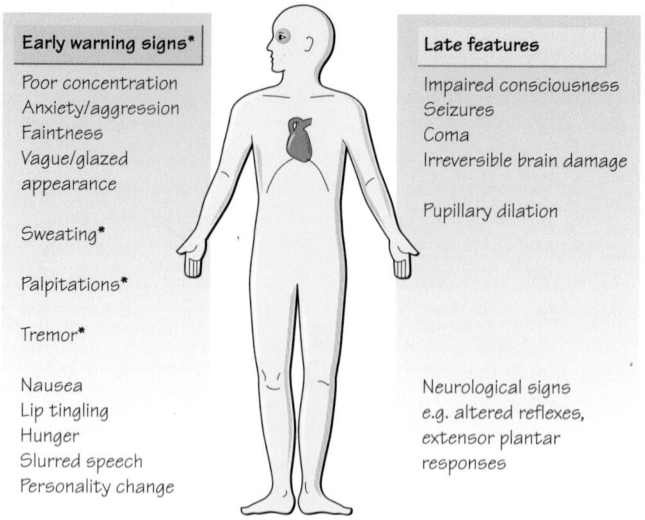

Early warning signs*
Poor concentration
Anxiety/aggression
Faintness
Vague/glazed appearance

Sweating*

Palpitations*

Tremor*

Nausea
Lip tingling
Hunger
Slurred speech
Personality change

Late features
Impaired consciousness
Seizures
Coma
Irreversible brain damage

Pupillary dilation

Neurological signs
e.g. altered reflexes, extensor plantar responses

* Early adrenergic signs may be lost in long-standing DM

Figure 50c   Ketogenesis in DKA

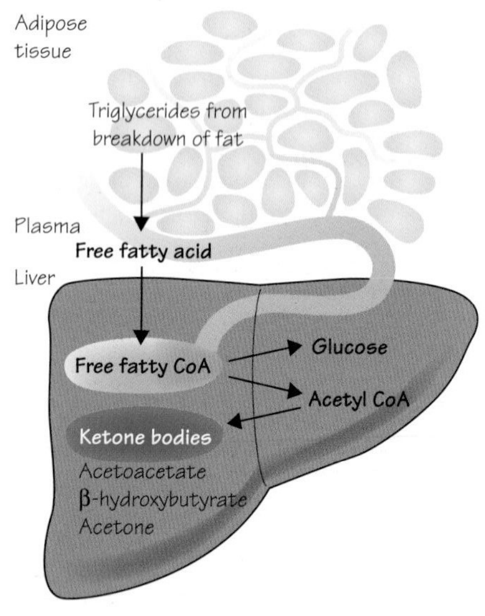

Adipose tissue

Triglycerides from breakdown of fat

Plasma
Liver

Free fatty acid

Free fatty CoA → Glucose

→ Acetyl CoA

Ketone bodies
Acetoacetate
β-hydroxybutyrate
Acetone

Figure 50e   Clinical features of DKA and investigations

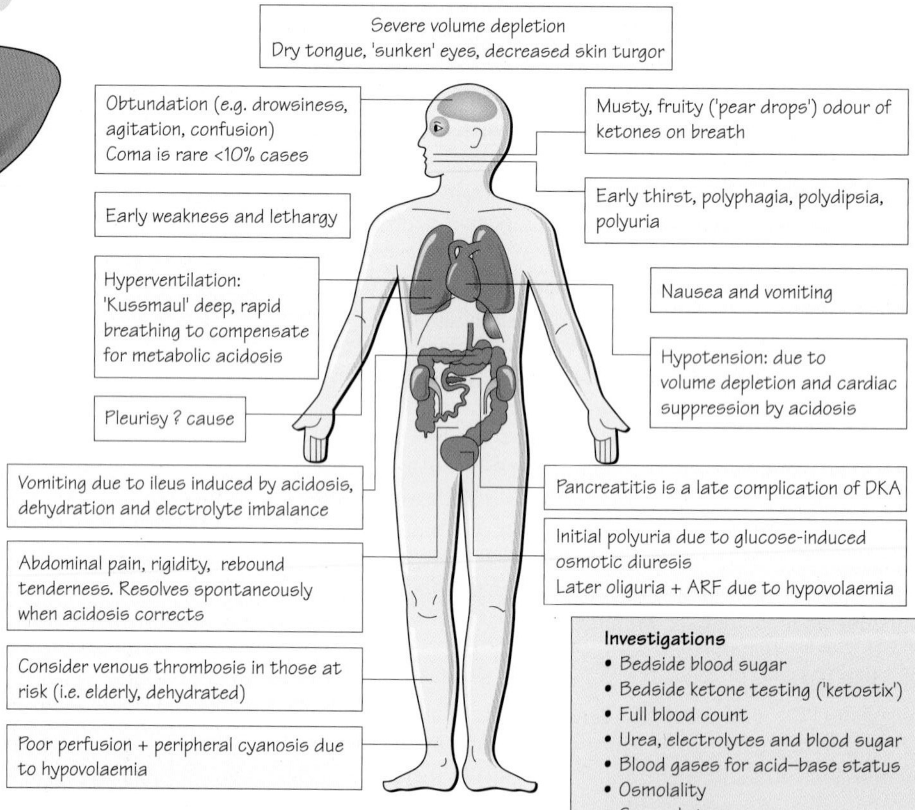

Severe volume depletion
Dry tongue, 'sunken' eyes, decreased skin turgor

Obtundation (e.g. drowsiness, agitation, confusion)
Coma is rare <10% cases

Musty, fruity ('pear drops') odour of ketones on breath

Early weakness and lethargy

Early thirst, polyphagia, polydipsia, polyuria

Hyperventilation: 'Kussmaul' deep, rapid breathing to compensate for metabolic acidosis

Nausea and vomiting

Pleurisy ? cause

Hypotension: due to volume depletion and cardiac suppression by acidosis

Vomiting due to ileus induced by acidosis, dehydration and electrolyte imbalance

Pancreatitis is a late complication of DKA

Abdominal pain, rigidity, rebound tenderness. Resolves spontaneously when acidosis corrects

Initial polyuria due to glucose-induced osmotic diuresis
Later oliguria + ARF due to hypovolaemia

Consider venous thrombosis in those at risk (i.e. elderly, dehydrated)

Poor perfusion + peripheral cyanosis due to hypovolaemia

Figure 50d   Initial management of DKA

Confirm diagnosis (investigations)
↓
Immediate, rapid fluid replacement with normal saline
↓
Start insulin therapy (bolus 4–8U iv), then sliding scale insulin infusion
↓
Beware K+
↓
Monitor / replace electrolytes
↓
Insulin rapidly corrects acidosis but consider bicarbonate if pH <7.1 with cardiovascular instability
↓
Assess co-existing problems and treat cause

Look for precipitating causes
• Infection (pneumonia, UTI)
• Myocardial infarct
• Pancreatitis
• Trauma
• Endocrine (e.g. thyrotoxicosis)

Monitor
• Hourly blood sugar
• Hourly vital signs
• 2-hourly U+E
• 2-hourly blood gases
• Flow chart records

Investigations
• Bedside blood sugar
• Bedside ketone testing ('ketostix')
• Full blood count
• Urea, electrolytes and blood sugar
• Blood gases for acid–base status
• Osmolality
• Serum ketones
• Blood cultures
• Cardiac enzymes
• Amylase (? spuriously elevated)
• Urine for microbiology
• ECG and chest radiograph
• Consider: neurological causes (i.e. lumbar puncture, head CT scan)

Critical Care Medicine at a Glance, Third Edition. Richard Leach. © 2014 John Wiley & Sons, Ltd. Published 2014 by John Wiley & Sons, Ltd.

Diabetes mellitus (DM) is a metabolic disorder characterized by hyperglycaemia (fasting blood sugar [BS] >7 mmol/L or >11.1 mmol/L 2 hours after a glucose challenge) due to insulin deficiency or resistance.

- **Type I DM** is rare (2/1000 population), usually presenting in young people (<30 years). Viral, autoimmune and genetic factors contribute to pancreatic β-islet cell damage and insulin deficiency. Hyperglycaemic symptoms (e.g. polyuria, weight loss, fatigue) progress to ketoacidosis if insulin therapy is not started.
- **Type II DM** occurs in older adults (>40 years) mainly due to insulin resistance (±deficiency). There is a strong genetic association but diet and obesity determine age of onset. Treatment is with diet ±oral hypoglycaemic agents including biguanides (e.g. metformin) and/or sulphonylureas (e.g. gliclazide). Insulin is required if BS control is poor and during illness.
- **Other causes of DM** include malnutrition, rare genetic and secondary DM (e.g. pancreatitis, endocrine disease, steroids).
- **Stress-induced hyperglycaemia** occurs during acute illness. Tight glycaemic control with insulin may improve outcome.

DM may present with end-organ damage (e.g. nephropathy) or life-threatening diabetic emergencies (see later).

Hypoglycaemia

Symptoms occur when BS is <2.2 mmol/L but the threshold is higher in poorly controlled DM. Sudden changes in mental state or neurological function should always raise suspicion. **Causes** are listed in Figure 50a; most are due to diabetic therapy. **Clinical features** (Figure 50b) include early 'adrenergic' symptoms (e.g. tremor, sweating), followed by progressive anxiety, confusion and seizures. Coma and neurological damage rapidly develop due to the brain's dependence on glucose metabolism.

Management: bedside BS measurement confirms hypoglycaemia. A glucose drink or 'carbohydrate snack' is given to alert patients. If conscious level is impaired, give intravenous (i.v.) glucose (e.g. 50 ml 20% dextrose). Severe or refractory hypoglycaemia (e.g. sulphonylurea overdose) may require glucagon (1 mg i.v./i.m.) or hydrocortisone therapy and admission for BS monitoring (±glucose infusions). When BS cannot be measured, consider giving glucose empirically. Supplemental thiamine prevents Wernicke's encephalopathy (i.e. ophthalmoplegia, ataxia, confusion) in malnourished patients (e.g. alcoholics).

Diabetic ketoacidosis

Diabetic ketoacidosis (DKA) occurs in type I DM due to insulin deficiency. Precipitants include infection (~30%), myocardial infarction (MI), surgery, pancreatitis and non-compliance. No cause is found in ~25%. **Pathogenesis:** insulin deficiency and stress hormones accelerate hepatic glucose production and prevent cellular glucose uptake. When hyperglycaemia (BS > 20 mmol/L) exceeds the renal glucose threshold, glycosuria causes an osmotic diuresis with water and electrolyte loss. Nausea and vomiting also prevent fluid intake, increasing dehydration. Insulin deficiency promotes intracellular lipolysis, and hepatic metabolism of released fatty acids produces ketones (e.g. β-hydroxybutyrate) and a metabolic acidosis (Figure 50c). **Mortality** is ~5%.

Clinical presentation (Figure 50e): ~10% of type I DM presents as DKA. Nausea, lethargy, thirst and polyuria often precede DKA, which may develop within hours. Presenting features are due to **severe volume depletion** (e.g. hypotension) and **metabolic acidosis** (e.g. hyperventilation).

Investigation (Figure 50e): bedside BS testing, arterial blood gases and urinary ketones are usually diagnostic. Laboratory tests assess dehydration, electrolyte imbalance and acidosis. The precipitating cause and co-morbidities (e.g. renal failure) must be established.

Management (Figure 50d): haemodynamic instability due to hypovolaemia, acidosis and rapid K$^+$ fluxes is potentially life-threatening during initial therapy.

- **Early fluid replacement** should be brisk. Give ~3–4 L normal (0.9%) saline (NS) in <6 hours (i.e. 1 L in 30 min, then 1 L over 1 hour, etc.) to correct hypovolaemia. Total fluid deficits of ~5–10 L and sodium losses of ~400 mmol are replaced over 48 hours. Monitor central venous pressure (CVP) if pulmonary oedema is a risk.
- **Insulin:** give a bolus (6–10 U i.v.), followed by an infusion (~6 U/h). BS often corrects before the acidosis but insulin must be continued until the acidosis has resolved by replacing NS with a 10% dextrose infusion to maintain BS (monitored hourly). Aim to reduce the BS by ~3–5 mmol/h because osmotic shifts during rapid BS correction can cause cerebral oedema.
- **Electrolyte replacement:** diuresis (±vomiting) cause severe K$^+$ depletion. However, initial serum K$^+$ levels are high due to acidosis-induced K$^+$ movement out of cells. Insulin therapy and correction of acidosis stimulates cellular K$^+$ uptake and a rapid fall in serum K$^+$. Hourly monitoring and K$^+$ supplements prevent profound hypokalaemia (±cardiac arrest). Correct hypomagnesaemia to prevent insulin resistance and arrhythmias. Phosphate supplements maintain tissue oxygenation.
- **Sodium bicarbonate therapy** is controversial. It may reduce oxygen delivery and cause hypokalaemia. However, in severe acidosis (pH < 7.1) with myocardial depression treatment may be unavoidable.
- **General measures** include antibiotics, heparin and oxygen.
- **The post-resuscitation phase** is often poorly managed and requires a diabetic specialist. When BS is <15 mmol/L, a dextrose infusion is commenced. Restart regular insulin regimes when ketoacidosis has resolved and nutrition is normal.

Hyperosmolar non-ketotic coma

Hyperosmolar non-ketotic coma (HONK) is uncommon but mortality is ~40%. It occurs in elderly type II DM with sufficient insulin production to prevent ketogenesis but not hyperglycaemia. Osmotic diuresis leads to severe dehydration and hyperosmolality. Metabolic acidosis is unusual.

- **Clinical features:** anorexia, malaise, polyuria and weakness progress slowly to confusion, seizures and coma. Diagnosis is based on BS (>40 mmol/L) and hyperosmolality (>330 mosm/L). Serum sodium is often >160 mmol/L.
- **Management:** despite severe fluid deficits (>10 L), slow rehydration with NS and gradual sodium and BS reductions (e.g. insulin 1 U/h) are essential to avoid sudden osmotic and electrolyte shifts, which may precipitate cerebral oedema and demyelination. Anticoagulation prevents dehydration-induced thromboembolic events.

Lactic acidosis

This is a rare complication of type II DM (e.g. metformin use, sepsis). It presents with hyperventilation, vomiting, drowsiness and coma. A high anion gap acidosis with normal BS and no ketones is characteristic. Prognosis is poor despite supportive and bicarbonate therapy.

Pearl of wisdom

Immediately check bedside blood sugar (BS) in every patient presenting with altered mental state

 **Endocrine emergencies**

Figure 51a Severe hyperthyroidism and thyrotoxic crisis

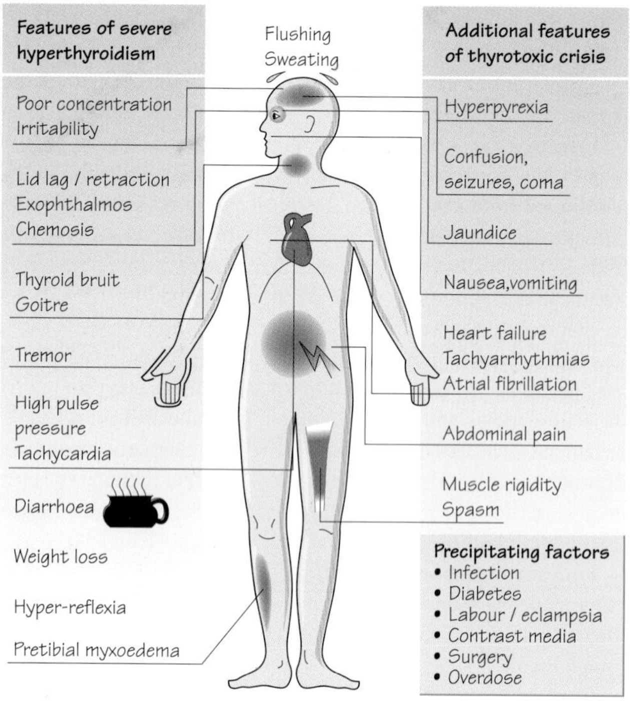

Features of severe hyperthyroidism

Flushing
Sweating

Poor concentration
Irritability

Lid lag / retraction
Exophthalmos
Chemosis

Thyroid bruit
Goitre

Tremor

High pulse pressure
Tachycardia

Diarrhoea

Weight loss

Hyper-reflexia

Pretibial myxoedema

Additional features of thyrotoxic crisis

Hyperpyrexia

Confusion, seizures, coma

Jaundice

Nausea, vomiting

Heart failure
Tachyarrhythmias
Atrial fibrillation

Abdominal pain

Muscle rigidity
Spasm

Precipitating factors
- Infection
- Diabetes
- Labour / eclampsia
- Contrast media
- Surgery
- Overdose

Figure 51b Severe hypothyroidism and 'myxoedema' coma

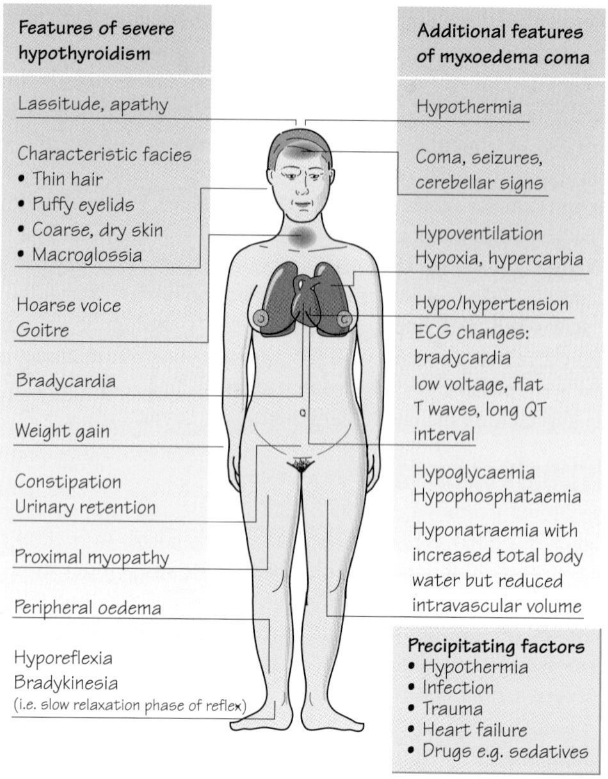

Features of severe hypothyroidism

Lassitude, apathy

Characteristic facies
- Thin hair
- Puffy eyelids
- Coarse, dry skin
- Macroglossia

Hoarse voice
Goitre

Bradycardia

Weight gain

Constipation
Urinary retention

Proximal myopathy

Peripheral oedema

Hyporeflexia
Bradykinesia
(i.e. slow relaxation phase of reflex)

Additional features of myxoedema coma

Hypothermia

Coma, seizures, cerebellar signs

Hypoventilation
Hypoxia, hypercarbia

Hypo/hypertension

ECG changes: bradycardia low voltage, flat T waves, long QT interval

Hypoglycaemia
Hypophosphataemia

Hyponatraemia with increased total body water but reduced intravascular volume

Precipitating factors
- Hypothermia
- Infection
- Trauma
- Heart failure
- Drugs e.g. sedatives

Figure 51c Causes of adrenal insufficiency

Adrenal gland destruction
- Autoimmune adrenalitis (Addison's disease)
- Surgical adrenalectomy, infarction
- Infection (e.g. TB, fungal, histoplasmosis, HIV)
- Infiltration (e.g. tumour, leukaemia, amyloidosis)
- Haemorrhage (e.g. anticoagulation, septicaemia)

Secondary (reduced pituitary ACTH secretion)
- Pituitary damage (e.g. adenoma, trauma)
- Pituitary infarction (e.g. postpartum haemorrhage)
- Pituitary haemorrhage (e.g. anticoagulation)
- Sudden exogenous steroid withdrawal

Rarely hypothalamic (reduced ACTH synthesis)
- Hypothalamic destruction (e.g. tumour, granuloma)

Drugs
- Inhibit steroid production (e.g. ketoconazole)
- Increase hepatic metabolism (e.g. rifampicin, phenytoin)

Relative adrenal insufficiency
- Critical illness

Figure 51d Acute adrenal (Addisonian) crisis

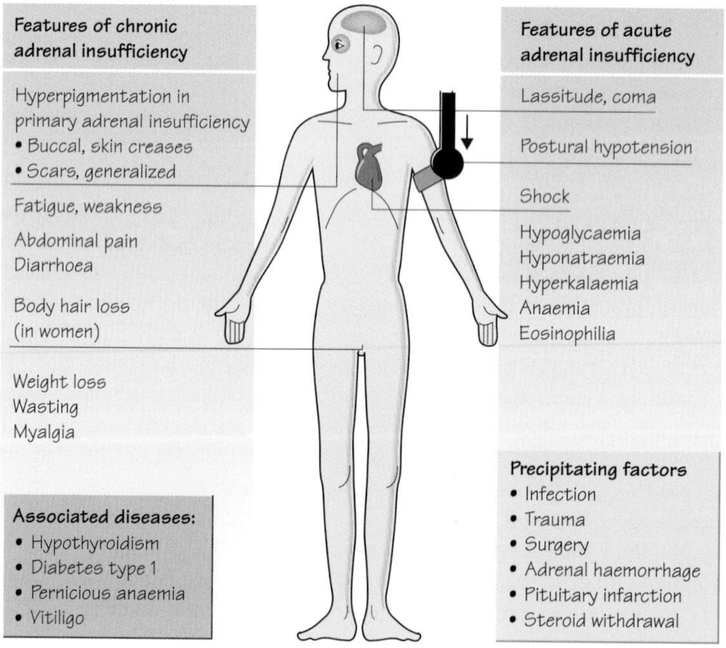

Features of chronic adrenal insufficiency

Hyperpigmentation in primary adrenal insufficiency
- Buccal, skin creases
- Scars, generalized

Fatigue, weakness

Abdominal pain
Diarrhoea

Body hair loss
(in women)

Weight loss
Wasting
Myalgia

Associated diseases:
- Hypothyroidism
- Diabetes type 1
- Pernicious anaemia
- Vitiligo

Features of acute adrenal insufficiency

Lassitude, coma

Postural hypotension

Shock

Hypoglycaemia
Hyponatraemia
Hyperkalaemia
Anaemia
Eosinophilia

Precipitating factors
- Infection
- Trauma
- Surgery
- Adrenal haemorrhage
- Pituitary infarction
- Steroid withdrawal

Figure 51e ACTH stimulation

Pituitary adrenal axis	Cortisol level	
	Baseline	Post ACTH
Normal	Normal	Increased
Primary adrenal failure	Low	Low
Secondary adrenal failure	Low	Increased
Critical Illness	Low/normal	Poor response

Thyroid emergencies

Thyrotoxic crisis (storm) is a hypermetabolic emergency (mortality ~20%). It affects <2% of thyrotoxic patients. Precipitants include infection, surgery, diabetes, labour, radioiodine therapy and iodinated contrast media. Thyroxine overdose and eclampsia are rare causes.

- **Clinical features** are those of severe hyperthyroidism (Figure 51a) with fever, weight loss (>15 kg), confusion and high output cardiac failure (~50%). Differential diagnosis includes sepsis, phaeochromocytoma, drug abuse and malignant hyperthermia.

- **Treatment** may be required before diagnostic confirmation.
  - **General management**: admit to ICU/HDU and treat precipitating causes. Control agitation with sedatives and correct dehydration, electrolyte disturbances and hypoglycaemia. Institute cooling but avoid aspirin (displaces T4 from binding protein). Dantrolene reduces fever due to extreme muscle activity (Chapter 23).
  - **High-dose beta-blockers** (e.g. propranolol) are the mainstay of therapy. They inhibit peripheral effects of thyroid hormone reducing tachycardia, hypertension, fever and tremor.
  - **Antithyroid drugs** block T4 synthesis. Propylthiouracil is preferred because it blocks T4 to T3 conversion but it can only be given enterally (e.g. nasogastric [NG] tube). Carbimazole is metabolized to methimazole. Onset of action is slow, but duration prolonged and it can be given by suppository. White cell suppression occurs with both drugs and therapy is stopped if sore throat develops.
  - **Hydrocortisone** inhibits T4 to T3 conversion.
  - **Iodine** (e.g. Lugol's solution), or lithium in allergic patients, prevents T4 release from the thyroid gland. Give antithyroid drugs 2 hours before iodine, which inhibits thyroid uptake.

Severe hypothyroidism (myxoedema coma) is precipitated by infection, illness or drugs (e.g. sedatives) in pre-existing hypothyroidism. It causes hypothermia, coma and hypotension. Elderly females with unrecognized hypothyroidism or patients who fail to take thyroxine replacement are often affected. It should be suspected in obtunded, hypothermic patients. Mortality is >50%.

- **Clinical features** are those of severe hypothyroidism (Figure 51b).
- **Investigation** may reveal anaemia, hypoglycaemia, hyponatraemia and electrocardiogram (ECG) changes (Figure 51b). In primary hypothyroidism, thyroid-stimulating hormone (TSH) is raised and T3/T4 is low. In pituitary failure (suspect when Na⁺ low), both TSH and T3/T4 are low.
- **Management**: rewarm, support ventilation and correct hypoglycaemia. Immediate treatment with T3 (5–20 μg i.v. slowly because ischaemic heart disease [IHD] can be unmasked; 6 hourly) may be required. Give corticosteroid therapy until pituitary or adrenal failure have been excluded.

Sick euthyroid syndrome occurs in severe illness but is not a thyroid disorder and should not be treated. Low T4 binding protein and altered T4 metabolism results in abnormal thyroid function tests (e.g. low total T4, normal free T4, low T3, normal TSH).

Adrenal emergencies

Adrenocortical insufficiency (AI) describes reduced cortisol (±aldosterone) production by the adrenal cortex. **Causes** are listed in Figure 51c. Primary adrenal insufficiency (PAI) follows adrenal damage (e.g. autoimmune adrenalitis; 'Addison's disease'). Secondary adrenal insufficiency (SAI) due to adrenocorticotrophic hormone (ACTH) deficiency follows pituitary or hypothalamic damage. Abrupt withdrawal of therapeutic steroids also causes AI due to suppression of ACTH secretion.

- **Clinical presentation** (Figure 51d) is either acute or chronic.
  - **Acute (Addisonian) crisis** is precipitated by stress (e.g. surgery) in patients with unrecognized, chronic AI. It also follows sepsis or adrenal haemorrhage in critical illness, or pituitary infarction after postpartum haemorrhage (Sheehan's syndrome). Always suspect acute AI in shock with hyponatraemia (±hyperkalaemia, hypoglycaemia) if the cause is not apparent. Characteristic features include apathy, postural hypotension and coma. In critical illness, 'relative AI' is common and steroid supplements may be beneficial.
  - **Chronic deficiency** (e.g. autoimmune adrenalitis) presents with fatigue, weakness, weight loss, fever and nausea. In PAI, hyperpigmentation is caused by excess pituitary melanocyte-stimulating hormone. Body hair loss in females is due to reduced adrenal androgen production.
- **Investigation:** hyponatraemia and hyperkalaemia are typical of aldosterone reduction in PAI. Hypoglycaemia, hypercalcaemia, eosinophilia and volume depletion with raised blood urea occur in all forms of AI. Immunology may reveal autoantibodies. **Adrenal function tests** must not delay cortisol replacement. A low baseline cortisol confirms AI. Cortisol levels 30 and 60 minutes after i.v. ACTH injection (short Synacthen test) indicate the cause (Figure 51e). ACTH is high in PAI and low in SAI.
- **Treatment** of shock (Chapters 7, 8) may require aggressive fluid therapy and inotropic support. High dose hydrocortisone (dexamethasone does not affect serum cortisol assays) is required as stress can increase cortisol levels 10 fold. Hyperkalaemia responds to fluid and steroid therapy and hypoglycaemia to glucose supplements. Treat infection with antibiotics. Mineralocorticoid replacement (e.g. fludrocortisone) is only needed in PAI.

Adrenocortical excess: cortisol is increased in Cushing's syndrome (e.g. steroid therapy, adrenal tumours) and Cushing's disease (e.g. ACTH secreting pituitary tumour). Characteristic features include a moon face, thin easily bruised skin, hypertension (~50%), diabetes (~10%), osteoporosis (~50%), central obesity and hypokalaemia (e.g. arrhythmias, weakness). Excess aldosterone secretion from an adrenal adenoma (Conn's syndrome) causes hypokalaemia, muscle weakness (e.g. post-operative ventilatory impairment) and hypertension.

Other endocrine emergencies

Hypopituitary crisis follows pituitary trauma, infiltration (e.g. tumour), haemorrhage or infarction. Reduced anterior pituitary hormone secretion causes adrenal and thyroid insufficiency and hypogonadism. Failure of posterior pituitary antidiuretic hormone release causes diabetes insipidus with thirst, dehydration and polyuria. Detailed pituitary–adrenal axis assessment and hormone replacement therapy are required.

Phaeochromocytomas are rare, benign (~90%), adrenal (~90%) tumours that release catecholamines. They are often familial or associated with other tumours (e.g. multiple endocrine neoplasia). Crises are precipitated by drugs, surgery or food (e.g. cheese). Features include headaches, sweating, flushing and arrhythmias. Hypertension may be sustained or labile. Raised plasma catecholamines or 24-hour urinary vanillyl mandelic acid (VMA) confirm the diagnosis. Treatment is with α-blockers (e.g. phenoxybenzamine), β-blockers and surgery.

Pearl of wisdom

Endocrine deficiency should be considered in obtunded, hypothermic patients or those whose condition fails to respond to appropriate therapy

52 Gastrointestinal haemorrhage

Figure 52a Age distribution of patients admitted with and dying from upper gastrointestinal bleeding

Bar chart: Number of patients (y-axis 0–200) vs Age (years) groups <30, 30–49, 50–69, >70. Legend: Survived, Died.

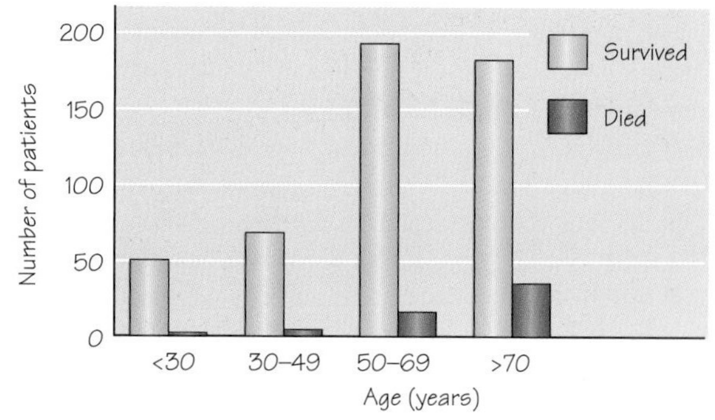

Figure 52b Causes of acute upper gastrointestinal haemorrhage

Drugs (e.g. NSAID, steroids, warfarin)/alcohol

Reflux oesophagitis

Mallory–Weiss tear (5%)

Oesophageal varices
Gastric varices — 15% (OV:GV 9:1)

Gastric carcinoma

60% (DU:GU 3:1)
Gastric ulcer
Duodenal ulcer

Acute gastric erosions (10%)

Rare causes
Angiodysplasia
Meckel's diverticulum
Dieulafoy Lesion
(rupture of a large arteriole in the stomach fundus)
Peutz-Jeghers syndrome
Osler-Weber-Rendu (HHT) syndrome

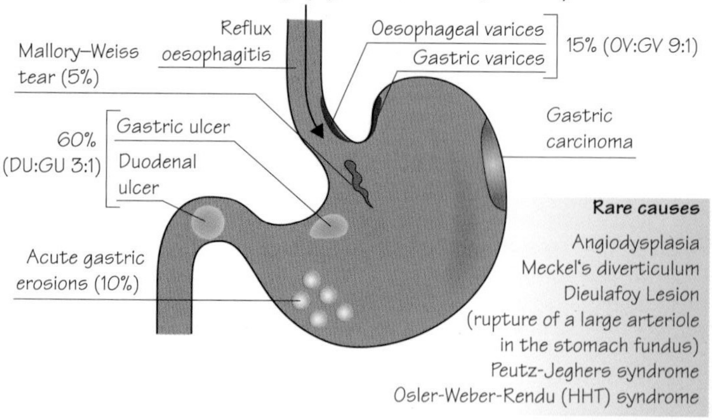

Figure 52c Use of the Sengstaken–Blakemore tube (SBT) to control variceal bleeding when other measures have failed (e.g. octreotide, sclerotherapy)

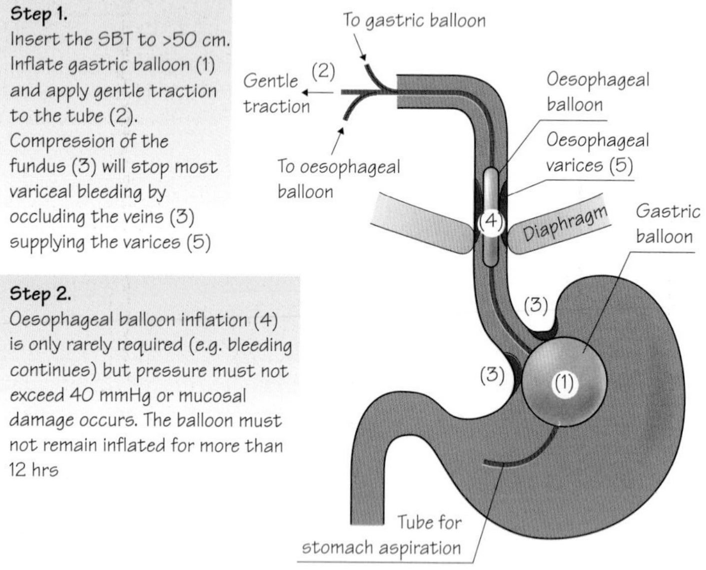

Step 1.
Insert the SBT to >50 cm. Inflate gastric balloon (1) and apply gentle traction to the tube (2). Compression of the fundus (3) will stop most variceal bleeding by occluding the veins (3) supplying the varices (5)

Step 2.
Oesophageal balloon inflation (4) is only rarely required (e.g. bleeding continues) but pressure must not exceed 40 mmHg or mucosal damage occurs. The balloon must not remain inflated for more than 12 hrs

To gastric balloon
Gentle traction (2)
To oesophageal balloon
Oesophageal balloon
Oesophageal varices (5)
Diaphragm
Gastric balloon
Tube for stomach aspiration

Figure 52d Risk of rebleeding based on OGD findings

Endoscopic finding	Risk
Likely to rebleed	
Visible spurting vessel	~80%
Non-bleeding vessel in an ulcer crater	~70%
Oesophageal varices	~50%
Clot over an ulcer crater	~30%
Ulcers >1cm or located on posterior duodenal wall (over the gastroduodenal artery) or on the lesser gastric curvature (left gastric artery)	
Less likely to rebleed	
Smooth ulcer base	<10%
Flat pigmented spots	<10%

Figure 51f Mesenteric angiogram showing angiodysplasia

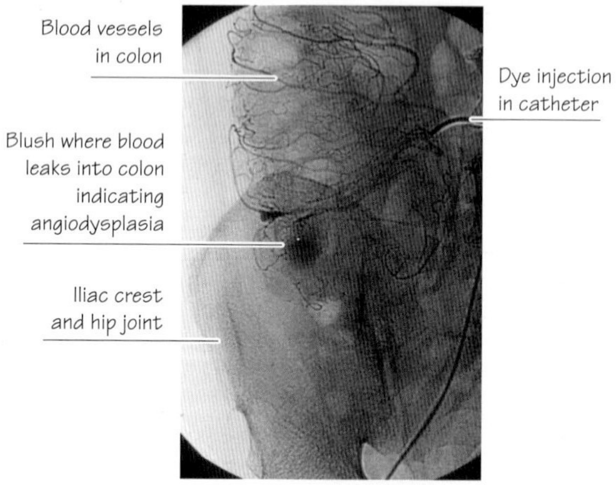

Blood vessels in colon

Dye injection in catheter

Blush where blood leaks into colon indicating angiodysplasia

Iliac crest and hip joint

Figure 51e Causes of lower gastrointestinal bleeding

Condition	Frequency
Angiomas	~35%
Carcinoma and polyps	~20%
Upper GI bleeding	~15%
Other causes (angiodysplasia, haemorrhoids)	~15%
Diverticular disease	~10%
Colitis (inflammatory, ischaemic)	~5%
Unknown causes	~15%

Upper gastrointestinal haemorrhage

Incidence: acute upper gastrointestinal (GI) bleeding affects ~1/1000 population. Most patients are >50 years old (Figure 52a). Stress-induced ulceration (±bleeding) occurs in <10% of acutely ill patients. **Causes** (Figure 52b) include peptic ulceration (~60%), gastritis/oesophagitis (10%) and oesophageal varices (15%). No cause is found in ~20%. Aspirin and non-steroidal anti-inflammatory drugs (NSAIDs) cause ~33% of gastritis and ulceration. Cirrhosis is the main cause of portal hypertension (PrHT). Oesophageal (±gastric, rectal, umbilical) varices develop when portal pressure is >12 mmHg. Acute variceal bleeding occurs in ~30% and causes >70% of upper GI bleeds in cirrhotics.

Clinical features

Common presentations include haematemesis (i.e. vomited blood; ~50–65%), melaena (i.e. black 'tarry' stool; ~65%) and shock (Chapter 7). Rectal blood clots occur in massive bleeds. Epigastric discomfort suggests peptic ulceration. Examine for stigmata of chronic liver disease (CLD), hepatosplenomegaly, mucocutaneous changes (e.g. hereditary haemorrhagic telangiectasia [HHT], Peutz–Jegher's syndrome) and bleeding disorders. Angiodysplasia is common in chronic renal failure (CRF). Gastro-oesophageal tears (Mallory–Weiss syndrome) follow previous retching or vomiting. Anorexia, weight loss, lymph nodes and an epigastric mass suggest gastric carcinoma. Aortoenteric fistula may follow aortic surgery. A drug history is essential (e.g. NSAIDs).

Investigation

- **Blood tests**: haemoglobin is initially normal because haemodilution occurs over many hours. Microcytic anaemia suggests previous chronic bleeding. A raised urea, due to the blood protein load, suggests upper rather than lower GI bleeding. Liver function and clotting tests assess liver damage and synthetic (e.g. albumin) and clotting function.
- **Diagnostic imaging**: air beneath the diaphragm on chest or abdominal radiography indicates viscus perforation. **Upper GI endoscopy**, within 12 hours, establishes the diagnosis, predicts re-bleeding risk and treats bleeding lesions endoscopically. **Angiography** is performed if endoscopy fails to locate the bleeding site (~20%).
- **Exploratory laparotomy** is occasionally required if bleeding persists despite negative investigations.

Management of upper gastrointestinal bleeding

- **Prophylaxis**: the risk of upper GI bleeding is reduced by enteral nutrition, gastric acid suppression (e.g. omeprazole) and mucosal coatings (e.g. sucralphate).
- **General management**: involve gastroenterologists and surgeons early. The priorities are:
  1 Resuscitation: protect the airway and give oxygen therapy. Blood transfusion follows initial fluid resuscitation(Chapters 8, 10). Monitor blood pressure, central venous pressure, arterial blood gases and urine output to guide resuscitation. Avoid nasogastric tubes in patients with varices.
  2 Identify and control active bleeding: correct clotting abnormalities (e.g. fresh frozen plasma [FFP], platelets, vitamin K), arrange urgent/early endoscopy and treat the cause.
  3 Prevent recurrence: identify rebleeding risk (Figure 52d).

Peptic ulcer management

Proton pump inhibitors (PPIs; e.g. pantoprazole) and H_2 receptor antagonists reduce gastric acid secretion and promote ulcer healing. Intravenous PPIs also reduce re-bleeding after endoscopic therapy. Eradication therapy (e.g. antibiotics and PPI) is indicated if *Helicobacter pylori* is detected. The value of tranexamic acid and octreotide is not established.
- **Endoscopic therapy**: electrocautery or epinephrine injection around a bleeding ulcer achieves haemostasis in >90%. It reduces re-bleeding, mortality and the need for emergency surgery.
- **Surgery** is required in severe haemorrhage or perforation despite the associated mortality (~20%). Usually, bleeding gastric ulcers require a Billroth gastrectomy and duodenal ulcers are over-sewn (±vagotomy and pyloroplasty). In high-risk cases, arterial embolization controls bleeding in ~50% but risks necrosis.

Management of oesophageal varices

Treat the underlying cause (e.g. cirrhosis) and associated liver failure (Chapter 54), which determine prognosis and the risk of variceal bleeding (Appendix 5).
- **Sclerotherapy**: endoscopic injection of a sclerosant (e.g. alcohol, ethanolamine) thromboses varices and controls bleeding in >90%. Complications include ulceration and stricture formation.
- **Endoscopic variceal ligation (banding)** is equally effective.
- **Pharmacotherapy**: terlipressin, a vasopressin analogue and splanchnic vasoconstrictor, lowers PrHT and controls variceal bleeding in >50% but risks cardiac ischaemia. Octreotide is also effective. Beta-blockade reduces PrHT and is used as prophylaxis.
- **Balloon tamponade** (e.g. Sengstaken–Blakemore tube; Figure 52c) is an effective temporizing measure to control massive bleeding.
- **Transjugular intrahepatic portal stents (TIPS)** decompress the portal system by placing a self-expanding stent over a wire passed from the hepatic vein (transjugular approach) through liver substance into the portal vein. Encephalopathy may ensue.
- **Surgery**: variceal ligation (e.g. transoesophageal stapling) or porto-caval shunting are occasionally required.

Prognosis

About 70% of upper GI bleeding stops spontaneously and mortality is ~5%. Poor prognostic features and risk factors for re-bleeding (Rockall Score; Appendix 4) include age >60 years, oesophageal varices (mortality ~30%), co-existing disease and persistent bleeding.

Lower gastrointestinal bleeding

Causes are listed in Figure 52e. Lower GI bleeding presents with either frank rectal bleeding or melaena (±shock). Abdominal examination may reveal a mass (e.g. neoplasia) or tenderness. A bruit suggests ischaemia. Angiodysplasia occurs in CRF, aortic stenosis and inherited vascular conditions like HHT. Initial investigation is as for upper GI bleeding but sequential diagnostic imaging includes sigmoidoscopy, colonoscopy if upper GI endoscopy is negative, mesenteric arteriography (Figure 52f), 'video-capsule' endoscopy, labelled red cell isotope scans or small bowel barium studies. Exploratory laparotomy may be needed if profuse undiagnosed bleeding persists.

Management

Most lower GI bleeding stops spontaneously (~80%) but recurs in ~25%.
- **General management** is as for upper GI bleeding.
- **Specific measures** include **colonoscopy** with electrocoagulation or laser therapy, which stops bleeding from polyps, angiodysplasia and colorectal carcinomas. **Elective surgery** is often required for lower GI bleeding. Severe, persistent but undiagnosed bleeding due to presumed angiodysplasia may require a right hemicolectomy although this is an unsatisfactory compromise. **Arterial embolization** may be used for vascular malformations and angiodysplasia (Figure 52f).

Pearl of wisdom

About 70% of upper gastrointestinal (GI) bleeding stops spontaneously regardless of the cause

53 Jaundice

Figure 53a Metabolism of bilirubin (steps 1-10)

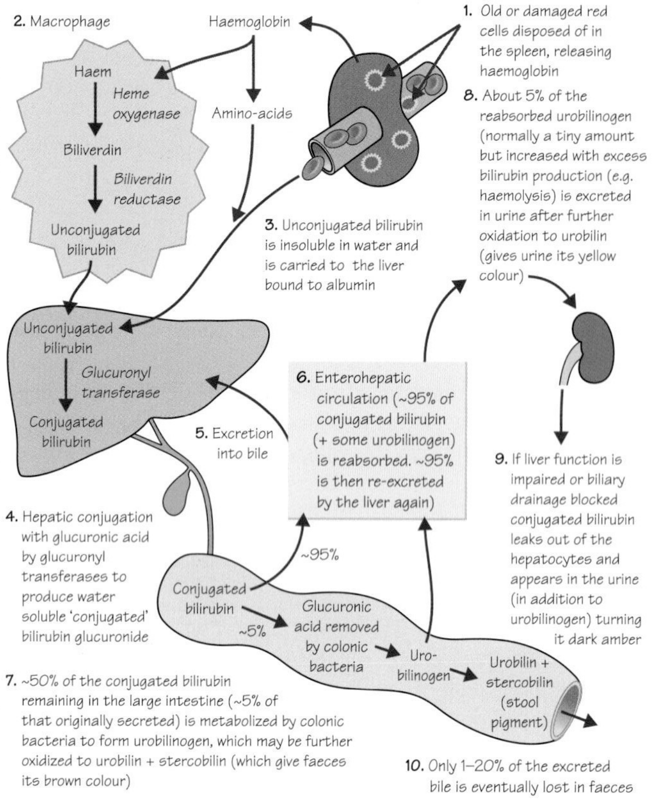

2. Macrophage

Haemoglobin

Haem
Heme oxygenase

Biliverdin
Biliverdin reductase

Unconjugated bilirubin

Amino-acids

1. Old or damaged red cells disposed of in the spleen, releasing haemoglobin

8. About 5% of the reabsorbed urobilinogen (normally a tiny amount but increased with excess bilirubin production (e.g. haemolysis) is excreted in urine after further oxidation to urobilin (gives urine its yellow colour)

3. Unconjugated bilirubin is insoluble in water and is carried to the liver bound to albumin

Unconjugated bilirubin
Glucuronyl transferase
Conjugated bilirubin

5. Excretion into bile

6. Enterohepatic circulation (~95% of conjugated bilirubin (+ some urobilinogen) is reabsorbed. ~95% is then re-excreted by the liver again)

9. If liver function is impaired or biliary drainage blocked conjugated bilirubin leaks out of the hepatocytes and appears in the urine (in addition to urobilinogen) turning it dark amber

4. Hepatic conjugation with glucuronic acid by glucuronyl transferases to produce water soluble 'conjugated' bilirubin glucuronide

Conjugated bilirubin

~95%

~5%

Glucuronic acid removed by colonic bacteria

Uro-bilinogen

Urobilin + stercobilin (stool pigment)

7. ~50% of the conjugated bilirubin remaining in the large intestine (~5% of that originally secreted) is metabolized by colonic bacteria to form urobilinogen, which may be further oxidized to urobilin + stercobilin (which give faeces its brown colour)

10. Only 1–20% of the excreted bile is eventually lost in faeces

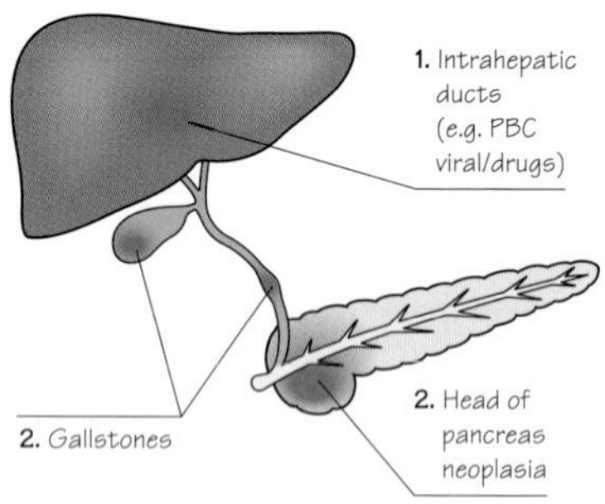

Figure 53b Causes and classification of jaundice

Pre-hepatic (haemolytic) jaundice
- Haemolytic anaemias (e.g. spherocytosis, pernicious anaemia, thalassaemia)
- Gilbert's syndrome (most common, inherited unconjugated hyperbilirubinaemia)
- Crigler-Najjar syndrome (rare autosomal recessive disorder of bilirubin metabolism, caused by deficient diphosphate glycosyltransferase)
- Trauma (haematoma, bruise reabsorption)

Hepatocellular (hepatic) jaundice
- Viral hepatitis (including type A and type B).
- Other infective causes (e.g. leptospirosis, brucellosis, Coxiella burnetii)
- Glandular fever
- Alcoholic hepatitis
- Drug-induced hepatitis (e.g. paracetamol; the most common)
- Hepatotoxic chemicals (e.g. phosphorous, carbon tetrachloride, phenol)
- Autoimmune hepatitis (10–20% of chronic hepatitis; an autoimmune disease of unknown cause, often in young women and associated with other autoimmune diseases (e.g. Grave's disease, systemic sclerosis, inflammatory bowel disease, rheumatoid arthritis)
- Decompensated cirrhosis

Cholestatic (obstructive) jaundice
1. **Extrahepatic cholestasis**
   - Gallstones (most common cause; common duct stone)
   - Bile duct strictures (benign, malignant)
   - Cancer of the head of the pancreas
   - Tumour of the ampulla of Vater
   - Pancreatitis (±pseudocysts)
   - Cancer of the gallbladder

2. **Intrahepatic cholestasis**
   - Primary biliary cirrhosis
   - Drugs (e.g. phenothiazines)
   - Primary sclerosing cholangiti
   - Dubin-Johnson syndrome: (autosomal recessive disorder characterized by conjugated hyperbilirubinaemia and deposition of pigment in hepatocytes)
   - Rotor's syndrome

Figure 53c Assessment of jaundice

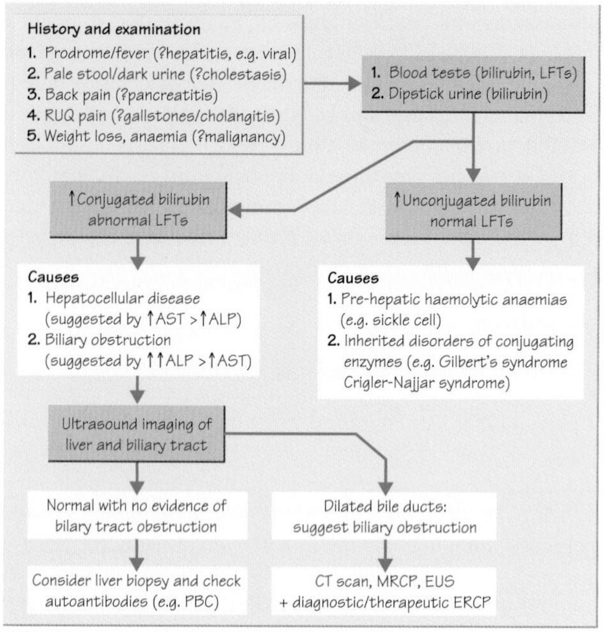

History and examination
1. Prodrome/fever (?hepatitis, e.g. viral)
2. Pale stool/dark urine (?cholestasis)
3. Back pain (?pancreatitis)
4. RUQ pain (?gallstones/cholangitis)
5. Weight loss, anaemia (?malignancy)

1. Blood tests (bilirubin, LFTs)
2. Dipstick urine (bilirubin)

↑Conjugated bilirubin abnormal LFTs

↑Unconjugated bilirubin normal LFTs

Causes
1. Hepatocellular disease (suggested by ↑AST >↑ALP)
2. Biliary obstruction (suggested by ↑↑ALP >↑AST)

Causes
1. Pre-hepatic haemolytic anaemia (e.g. sickle cell)
2. Inherited disorders of conjugating enzymes (e.g. Gilbert's syndrome Crigler-Najjar syndrome)

Ultrasound imaging of liver and biliary tract

Normal with no evidence of biliary tract obstruction

Dilated bile ducts: suggest biliary obstruction

Consider liver biopsy and check autoantibodies (e.g. PBC)

CT scan, MRCP, EUS + diagnostic/therapeutic ERCP

RUQ = right upper quadrant, LFTs = liver function tests, AST = aspartate transaminase, ALP = alkaline phosphatase, PBC = primary biliary cirrhosis, CT = computer tomography, MRCP = magnetic resonance cholangiopancreatography, EUS = endoscopic ultrasound scan, ERCP = endoscopic retrograde pancreatic cholangiography

Pearl of wisdom

Beware inadvertent paracetamol overdose as a cause of accidental liver injury and hepatocellular jaundice

Figure 53d Causes of biliary obstruction

1. Intrahepatic ducts (e.g. PBC viral/drugs)

2. Gallstones

2. Head of pancreas neoplasia

Figure 53e Causes of acute and chronic jaundice

	Acute	Chronic
Hepatocellular ('hepatic') jaundice	**Causes of acute hepatitis** • Viral hepatitides (e.g. A, B, EBV) • Other infective causes (e.g. leptospirosis) • Drug reactions (e.g. paracetamol) • Budd-Chiari syndrome	**Causes of chronic liver disease** • Alcoholic liver disease • Chronic viral hepatitides (e.g. B, C) • Autoimmune hepatitis • Haemochromatosis • Drug induced (e.g. methotrexate)
Cholestatic ('obstructive') jaundice	**Biliary obstruction** • Gallstones • Other biliary causes (e.g. cholangitis) • Drugs • Pancreatitis • Pancreatic cancer	**Chronic biliary disease** • Primary biliary cirrhosis • Primary sclerosing cirrhosis • Bile duct strictures (e.g. benign, malignant) • Inherited disorders (e.g. Dubin-Johnson syndrome)

EBV = Epstein Barr virus (glandular fever)

Definition

Jaundice describes a yellow discolouration in tissues (e.g. skin) caused by bilirubin accumulation. It becomes apparent when serum bilirubin is >35 μmol/L (normal 3–20 μmol/L). Jaundice can occur transiently in acute illness (e.g. hepatitis A) or chronically in end-stage disease (e.g. cirrhosis).

Critical Care Medicine at a Glance, Third Edition. Richard Leach. © 2014 John Wiley & Sons, Ltd. Published 2014 by John Wiley & Sons, Ltd.

Aetiology

Jaundice is due to impaired bilirubin metabolism (Figures 53a and 53b). It is classified as:

- **Pre-hepatic jaundice**: is due to haemolytic anaemia (e.g. sickle cell disease) or inherited disorders of conjugating enzymes (e.g. Gilbert's, Crigler–Najjar syndromes). Gilbert's syndrome is the most common inherited unconjugated hyperbilirubinaemia, affecting ~5% of the population. It causes mild, insignificant jaundice, worse during fasting. **Investigation** reveals raised serum unconjugated bilirubin. As liver and enterohepatic function are normal, urobilinogen production and hence urinary urobilinogen increase (Figure 53a). Unconjugated bilirubin is not water soluble (i.e. not found in urine). Consequently, an increase in urinary urobilinogen, with no urinary bilirubin, suggests haemolytic jaundice.

- **Hepatocellular jaundice**: is due to liver disease. Causes include acute (e.g. hepatitis A, glandular fever) or chronic (e.g. autoimmune, hepatitis C) hepatitis, cirrhosis, hepatotoxicity (e.g. carbon tetrachloride), drug-related (e.g. paracetamol) and alcoholic liver disease. Primary biliary cirrhosis (PBC) impairs excretion of conjugated bilirubin. Newborn neonatal jaundice is common because bilirubin conjugation/excretion mechanisms do not mature for ~2 weeks. Cholestasis occurs in all forms of hepatocellular jaundice. **Laboratory findings** depend on the cause. Bilirubin metabolism is affected at all stages including uptake, conjugation and excretion into biliary canaliculi (i.e. inflammatory obstruction). Both unconjugated and conjugated bilirubin serum concentrations rise but, because excretion is most impaired, conjugated hyperbilirubinaemia predominates. Conjugated bilirubin, which did not enter the intestine gives urine its dark, amber color (Figure 53a).

- **Cholestatic (obstructive) jaundice**: is due to impaired biliary drainage. **Extrahepatic causes** include obstruction of the common bile duct by gallstones (most common), strictures, head of pancreas cancer, pancreatitis and cholangiocarcinoma. **Intrahepatic causes** include PBC, drugs (e.g. phenothiazines), primary sclerosing cholangitis and rare inherited disorders of conjugated hyperbilirubinaemia (e.g. Dubin–Johnson syndrome). Obstructive jaundice is suggested by pale stools (bile pigments colour faeces) and dark urine (also present in hepatocellular jaundice). Severe itching is due to skin bile salt deposition. Serum cholesterol is elevated. **Laboratory findings**: in complete bile duct obstruction, no urobilinogen is found in the urine, because bilirubin has no access to the intestine where it is converted to urobilinogen before reabsorption (Figure 53a). Hence, urinary conjugated bilirubin without urinary urobilinogen suggests obstructive jaundice.

Assessment (Figure 53c)

A comprehensive history and examination aid diagnosis.

- Initially assess symptom duration to establish if the presentation is acute or chronic. A prodromal flu-like illness suggests viral hepatitis; sudden pain with jaundice indicates gallstones; and fever (±rigors) occurs in ascending cholangitis. Slowly progressive, painless jaundice with weight loss suggests carcinoma. For unknown reasons, pruritus may occur before jaundice. Review previous chronic liver disease (CLD), hepatitis (e.g. chronic active hepatitis), biliary surgery or malignancy (e.g. bowel).
- Exclude liver failure and hepatic encephalopathy.
- Assess urine and stool colour; in viral hepatitis and obstructive jaundice, dark urine and/or pale stool may precede jaundice.

- Review travel/contact history, sexual orientation, family history (e.g. Gilbert's syndrome), alcohol intake, previous blood transfusions, medications (e.g. inadvertent paracetamol overdose) and illicit drug use. Drugs associated with jaundice include amitriptyline, chlorpromazine, erythromycin, halothane, imipramine, indomethacin, isoniazid, rifampicin, salicylates, sulphonamides and oral contraceptive pills. Occupational history may be important (e.g. leptosporosis in sewerage workers).

Examination

Jaundice severity is less important than detecting CLD and liver failure. Signs of CLD include spider naevi, liver palms (thenar/hypothenar erythema), gynaecomastia, testicular atrophy, finger clubbing and peripheral oedema. Splenomegaly and ascites suggest portal hypertension (e.g. cirrhosis). The liver is tender and slightly enlarged in viral hepatitis, smoothly enlarged in obstructive jaundice and has a firm edge in cirrhosis. An irregular liver edge suggests malignancy. A yellow-green 'tinge' characterises severe obstructive jaundice (due to biliverdin). If the gallbladder is palpable, the cause of the jaundice is unlikely to be a stone (Courvoisier's sign); suspect pancreatic malignancy. Encephalopathy (±'flapping' tremor) indicates liver failure (Chapter 54).

Investigation (Figure 53c)

'Haemolytic' jaundice is easily recognized but differentiating hepatic and obstructive jaundice is difficult because they often co-exist. **Blood tests** may indicate haemolysis (e.g. raised lactate dehydrogenase) or CLD (e.g. thrombocytopenia, low urea). In CLD, low albumin or sodium (not due to diuretics) and raised INR are poor prognostic signs. **Liver function tests** differentiate between 'hepatocellular' (transaminases (i.e. aspartate transaminase [AST], alanine transaminase [ALT]) >alkaline phosphatase [ALP]) and 'cholestatic' jaundice (ALP or gamma-glutamyl transferase >transaminases). However, the picture is often mixed. Normal transaminases suggest haemolysis or Gilbert's syndrome. The implications of unconjugated/conjugated bilirubin, urinary bilirubin and urobilinogen are discussed earlier. Clinical jaundice with normal serum and urinary bilirubin suggests excess vitamin A or serum carotene (e.g. carrots). **Coagulation**: impaired by vitamin K malabsorption. **Viral/hepatitis serology** is diagnostic of acute hepatitis A (i.e. IgM) or hepatitis B (i.e. surface antigen [HbsAg]). Hepatitis C rarely causes acute hepatitis but often results in CLD. **Autoantibodies** aid diagnosis (e.g. antinuclear [20–50% PBC positive], antimitochondrial (90–95% PBC positive). **Alpha-1-antitrypsin deficiency** causes cirrhosis and emphysema. **Elevated ferritin** indicates haemochromatosis. **Imaging**: abdominal ultrasound detects liver abnormalities, hepatosplenomegaly, gallstones, biliary obstruction and intrahepatic disease (e.g. metastases). Magnetic resonance cholangiopancreatography (MRCP) and endoscopic ultrasound (EUS) define biliary anatomy before endoscopic intervention in obstructive jaundice. Endoscopic retrograde choledochopancreatography (ERCP) determines if biliary obstruction is intraluminal (e.g. gallstones) or extraluminal (e.g. pancreatic cancer) and is combined with interventional procedures to relieve obstruction. **Liver biopsy/histology** (percutaneous, laproscopic) confirms the cause of 'hepatic' (e.g. cirrhosis) and some 'cholestatic' jaundice (e.g. PBC).

Management (e.g. the need for hospital admission) depends on the underlying condition and whether there is associated liver failure (Chapter 54).

 **Acute liver failure**

Figure 54a Clinical features and complications

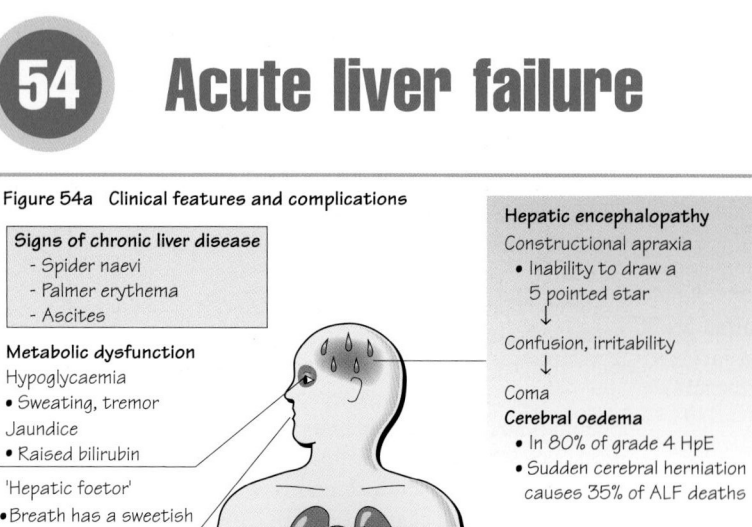

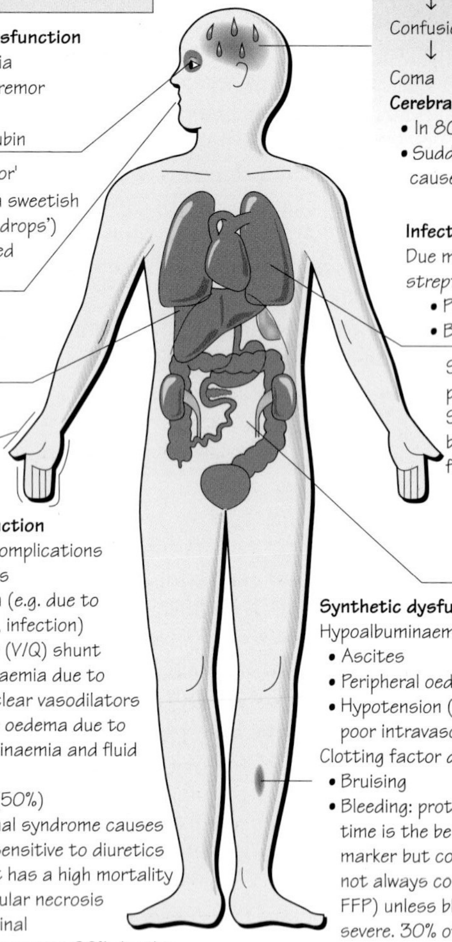

Signs of chronic liver disease
- Spider naevi
- Palmer erythema
- Ascites

Metabolic dysfunction
Hypoglycaemia
• Sweating, tremor
Jaundice
• Raised bilirubin

'Hepatic foetor'
• Breath has a sweetish smell ('pear drops') due to exhaled mercaptans

Right upper quadrant tenderness

Tremor and 'liver flap'

Hepatic encephalopathy
Constructional apraxia
• Inability to draw a 5 pointed star
↓
Confusion, irritability
↓
Coma

Cerebral oedema
• In 80% of grade 4 HpE
• Sudden cerebral herniation causes 35% of ALF deaths

Infection
Due mainly to staphylococci, streptococci, Gm –ve bacilli
• Pneumonia
• Bacteraemia

Spontaneous bacterial peritonitis (SBP):
SBP diagnosis confirmed by aspirating peritoneal fluid which reveals:
• Leukocytes >500/mm^3
• pH <7.3
• Raised lactate
• Bacteria (Gm –ve rods)

Synthetic dysfunction
Hypoalbuminaemia
• Ascites
• Peripheral oedema
• Hypotension (due to poor intravascular filling)
Clotting factor deficiency
• Bruising
• Bleeding: prothrombin time is the best prognostic marker but coagulopathy is not always corrected (e.g. FFP) unless bleeding is severe. 30% of ALF cases die with clotting disorders including GI bleeding

Organ dysfunction
Respiratory complications
• Atelectasis
• Pneumonia (e.g. due to aspiration, infection)
• Pulmonary (V/Q) shunt with hypoxaemia due to failure to clear vasodilators
• Pulmonary oedema due to hypoalbuminaemia and fluid overload
Renal failure (50%)
• Hepatorenal syndrome causes oliguria insensitive to diuretics or fluids. It has a high mortality
• Acute tubular necrosis
Gastrointestinal
• GI bleeding causes 20% deaths and precipitates shock and HpE

HpE= hepatic encephalopathy; GI=gastrointestinal;
ALF= acute liver failure; Gm –ve=Gram negative

Figure 54b Causes of acute liver failure

Viral hepatitis (40–70%)	Chemical toxins (5%)
Hepatitis A, B, C, δ	Carbon tetrachloride
Cytomegalovirus	Benzene/ethanol
Epstein-Barr virus	Ethylene glycol
Varicella-zoster virus	Phosphorus
	Ethanol

Drug related (20%)	Others (10%)
Halothane	Toxic mushrooms:
Paracetamol*	- Amanita phalloides
Amphetamine / 'Ecstasy'	Reye's syndrome
Isoniazid / Rifampicin	Wilson's disease
Anabolic steroids	Autoimmune hepatitis
Phenytoin / Na Valproate	Budd-Chiari syndrome
Methyldopa	Galactosaemia

* Incidence of paracetamol induced ALF is much higher in the UK

Figure 54c Investigations

2-to 4-hourly	Blood sugar, gases, acid-base
Daily	FBC, biochemistry, clotting, ECG, CXR
As required	Microbiology (e.g. blood cultures), CT scan, ammonia levels, liver biopsy
To establish aetiology	Serology (e.g. viral hepatitis), drug screen (e.g. paracetamol), plasma caeroplasmin for Wilson's disease Abdominal ultrasound, EEG

Figure 54e Pathogenesis of spontaneous bacterial peritonitis

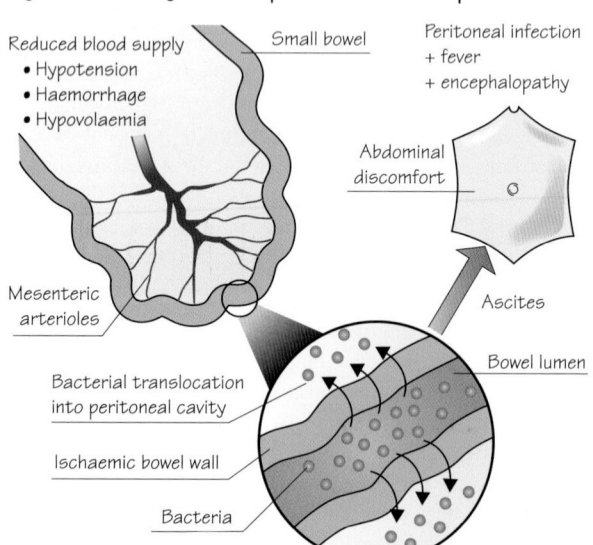

Reduced blood supply
• Hypotension
• Haemorrhage
• Hypovolaemia

Small bowel

Peritoneal infection
+ fever
+ encephalopathy

Abdominal discomfort

Ascites

Bowel lumen

Mesenteric arterioles

Bacterial translocation into peritoneal cavity

Ischaemic bowel wall

Bacteria

Figure 54d Grades of hepatic encephalopathy

Grade	Mental status	Liver flap	EEG
1	Altered mood, slow mentation	None	Normal
2	Drowsiness, inappropriate behaviour, confusion, slurred speech	Present	Becomes abnormal
3	Severe confusion, semi-stuporose but responds to simple commands	Present (if cooperates)	Always abnormal
4	Comatose but may respond to pain	Absent	Always abnormal

Classification

- **Primary acute liver failure (ALF; fulminant hepatic failure)** is defined as potentially reversible liver injury with hepatic encephalopathy (HpE), coagulopathy and jaundice developing within 4 weeks in a previously healthy person. Hyperacute liver failure describes encephalopathy within 7 days of onset of jaundice. It is fatal in 40–85% of cases. The most common causes (Figure 54b) are viral hepatitis (40–70%) and paracetamol toxicity (5–40%). Hepatitis A (5–30%) and B (25–75%) are the main viral causes but the risk of developing ALF in viral hepatitis is <1%. Paracetamol poisoning is discussed in Chapter 70.
- **Secondary acute liver failure** is more frequent and occurs when acute illness causes decompensation in pre-existing chronic liver disease (CLD; e.g. cirrhosis). Potential precipitants include ischaemia (e.g. shock, sepsis, thrombosis) and liver toxins (e.g. drugs, total parenteral nutrition [TPN]).

Clinical features

Biochemical and central nervous system (CNS) dysfunction are the hallmarks of ALF. Figure 54a illustrates these features (and those of CLD), which are due to:

- **Metabolic dysfunction**: reduced hepatic gluconeogenesis and raised insulin levels cause hypoglycaemia in ~40% of cases. Inadequate lactate metabolism causes lactic acidosis in ~50% of late ALF. Liver function tests (e.g. bilirubin, serum transaminases >2000 IU/L) and ammonia levels are usually raised. Clinically, 'hepatic foetor' and jaundice are often detected. Electrolyte disturbances (e.g. hyponatraemia, hypokalaemia) and secondary hyperaldosteronism are common.
- **Synthetic dysfunction** includes hypoalbuminaemia and clotting factor deficiencies. Gastrointestinal (GI) bleeding causes ~20% of deaths (Chapter 52), and often precipitates shock and HpE.
- **Reduced immunity**: although fever and leukocytosis only affect ~30%, phagocytic dysfunction causes infection (e.g. pneumonia) in ~80% and fatal sepsis in ~15% of ALF cases.
  - **Spontaneous bacterial peritonitis (SBP)** is due to splanchnic hypoperfusion, which impairs bowel wall integrity, allowing bacterial translocation and peritoneal infection (Figure 54e). Characteristic features are fever, abdominal discomfort, encephalopathy, sudden renal impairment, weight gain or ascites. The diagnosis is confirmed if aspirated peritoneal fluid reveals bacteria, typically gram-negative rods (e.g. *E. coli*), but a leukocyte count >500/mm³, pH < 7.3 or raised lactate are also indications for treatment. Blood cultures are positive in ~50%. Untreated SBP is fatal in 70–90%.
- **Organ dysfunction** (Figure 54a) including respiratory complications (e.g. pneumonia, shunt, oedema), renal failure (e.g. hepatorenal syndrome, acute tubular necrosis [ATN]) and cerebral oedema may progress to multi-organ failure.
- **Hepatic encephalopathy** arises when toxin-laden portal blood bypasses the liver and is shunted into the systemic circulation. It is the most common cause of death.
  - **Precipitating factors** include upper GI bleeding, which increases gut protein (i.e. blood) with associated bacterial ammonia formation; intravascular volume depletion, which reduces hepatic perfusion (e.g. diuretics); renal failure, which impairs toxin/drug clearance; and infection.
  - **Clinical features**: early signs are irritability and confusion. Drowsiness and coma develop over hours to weeks. Exclude reversible causes (e.g. hypoglycaemia, sedatives). Tremor, liver 'flap' and sustained clonus may be elicited.
  - **Diagnosis** is clinical, supported by elevated ammonia levels and specific electroencephalogram (EEG) findings (e.g. high

amplitude δ and triphasic waves), although most EEGs show non-specific diffuse slowing. HpE grades (Figure 54d) are of limited value because of fluctuations in coma level.

Management

Management is mainly supportive but early involvement of a specialist liver unit is essential. Figure 54c lists appropriate investigations. In survivors, liver regeneration may be associated with complete recovery.

- **General**: glucose infusions (i.e. 10% dextrose) prevent hypoglycaemia. Potassium supplements may be required. Infection must be treated (e.g. broad-spectrum antibiotics, antifungals) promptly but prophylactic antibiotics are ineffective. Antacids prevent stress ulceration but H₂ blockers and proton pump inhibitors (PPIs) can cause CNS side-effects due to impaired drug metabolism.
  - **Nutrition**: avoid high-protein diets and limit sodium intake. Branched-chain amino acids in TPN minimize HpE. Supplement vitamin K, thiamine and folate.
- **Cardiorespiratory support**: the circulation is often hyperdynamic, vasodilated and volume depleted. Careful resuscitation (e.g. central venous pressure [CVP] monitored) maintains organ perfusion but avoids pulmonary and cerebral oedema due to excessive fluid. Hypoxaemia (e.g. ventilation/perfusion [V/Q] mismatch), inadequate ventilation (e.g. ascitic diaphragmatic splinting) and HpE (e.g. aspiration risk) may require mechanical ventilation.
  - **Ascites, oedema (±hypokalaemia)** require fluid restriction, a low salt diet and potassium-sparing diuretics (e.g. spironolactone).
  - **Coagulopathy**: vitamin K, platelets and fresh frozen plasma (FFP) are given for active bleeding and invasive procedures but not prophylaxsis.
  - **Cerebral oedema** is transiently reduced by hyperventilation and mannitol therapy (Chapter 72) but survival is not improved.
- **Encephalopathy** is prevented by avoiding sedation and correcting precipitating factors. Bacterial generation and bowel absorption of nitrogenous toxins are reduced with a low-protein diet (<40 g/day), laxatives (e.g. lactulose) to reduce bowel transit time (e.g. GI bleeding) and non-absorbable antibiotics (e.g. neomycin) to sterilize the bowel. Convulsions are treated aggressively (Chapter 60).
- **Specific therapies** are limited.
  - **N-acetylcysteine** benefits most patients but is essential in paracetamol-induced ALF (Chapter 70).
  - **Liver transplantation** is a last resort with 1-year survivals between 50% and 75%. It has a limited but definite role in paracetamol-induced ALF but is less successful in alcohol-related ALF (Appendix 6). Limited organ availability means that ~50% of candidates die awaiting a donor.

Prognosis

Overall, ALF survival rates are 20–30%. Mortality depends on cause (i.e. hepatitis A ~33–55%; paracetamol-induced ~47–65%; hepatitis B ~61–76%; and non-A, non-sB hepatitis >85%), age (i.e. worse if >40 years) and HpE grade. Other poor prognostic factors are bilirubin level (>300 μmol/L), metabolic acidosis (pH < 7.3), prothrombin time (>3.5) and organ failure (e.g. renal).

Pearl of wisdom
Viral hepatitis rarely causes acute liver failure (<1%), but because it is common it accounts for ~50% of acute liver failure (ALF)

55 Acute pancreatitis

Figure 55a Contrast-enhanced scan of pancreas

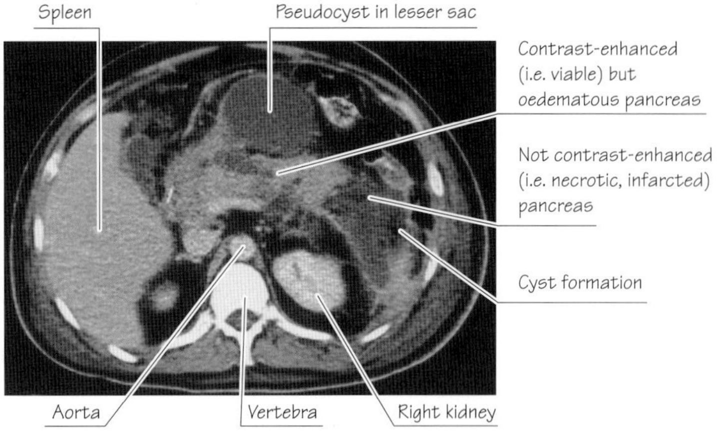

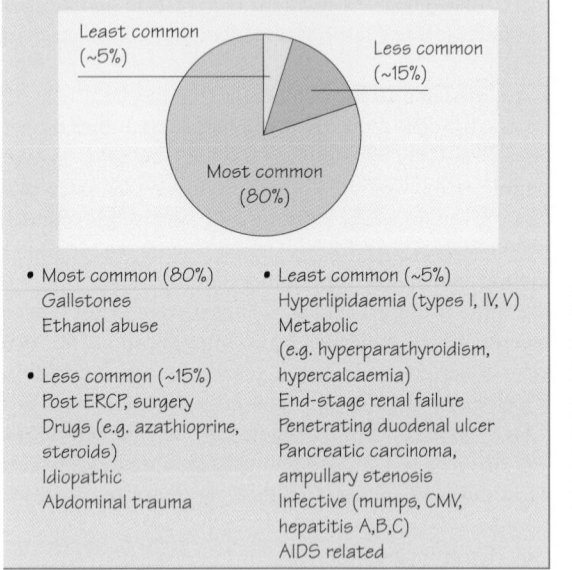

Spleen
Pseudocyst in lesser sac
Contrast-enhanced (i.e. viable) but oedematous pancreas
Not contrast-enhanced (i.e. necrotic, infarcted) pancreas
Cyst formation
Aorta
Vertebra
Right kidney

Figure 55b Adverse prognostic features of acute pancreatitis

Ranson's Score parameters

On admission	Within 48 h of admission
Age >55 years	Decrease in Hct >10%
WBC >16000/mm^3	Rise in urea >5 mg/dL (1.8 mmol/L)
Glucose >11 mmol/L	Calcium <8 mg/dL (2.0 mmol/L)
AST > 250 IU/L	P_aO_2 <8 kPa (60 mmHg)
LDH > 400 IU/L	Base deficit >4 mmol/L
	Fluid deficit >6L

Ranson's Score predicts outcome

No. risk factors	Mortality
0–2	<1%
3–4	~15%
5–6	~40%
>6	~80%

Glasgow criteria (Imrie's score) uses 8 of Ranson's original variables (LDH, base deficit and fluid deficit excluded) without losing predictive power

Figure 55c Causes of acute pancreatitis

Least common (~5%)
Less common (~15%)
Most common (80%)

- Most common (80%)
  Gallstones
  Ethanol abuse

- Less common (~15%)
  Post ERCP, surgery
  Drugs (e.g. azathioprine, steroids)
  Idiopathic
  Abdominal trauma

- Least common (~5%)
  Hyperlipidaemia (types I, IV, V)
  Metabolic (e.g. hyperparathyroidism, hypercalcaemia)
  End-stage renal failure
  Penetrating duodenal ulcer
  Pancreatic carcinoma, ampullary stenosis
  Infective (mumps, CMV, hepatitis A,B,C)
  AIDS related

Figure 55d Clinical features and complications

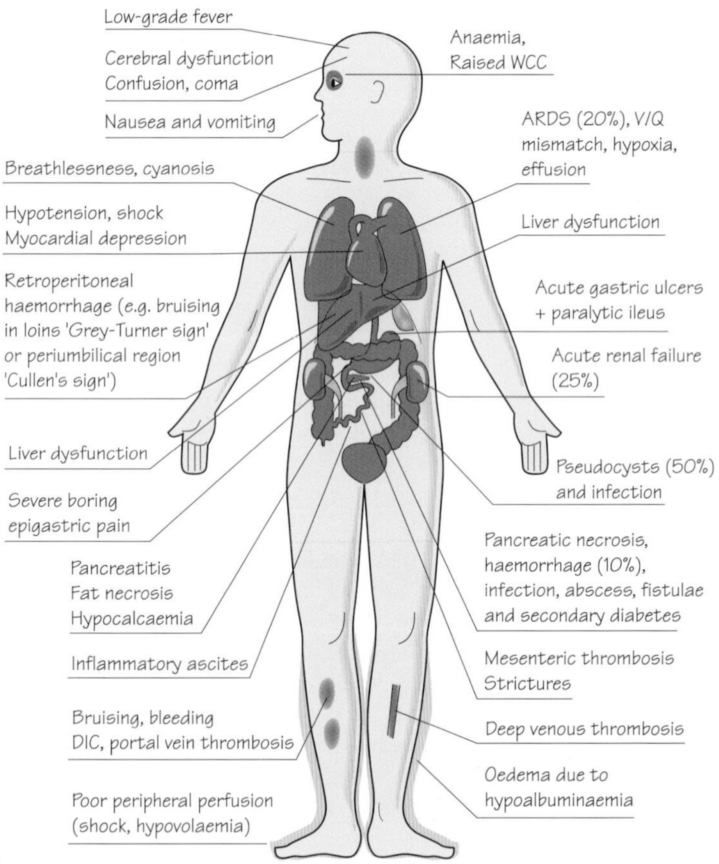

Clinical features

Low-grade fever
Cerebral dysfunction Confusion, coma
Nausea and vomiting
Breathlessness, cyanosis
Hypotension, shock Myocardial depression
Retroperitoneal haemorrhage (e.g. bruising in loins 'Grey-Turner sign' or periumbilical region 'Cullen's sign')
Liver dysfunction
Severe boring epigastric pain
Pancreatitis Fat necrosis Hypocalcaemia
Inflammatory ascites
Bruising, bleeding DIC, portal vein thrombosis
Poor peripheral perfusion (shock, hypovolaemia)

Complications

Anaemia, Raised WCC
ARDS (20%), V/Q mismatch, hypoxia, effusion
Liver dysfunction
Acute gastric ulcers + paralytic ileus
Acute renal failure (25%)
Pseudocysts (50%) and infection
Pancreatic necrosis, haemorrhage (10%), infection, abscess, fistulae and secondary diabetes
Mesenteric thrombosis Strictures
Deep venous thrombosis
Oedema due to hypoalbuminaemia

Figure 55e CT scan assessment of pancreatitis severity

Grade of pancreatitis		Degree of pancreatic necrosis	
Normal pancreas	0	No necrosis	0
Pancreatic enlargement	1	Necrosis 33% pancreas	2
Inflammation of pancreas	2	Necrosis 50% pancreas	4
One fluid collection	3	Necrosis >50% pancreas	6
>1 fluid collection	4		

Total score	
Score <3 = mortality <5%	0–10
Score 7–10 = mortality >15%	

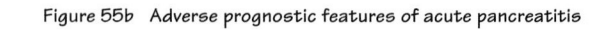

Critical Care Medicine at a Glance, Third Edition. Richard Leach. © 2014 John Wiley & Sons, Ltd. Published 2014 by John Wiley & Sons, Ltd.

cute pancreatitis is either clinically mild (75%) or severe (25%). Mild pancreatitis usually resolves with analgesia and fluid therapy. In severe pancreatitis, prompt identification and management of organ failure and local complications (e.g. necrosis) improves outcome. However, mortality is still ~25%.

Aetiology

- *Causes:* gallstones and alcohol cause 80% of cases (Figure 55c).
- *Pathogenesis:* ductal obstruction (e.g. gallstones) with biliary reflux into the pancreas or cytotoxic injury (e.g. alcohol) initiates pancreatic auto-digestion by the enzymes trypsin, lipase and elastase.
- *Histology:* Acute pancreatitis is classified as oedematous (~75%) or necrotizing (~25%). Failure of contrast enhancement on CT scan identifies necrotic tissue (Figure 55a).

Clinical features (Figure 55d)

Pancreatitis presents with severe, 'boring' epigastric and/or back pain. Nausea, vomiting and low-grade fever are common. Pain and fluid loss cause tachycardia, hypotension and shock. Acute lung injury may cause respiratory distress. Peritonitis is unusual because the pancreas is retroperitoneal but abdominal tenderness and ileus-induced distension are common. Bruising in the loins (Grey–Turner's sign) and around the umbilicus (Cullen's sign) are rare features of retroperitoneal haemorrhage.

There are two clinical phases during severe pancreatitis:
1 The early phase (0–14 days) is due to inflammation (i.e. cytokines, systematic inflammatory response syndrome [SIRS]) and fluid shifts. Shock, acute respiratory distress syndrome [ARDS], acute kidney injury, coagulopathy, fat necrosis and hypocalcaemia occur.
2 The late phase is associated with local complications (e.g. pancreatic necrosis, infection (±abscess), pseudocyst, fistula, ascites, strictures, ileus, portal vein thrombosis, diabetes).

Investigation

- **Laboratory**: raised white cell count (WCC), uraemia, hypocalcaemia, hypoglycaemia and hypoalbuminaemia are common. Serum amylase levels 3–5 times normal strongly suggest pancreatitis. However, the amylase level has little prognostic value because it is raised in many abdominal emergencies or normal in 30% of confirmed pancreatitis. Raised serum lipase is more specific but not widely available.
- **Radiological**: abdominal X-rays show localized ileus (e.g. 'sentinel loop') and calcification in chronic pancreatitis. Abdominal ultrasound scans detect gallstones, biliary duct dilation and pancreatic pseudocysts. CT scans best visualize the pancreas (e.g. oedema) and associated complications (e.g. necrosis) but only confirm the cause in ~25%.

Prognosis

Mortality is ~10% in sterile and ~35% in infected pancreatitis. **Early deaths** (<14 days) are due to inflammation (e.g. multi-organ failure [MOF]); **late deaths** to infection, which occurs in 40–60% of necrotizing pancreatitis. Infection risk increases with the amount of necrosis and time from onset.

Severity assessment: scoring systems (e.g. APACHE II) assess severity and prognosis. Of the specific scoring systems, Ranson's criteria are most commonly used (Figure 55b). Prognostic factors include: (a) **Cause (i.e. cytotoxic vs gallstone)**: death occurs early in alcohol-induced (i.e. inflammatory) and later in gallstone-induced (i.e. sepsis-related) pancreatitis. Mortality is ~50% if gallstones are not removed. Pancreatic haemorrhage carries the worst prognosis; (b) **Histology (i.e. oedematous vs necrotic)**: necrosis increases mortality (Figure 55e); (c) **Pancreatic infection**: serial procalcitonin measurement and CT-guided fine needle aspiration reliably detect onset of infection in necrotic pancreatic tissue. (d) **MOF**: number of organ failures correlates with mortality.

Management

Uncomplicated, oedematous pancreatitis management includes:
1 Fluid resuscitation and electrolyte replacement: correct hypovolaemia due to oedema, ileus and vomiting with balanced crystalloid solutions. Vasopressors may be needed to maintain blood pressure (BP) in patients with shock.
2 Nutrition: initially withhold oral feeding to reduce pancreatic enzyme release. Initiate nasogastric tube drainage. Nutritional support is of little value in uncomplicated pancreatitis. However, in severe pancreatitis, early enteric feeding through a naso-jejunal tube is well tolerated and reduces infectious complications. Parenteral nutrition is only justified if enteral feeding fails.
3 Pain control can be difficult. Theoretical concerns that morphine may evoke ampullary spasm are probably unjustified.
4 Prophylactic antibiotics are given in gallstone-induced pancreatitis (i.e. high risk of biliary tract infection) and all cases with shock, but are not required in other cases.
5 Stress-ulcer prophylaxis (e.g. proton pump inhibitors) reduces peptic ulceration but pancreatitis is unaffected.
6 Early gallstone extraction reduces mortality, infective complications and severity of pancreatitis. Endoscopic retrograde choledochopancreatograhy (ERCP) is as successful as surgery if accomplished within 48 hours.
7 Non-specific sepsis measures include glucose control and steroids for relative adrenocortical insufficiency (Chapter 25).

Severe necrotizing pancreatitis is treated as above; but, as infected necrosis substantially increases mortality, prevention and treatment of infection are essential.
1 Antibiotic therapy reduces infection and late mortality in necrotizing pancreatitis. Start high-dose cefuroxime or meropenem when necrosis is confirmed and continue for 10–14 days.
2 Radiological percutaneous drainage of infected collections may avoid the need for surgery.
3 Surgery does not reduce mortality in sterile necrotizing pancreatitis but may be considered later in patients with infected necrosis who have not improved with antibiotic therapy.
4 Somatostatin and octreotide may be used to reduce pancreatic secretions but there is no evidence of benefit.

Complications and long-term sequelae

Complications are illustrated in Figure 55d. **Pseudocysts** (i.e. collections of pancreatic secretions) occur in ~20% of cases. Indications for drainage are pain, size >6 cm, gastric outlet obstruction and infection or haemorrhage.

Chronic pancreatitis follows recurrent pancreatitis and causes chronic pain, pancreatic calcification, and impaired endocrine and exocrine pancreatic function (e.g. diabetes, malabsorption).

Pearl of wisdom
Start high-dose antibiotics when necrotic pancreatitis is confirmed to avoid infection and reduce late mortality

56 Vomiting and intestinal obstruction

Figure 56a Causes of vomiting

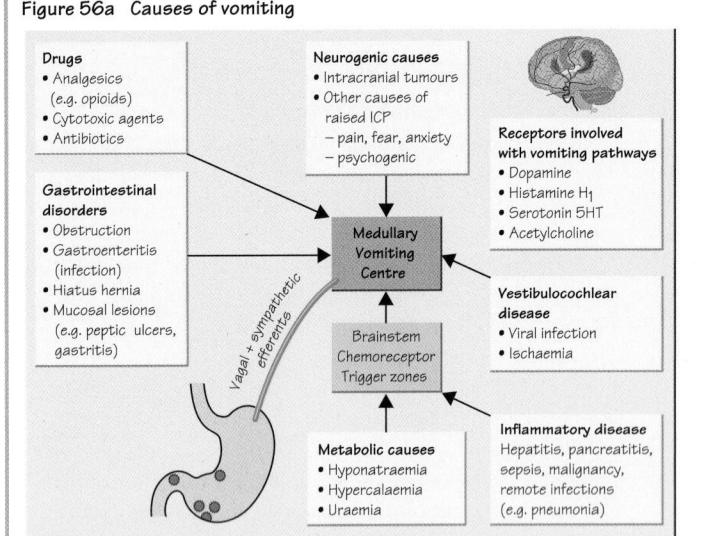

Drugs
• Analgesics (e.g. opioids)
• Cytotoxic agents
• Antibiotics

Neurogenic causes
• Intracranial tumours
• Other causes of raised ICP
  – pain, fear, anxiety
  – psychogenic

Receptors involved with vomiting pathways
• Dopamine
• Histamine H₁
• Serotonin 5HT
• Acetylcholine

Gastrointestinal disorders
• Obstruction
• Gastroenteritis (infection)
• Hiatus hernia
• Mucosal lesions (e.g. peptic ulcers, gastritis)

Medullary Vomiting Centre

Vagal + sympathetic efferents

Brainstem Chemoreceptor Trigger zones

Vestibulocochlear disease
• Viral infection
• Ischaemia

Metabolic causes
• Hyponatraemia
• Hypercalaemia
• Uraemia

Inflammatory disease
Hepatitis, pancreatitis, sepsis, malignancy, remote infections (e.g. pneumonia)

ICP = intracranial pressure

Figure 56b Assessment of vomiting

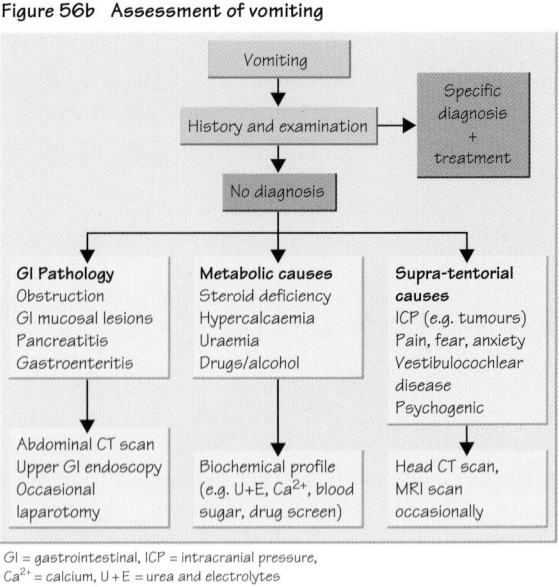

Vomiting

History and examination → Specific diagnosis + treatment

No diagnosis

GI Pathology
Obstruction
GI mucosal lesions
Pancreatitis
Gastroenteritis
↓
Abdominal CT scan
Upper GI endoscopy
Occasional laparotomy

Metabolic causes
Steroid deficiency
Hypercalcaemia
Uraemia
Drugs/alcohol
↓
Biochemical profile (e.g. U+E, Ca²⁺, blood sugar, drug screen)

Supra-tentorial causes
ICP (e.g. tumours)
Pain, fear, anxiety
Vestibulocochlear disease
Psychogenic
↓
Head CT scan, MRI scan occasionally

GI = gastrointestinal, ICP = intracranial pressure,
Ca²⁺ = calcium, U + E = urea and electrolytes

Figure 56c Causes of intestinal obstruction

Small bowel obstruction
• *Adhesions* (~60%)
• *Strangulated herniae* (20%)
• *Volvulus* (5%)
• *Strictures* (e.g. Crohn's disease, NSAID)
• *Extrinsic malignancy* (e.g. pancreas)
• *Intrinsic malignancy* (5%; but usually in caecum)

Large bowel obstruction (LBO)
• *Colorectal malignancy* (>90%)
  (typically >70 years old; distal tumours most likely to obstruct; often advanced with distant metastases in 25%; perforations can occur at the site of tumour or dilated caecum)
• *Sigmoid/caecal volvulus* (rotation of gut on its mesenteric axis, 75% sigmoid (5% LBO) + 25% caecal colon; occurs mainly in older or psychiatrically unwell patients; 10x as common in Africa as Europe/USA).

Ileus (pseudo-obstruction; paralytic ileus; with large (± small) bowel dilation)
• *Postoperative* ↓by reducing bowel handling
• *Medical conditions* (e.g. electrolyte disturbance, DKA, chest infection, trauma, MI, stroke, AKI, hypothyroidism)

Miscellaneous causes
• *Bodypackers* (i.e. swallowed packets of illicit drugs; associated with intoxication if packets rupture)
• *Severe constipation* (i.e. faecal impaction)
• *Gallstone ileus* (i.e. blockage by a large gallstone)
• *Crohn's disease* (i.e. due to strictures)
• *External compression* (e.g. gynaecological tumours)

Childhood causes
• *Congenital gastrointestinal malformations*
• *Hirschsprung's disease*
• *Intussusception*
• *Childhood volvulus and mid-gut rotations*
• *Meconium ileus in cystic fibrosis*

NSAID = non-steroidal anti-inflammatory drugs,
DKA = diabetic ketoacidosis; MI=myocardial infarction;
AKI = acute kidney injury

Pearl of wisdom

Sigmoid volvulus and bowel obstructions due to adhesions can be treated conservatively in over 65% of cases

Figure 56f Royal College of Physicians

'Ten Top Tips' for Nil-by-Mouth orders

1. A 'Nil by Mouth' (NBM) protocol should be initiated when NBM for >8-24 hours
2. The protocol should include:
   • Reason for NBM (e.g. procedure, unsafe swallow)
   • Document plan for alternative hydration, nutrition + medication needs
   • Time, date + person responsible for review of NBM plan
   • Clear signage that the patient is NBM
3. NBM should be documented in medical and nursing notes
4. Reason for NBM and review time should be discussed with the patient
5. NBM orders should be reviewed at least every 24 hours (e.g. by the clinician in charge)
6. NBM patients require regular mouth care and sips of water are allowed if there is no risk of aspiration
7. No NBM orders should be made until investigations or procedures have been booked
8. When investigations or procedures are cancelled, patients should be offered oral food and fluids immediately, and until rebooking
9. Relatives and carers should be informed about, and involved in, NBM decisions
10. While NBM review all medications daily
    • Stop oral medications
    • Diabetic patients are at particular risk: assess oral + insulin regimes

Figure 56d Key clinical features of intestinal obstruction

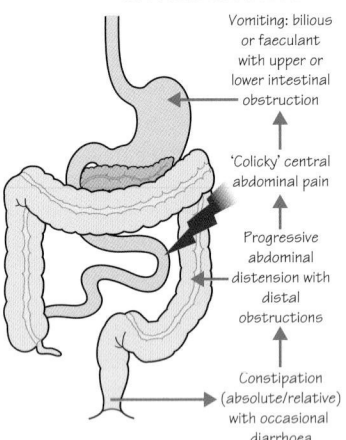

Vomiting: bilious or faeculant with upper or lower intestinal obstruction

'Colicky' central abdominal pain

Progressive abdominal distension with distal obstructions

Constipation (absolute/relative) with occasional diarrhoea

Figure 56e Abdominal X-ray of small bowel obstruction

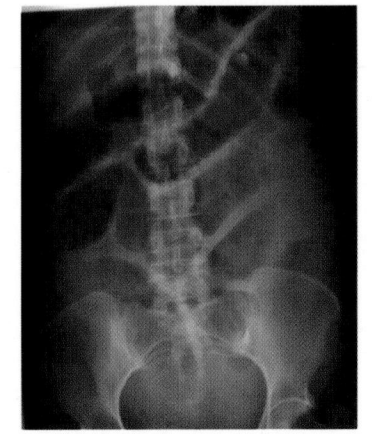

Critical Care Medicine at a Glance, Third Edition. Richard Leach. © 2014 John Wiley & Sons, Ltd. Published 2014 by John Wiley & Sons, Ltd.

Vomiting

Vomiting is common and often associated with diarrhoea (Chapter 57). The brainstem 'vomiting centre' (Figure 56a) receives input from:

- Cerebral receptors (e.g. dopamine, histamine [H_1]) activated by raised intracranial pressure (ICP), pain or anxiety.
- Brainstem chemoreceptors activated by drugs (e.g. opiods) or metabolic stimuli (e.g. uraemia).
- Afferent vagal or sympathetic nerves originating in the inner ear motion centres or gastrointestinal (GI) tract (e.g. stomach).

Most vomiting is rapidly self-limiting (e.g. travel sickness, gastro-enteritis) but investigation is required if vomiting is severe, persistent or associated with other symptoms (e.g. morning headache). Initial assessment identifies self-limiting causes requiring symptomatic therapy. If the diagnosis is unclear, investigation excludes metabolic, GI and supratentorial causes (Figure 56b).

History and examination

These assess duration, severity and progress of symptoms (i.e. is the vomiting getting worse?); potential food poisoning (e.g. unrefrigerated/street foods, travel); new medications (e.g. 'over-the-counter' preparations); nausea, thirst, polyuria or oliguria; GI causes (e.g. recent surgery, Crohn's disease); tinnitus, vertigo, deafness or loss of balance and features of raised ICP. Examination may reveal dehydration (e.g. postural blood pressure [BP] drop), abdominal distension or mechanical obstruction (see later).

Investigation

Clinical evaluation guides investigation. **Routine blood tests** include electrolytes, amylase, renal and liver function, and morning cortisol (±short Synacthen test) to exclude hypoadrenalism. **Imaging** includes chest radiography (CXR) (i.e. aspiration, neoplasm), abdominal X-ray and abdominal CT scan (±small bowel 'contrast') to detect the cause and site of intestinal obstruction (e.g. pancreatic tumour). Head CT scan excludes raised ICP when no other cause is identified. In persistent vomiting, **endoscopy** detects upper GI strictures and the cause (e.g. duodenal ulcer).

Management

Treat the underlying cause. If mechanical obstruction has been excluded, consider empirical antiemetic therapy. Metoclopramide and prochlorperazine are commonly used but occasionally cause neurological side-effects (e.g. dyskinesia). Domperidone does not cross the blood brain barrier and is useful for prolonged 'as needed' therapy. Centrally acting serotonin antagonists (e.g. ondansetron) are effective but expensive.

Intestinal obstruction

Intestinal obstruction causes 20% of admission abdominal pain, of which ~80% are small bowel obstructions (SBOs). Causes are reported in Figure 56c. Colorectal cancers present with large bowel obstruction (LBO) in 16% of cases. Ileus implies non-mechanical obstruction (e.g. bowel 'paralysis').

Clinical features: typically pain is central, intermittent and 'colicky' with progressively increasing severity. Severe pain or tenderness suggests ischaemia or perforation. Vomiting is 'bilious' (i.e. green/yellow) in upper, and faeculant (i.e. brown) in lower, GI obstruction. Abdominal distension is marked in lower GI obstructions (e.g. sigmoid volvulus). Absolute constipation occurs early in low GI obstructions, often with preceding bowel habit changes (i.e. blood, diarrhoea, constipation). In 'paralytic' ileus, bowel movement and flatus are absent. Onset may be acute (e.g. sigmoid volvulus) or gradual (e.g. bowel malignancy). Anorexia, weight loss and progressive pain suggest progressive pathology (e.g. GI neoplasms). Previous history suggests potential causes (e.g. oesophageal stricture in prolonged gastric reflux). Recent abdominal surgery may cause paralytic ileus or complications, whereas previous surgery causes adhesions.

Examination reveals pyrexia (i.e. perforation), lymphadenopathy, strangulated hernias (e.g. femoral, inguinal), scars from previous abdominal surgery (i.e. adhesions) and dehydration due to vomiting or failure of fluid absorption (e.g. postural hypotension, tachycardia, oliguria). Abdominal distension is common with paralytic ileus or distal obstructive lesions. Absent bowel sounds suggest paralytic ileus but in most cases, bowel sounds increase and have a 'tinkling' quality. A succession splash on abdominal movement suggests gastric outflow obstruction. Palpable masses may be inflammatory or malignant. Rebound tenderness suggests perforation. Rectal examination (±sigmoidoscopy) detects causes of LBO.

Investigations confirm the cause and metabolic consequences of intestinal obstruction. **Routine blood (±blood gas) analysis** assesses the effects of vomiting and intestinal obstruction on electrolyte homeostasis, renal function and acid–base balance (e.g. gastric outflow obstruction causes hypokalaemic, hypochloraemic alkalosis). **Abdominal X-ray** (60% sensitivity) reveals dilated bowel ('ladder-like' in SBO), fluid levels on erect films and occasionally the level of obstruction (Figure 56d). **Ultrasound** reliably excludes obstruction in ~89% of cases. **Abdominal CT scans** (±water soluble contrast) aid intraluminal and extraluminal (e.g. pancreatic tumour) diagnosis. **Endoscopy** detects upper and lower GI lesions. **Barium-contrast imaging** (e.g. 'barium swallow'; 'barium enema') is also useful.

Management should involve a GI surgeon.

- **Conservative management**: institute a 'nil by mouth' order (Figure 56f). Insert a large bore nasogastric tube (Appendix 7) to drain obstructed GI contents (i.e. ~2 L/day of upper GI secretions) and prevent aspiration. Monitor haemodynamic parameters, fluid balance and urine output. Large volumes of intravenous fluids and electrolytes may be required for resuscitation and to correct previous depletions. This reduces operative risks and facilitates recovery of bowel function in paralytic ileus. Limit opiate therapy in pain management because this inhibits intestinal motility and prolongs post-operative ileus. In 'pseudo-obstruction', consider cautious use of neostigmine and colonoscopy for decompression.
- **Laparotomy** may be required before a diagnosis is established or if conservative management fails. It is not possible to predict who will need surgery. If possible, await full resuscitation, but early surgery may be necessary if the patient is toxic (e.g. peritonitis). Obstructions due to adhesions resolve with conservative therapy in 65% of cases. Caecum/terminal ileum volvulus (~25% of volvulus cases) often require surgery (or colonoscope decompression) whereas ~80% of sigmoid volvulus (~75% of volvulus cases) is treated conservatively (e.g. flatus tube). A palpable mass or failure to improve are relative indications to intervene surgically.

Prognosis

SBO mortality is 8% or 25% if surgery occurs before or after 36 hours respectively. Sigmoid volvulus recurs within 2 years in >50%. Prognosis in advanced colonic cancer is poor and ~25% of patients presenting with obstruction have distant metastases.

57 Diarrhoea

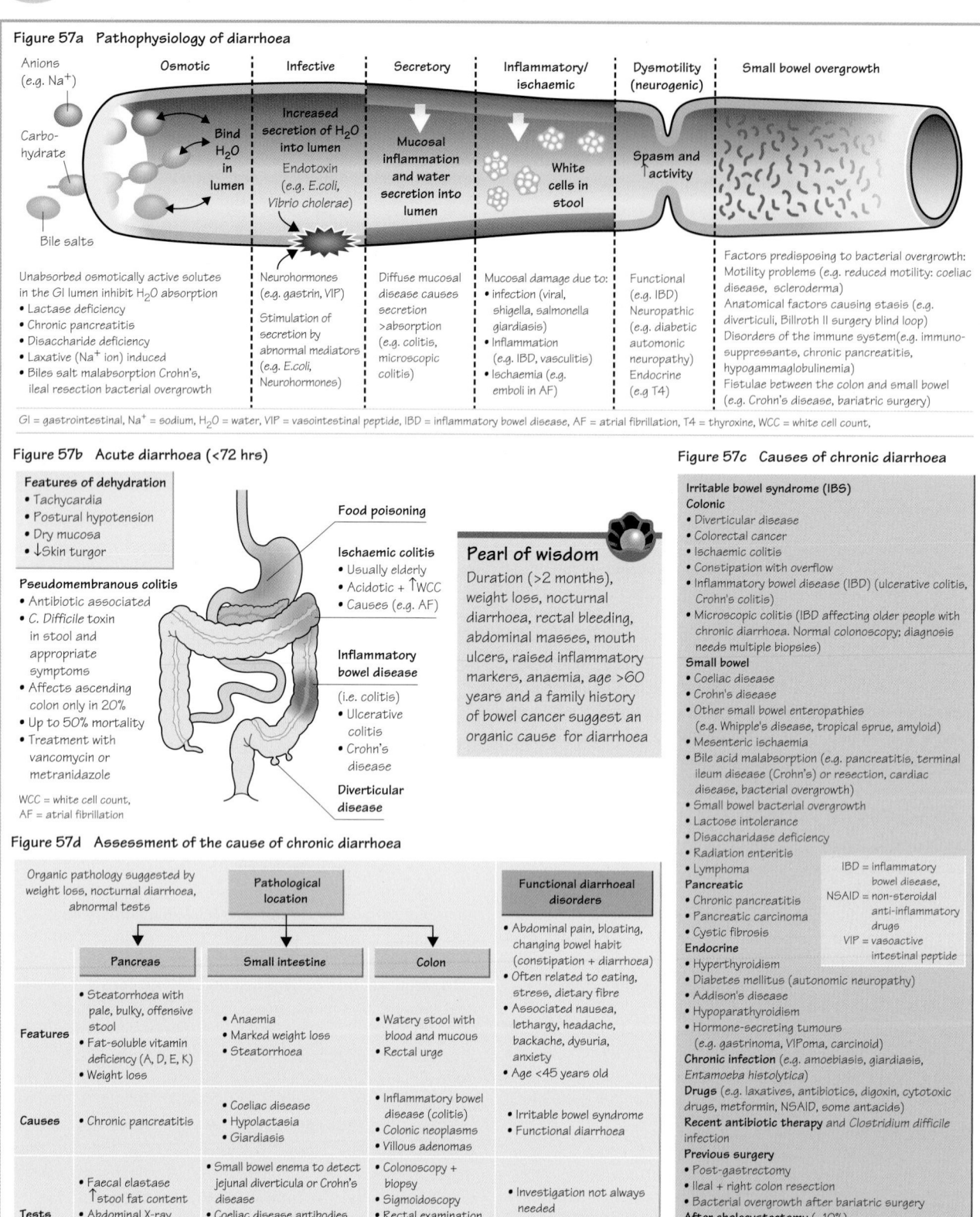

Figure 57a Pathophysiology of diarrhoea

	Osmotic	Infective	Secretory	Inflammatory/ischaemic	Dysmotility (neurogenic)	Small bowel overgrowth
Anions (e.g. Na⁺)	Bind H_2O in lumen	Increased secretion of H_2O into lumen. Endotoxin (e.g. E.coli, Vibrio cholerae)	Mucosal inflammation and water secretion into lumen	White cells in stool	Spasm and ↑activity	

Carbohydrate

Bile salts

Unabsorbed osmotically active solutes in the GI lumen inhibit H_2O absorption
• Lactase deficiency
• Chronic pancreatitis
• Disaccharide deficiency
• Laxative (Na⁺ ion) induced
• Biles salt malabsorption Crohn's, ileal resection bacterial overgrowth

Neurohormones (e.g. gastrin, VIP)

Stimulation of secretion by abnormal mediators (e.g. E.coli, Neurohormones)

Diffuse mucosal disease causes secretion >absorption (e.g. colitis, microscopic colitis)

Mucosal damage due to:
• infection (viral, shigella, salmonella giardiasis)
• Inflammation (e.g. IBD, vasculitis)
• Ischaemia (e.g. emboli in AF)

Functional (e.g. IBD) Neuropathic (e.g. diabetic automonic neuropathy) Endocrine (e.g T4)

Factors predisposing to bacterial overgrowth:
Motility problems (e.g. reduced motility: coeliac disease, scleroderma)
Anatomical factors causing stasis (e.g. diverticuli, Billroth II surgery blind loop)
Disorders of the immune system(e.g. immunosuppressants, chronic pancreatitis, hypogammaglobulinemia)
Fistulae between the colon and small bowel (e.g. Crohn's disease, bariatric surgery)

GI = gastrointestinal, Na⁺ = sodium, H_2O = water, VIP = vasointestinal peptide, IBD = inflammatory bowel disease, AF = atrial fibrillation, T4 = thyroxine, WCC = white cell count.

Figure 57b Acute diarrhoea (<72 hrs)

Features of dehydration
• Tachycardia
• Postural hypotension
• Dry mucosa
• ↓Skin turgor

Pseudomembranous colitis
• Antibiotic associated
• C. Difficile toxin in stool and appropriate symptoms
• Affects ascending colon only in 20%
• Up to 50% mortality
• Treatment with vancomycin or metranidazole

WCC = white cell count,
AF = atrial fibrillation

Food poisoning

Ischaemic colitis
• Usually elderly
• Acidotic + ↑WCC
• Causes (e.g. AF)

Inflammatory bowel disease
(i.e. colitis)
• Ulcerative colitis
• Crohn's disease

Diverticular disease

Pearl of wisdom

Duration (>2 months), weight loss, nocturnal diarrhoea, rectal bleeding, abdominal masses, mouth ulcers, raised inflammatory markers, anaemia, age >60 years and a family history of bowel cancer suggest an organic cause for diarrhoea

Figure 57c Causes of chronic diarrhoea

Irritable bowel syndrome (IBS)
Colonic
• Diverticular disease
• Colorectal cancer
• Ischaemic colitis
• Constipation with overflow
• Inflammatory bowel disease (IBD) (ulcerative colitis, Crohn's colitis)
• Microscopic colitis (IBD affecting older people with chronic diarrhoea. Normal colonoscopy; diagnosis needs multiple biopsies)
Small bowel
• Coeliac disease
• Crohn's disease
• Other small bowel enteropathies (e.g. Whipple's disease, tropical sprue, amyloid)
• Mesenteric ischaemia
• Bile acid malabsorption (e.g. pancreatitis, terminal ileum disease (Crohn's) or resection, cardiac disease, bacterial overgrowth)
• Small bowel bacterial overgrowth
• Lactose intolerance
• Disaccharidase deficiency
• Radiation enteritis
• Lymphoma
Pancreatic
• Chronic pancreatitis
• Pancreatic carcinoma
• Cystic fibrosis
Endocrine
• Hyperthyroidism
• Diabetes mellitus (autonomic neuropathy)
• Addison's disease
• Hypoparathyroidism
• Hormone-secreting tumours (e.g. gastrinoma, VIPoma, carcinoid)
Chronic infection (e.g. amoebiasis, giardiasis, Entamoeba histolytica)
Drugs (e.g. laxatives, antibiotics, digoxin, cytotoxic drugs, metformin, NSAID, some antacids)
Recent antibiotic therapy and Clostridium difficile infection
Previous surgery
• Post-gastrectomy
• Ileal + right colon resection
• Bacterial overgrowth after bariatric surgery
After cholecystectomy (~10%)
Alcohol abuse
Immunodeficiency
Factitious diarrhoea (±eating disorder)

IBD = inflammatory bowel disease, NSAID = non-steroidal anti-inflammatory drugs, VIP = vasoactive intestinal peptide

Figure 57d Assessment of the cause of chronic diarrhoea

Organic pathology suggested by weight loss, nocturnal diarrhoea, abnormal tests

Pathological location

Functional diarrhoeal disorders
• Abdominal pain, bloating, changing bowel habit (constipation + diarrhoea)
• Often related to eating, stress, dietary fibre
• Associated nausea, lethargy, headache, backache, dysuria, anxiety
• Age <45 years old

	Pancreas	Small intestine	Colon	
Features	• Steatorrhoea with pale, bulky, offensive stool • Fat-soluble vitamin deficiency (A, D, E, K) • Weight loss	• Anaemia • Marked weight loss • Steatorrhoea	• Watery stool with blood and mucous • Rectal urge	
Causes	• Chronic pancreatitis	• Coeliac disease • Hypolactasia • Giardiasis	• Inflammatory bowel disease (colitis) • Colonic neoplasms • Villous adenomas	• Irritable bowel syndrome • Functional diarrhoea
Tests	• Faecal elastase ↑stool fat content • Abdominal X-ray (? calcification) • Pancreatic CT scan	• Small bowel enema to detect jejunal diverticula or Crohn's disease • Coeliac disease antibodies • Endoscopy with biopsies (e.g. coeliac) and aspirations (e.g. giardiasis)	• Colonoscopy + biopsy • Sigmoidoscopy • Rectal examination • Contrast enemas for diverticulae, fistulae	• Investigation not always needed • Negative tests supports the diagnosis

Definition: diarrhoea is the abnormal passage of 'loose' stools >3 times/day (and/or a stool volume >200 g/day). *Acute diarrhoea* lasts <4 weeks and is more common in travellers, older people, the immunocompromised and homosexual men. UK incidence is ~1 episode/adult/year. *Chronic diarrhoea* lasts >4 weeks and requires further investigation. Prevalence, without abdominal pain, is ~4% in developed countries.

Acute diarrhoea

Infective causes are usually short-lived (<72 h) and often due to food poisoning.

- *Infective gastroenteritis* may be viral (30–40%; e.g. norovirus [the most common cause], rotavirus), bacterial (e.g. *Campylobacter* spp., *Salmonella* spp., *Staph. aureus* toxins) or parasitic (e.g. amoebiasis, *Giardia lamblia*). Poor personal hygiene and lack of sanitation increase the incidence.
- *Pseudomembranous colitis* due to *Clostridium difficile* infection is common in older people following antibiotic therapy (Chapter 26). Other infective causes of bloody diarrhoea include cytomegalovirus, *Campylobacter jejuni*, *E.coli* O157, *Vibrio parahaemolyticus*, *Shigella* spp., *Yersinia* spp. and schistosomiasis.
- *Travellers' diarrhoea* affects ~40% of 'Western' tourists to tropical/semi-tropical destinations (e.g. Latin America, Africa, Southern Asia). Bacterial infection, especially *E.coli*, causes most (~60–85%) cases, parasites ~10% and viruses ~5%.

Non-infective causes are less common including:

- *Early chronic causes* (e.g. inflammatory bowel disease [IBD]).
- *Drugs* include antibiotics, digoxin, metformin, proton pump inhibitors, non-steroidal anti-inflammatory drugs (NSAIDs), allopurinol, cytotoxic drugs, serotonin reuptake inhibitors, statins, theophylline, thyroxine and some antacids.
- *Constipation* with 'overflow diarrhoea'.
- *Other causes*: ischaemic colitis, diverticulitis, hyperthyroidism, anxiety, allergy, appendicitis, radiation enteritis, VIPoma.

History: determine diarrhoea frequency, severity, quantity, character (i.e. watery) and presence of blood. Review associated features including vomiting, weight loss, dehydration and nocturnal symptoms. Consider underlying causes and factors associated with infection (e.g. fever, recent travel, contacts, takeaway/restaurant food). Assess recent hospital admissions, medications and antibiotic therapy. *C. difficile* occurs 2–30 days after antibiotics, especially cephalosporins. Identify factors like stress, radiotherapy and bowel ischaemia. *Complications* associated with diarrhoea include reactive arthritis, septicaemia, irritable bowel syndrome (IBS), lactose intolerance and poor drug absorption.

Examination: Assess hydration because many patients are volume depleted and require fluid resuscitation. Fever suggests infection, but may occur with severe colitis. Chronic IBD is associated with clubbing, mouth ulcers, weight loss and koilonychias. Assess abdominal tenderness and perform a rectal examination, especially in patients >50 years old (i.e. faecal impaction, colorectal cancer). Rectal biopsy and sigmoidoscopy may be useful.

Investigation is not always required. *Blood tests* may suggest infection or chronic conditions. *Stool cultures* identify responsible organisms. Send culture specimens if the patient is unwell, immunocompromised, has bloody stool, after third-world travel (and request ova, cysts and parasites), if the cause is uncertain or the diarrhoea persists (i.e. >1 week). Request *C. difficile* if the patient

has recently received antibiotics or hospitalization (5% of normal people are positive; review with toxin results). Pathogens routinely checked for include *Campylobacter* spp., *E.coli* O157, *Salmonella* spp. and *Shigella* spp. *Abdominal X-rays* may suggest colitis. Consider further investigation if an underlying chronic cause is suspected.

Management is supportive. It addresses fluid and electrolyte depletion and rests the GI tract. Antibacterial drugs are often unnecessary but may be required in systemic infections, campylobacter enteritis, shigellosis and salmonellosis. Metronidazole or vancomycin may be required for *C.difficile* infection (Chapter 26). Ciprofloxacin is used for prophylaxis and treatment of travellers' diarrhoea. Antimotility drugs reduce symptoms and antispasmodics are useful for treating abdominal cramps. Consider steroids in IBD. Notify local health protection units if there is a suspected public health hazard (e.g. food handlers). *Prognosis*: most cases improve rapidly (i.e. rotavirus 3–8 days, norovirus ~2 days, *Campylobacter* spp. and *Salmonella* spp. 2–7 days). *Giardia* spp. infection may persist and cause chronic diarrhoea.

Chronic diarrhoea

Causes of chronic diarrhoea are listed in Figure 57c. Common causes include IBS, constipation, coeliac disease, IBD, drugs, chronic pancreatitis and, in tropical areas, chronic infection (e.g. giardiasis). Less common causes include lactose intolerance, thyrotoxicosis and rare endocrine tumours.

History and examination aid assessment of cause (Figure 57d). Organic disease requiring prompt investigation is suggested if diarrhoea is of <2 months' duration, nocturnal or continuous (i.e. not intermittent) and associated with weight loss, rectal bleeding, raised inflammatory markers, iron deficiency anaemia, abdominal masses, mouth ulcers, age > 60 years or family history of bowel cancer. *Malabsorption* causes steatorrhoea (i.e. bulky foul-smelling pale stools) and examination may reveal koilonychia, glossitis, chelitis, mouth ulcers and bruising (due to fat soluble vitamin deficiency). Most colonic, inflammatory or secretory diarrhoeas present with 'liquid' stools and bloody/mucous discharge. Abdominal examination should include rectal and sigmoidoscopy examinations. *Functional bowel disturbance* is characterized by features of IBS (i.e. age < 45 years, normal physical examination and the absence of features of organic disease).

Investigations include *blood tests* for anaemia, inflammatory markers (e.g. C-reactive protein), liver function including albumin, indicators of malabsorption (e.g. calcium, vitamin B_{12}, folate), thyroid function, coeliac antibody tests (e.g. endomysial antibody); rarely, gut hormones (e.g. gastrin). *Stool (×3)* for culture and ova, cysts and parasites if there is an appropriate travel history. Consider *C. difficile* if relapse is a possibility. *Faecal elastase/chymotrypsin* are low in exocrine pancreatic deficiency (±faecal fat levels raised). *Hydrogen breath tests* detect small bowel overgrowth or hypolactasia. *Imaging*: abdominal CT scan identifies pancreatitis and contrast studies, diverticulae and strictures. *Endoscopy* (±biopsies, aspiration) confirms coeliac disease, IBD, giardiasis and bowel tumours.

Management: depends on the cause. Consider symptomatic therapy with antimotility drugs (e.g. loperamide) but only when a diagnosis has been made and there are no contraindications.

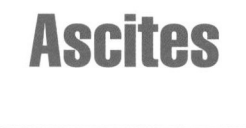

58 Ascites

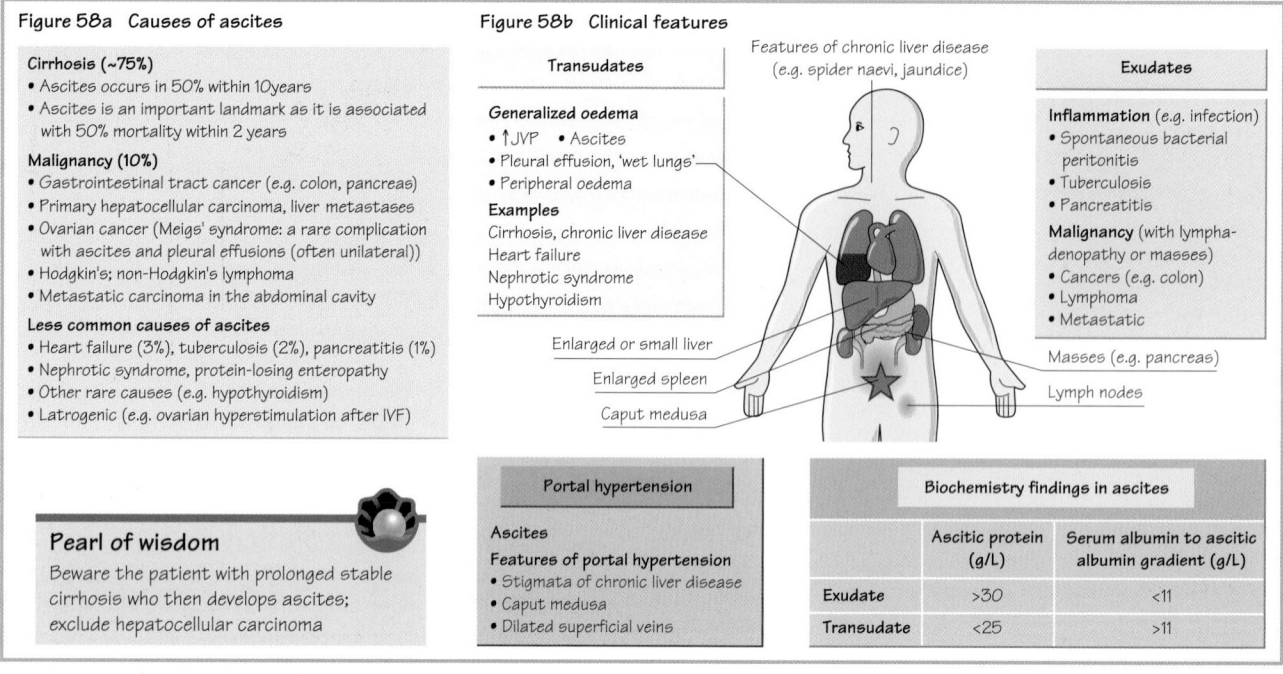

Figure 58a   Causes of ascites

Cirrhosis (~75%)
- Ascites occurs in 50% within 10 years
- Ascites is an important landmark as it is associated with 50% mortality within 2 years

Malignancy (10%)
- Gastrointestinal tract cancer (e.g. colon, pancreas)
- Primary hepatocellular carcinoma, liver metastases
- Ovarian cancer (Meigs' syndrome: a rare complication with ascites and pleural effusions (often unilateral))
- Hodgkin's; non-Hodgkin's lymphoma
- Metastatic carcinoma in the abdominal cavity

Less common causes of ascites
- Heart failure (3%), tuberculosis (2%), pancreatitis (1%)
- Nephrotic syndrome, protein-losing enteropathy
- Other rare causes (e.g. hypothyroidism)
- Iatrogenic (e.g. ovarian hyperstimulation after IVF)

Pearl of wisdom
Beware the patient with prolonged stable cirrhosis who then develops ascites; exclude hepatocellular carcinoma

Figure 58b   Clinical features

Features of chronic liver disease (e.g. spider naevi, jaundice)

Transudates

Generalized oedema
- ↑JVP   • Ascites
- Pleural effusion, 'wet lungs'
- Peripheral oedema

Examples
Cirrhosis, chronic liver disease
Heart failure
Nephrotic syndrome
Hypothyroidism

Enlarged or small liver
Enlarged spleen
Caput medusa

Exudates

Inflammation (e.g. infection)
- Spontaneous bacterial peritonitis
- Tuberculosis
- Pancreatitis

Malignancy (with lymphadenopathy or masses)
- Cancers (e.g. colon)
- Lymphoma
- Metastatic

Masses (e.g. pancreas)
Lymph nodes

Portal hypertension

Ascites
Features of portal hypertension
- Stigmata of chronic liver disease
- Caput medusa
- Dilated superficial veins

Biochemistry findings in ascites

	Ascitic protein (g/L)	Serum albumin to ascitic albumin gradient (g/L)
Exudate	>30	<11
Transudate	<25	>11

Definition: ascites is a pathological accumulation of fluid in the peritoneal cavity. Clinical detection requires ~1500 mls but ultrasound detects volumes ≥500 mls. Ascites is:
- **Exudative**, if protein content is raised due to inflammation (e.g. infection) or malignancy.
- **Transudative**, if due to portal hypertension and/or impaired renal sodium clearance with fluid retention.

Causes (Figure 58a)

Ascites is usually due to decompensated chronic liver disease (CLD) or intra-abdominal malignancy.
- **Cirrhosis** causes ~75% of ascites and ~50% of cirrhotic patients develop ascites within 10 years. Ascites is associated with worse prognosis (5-year survival rate ~55%). Exclude hepatocellular carcinoma if ascites occurs in long-standing stable cirrhosis.
- **Malignancy** accounts for ~10% of ascites. It includes gastrointestinal (GI) tract (e.g. colon, stomach), liver (e.g. primary, metastatic), ovarian and metastatic malignancy.

Clinical features and investigation

A comprehensive history may be suggestive but few features distinguish between the different causes of ascites. Clinical features are illustrated in Figure 58b. Inspection reveals abdominal distension in gross ascites and 'shifting dullness' in less severe cases. Useful investigations include:
- **Blood tests**: biochemical and coagulation profiles may suggest cirrhosis (e.g. abnormal liver function and clotting tests, hypoalbuminaemia, low platelets). Consider tumour markers if malignancy is suspected (e.g. α-fetoprotein – hepatoma).
- **Ascitic fluid examination**: check colour (straw-coloured in cirrhosis; cloudy in infection; blood-stained in malignancy), white cell count (WCC) >250 ml diagnostic of bacterial peritonitis even without an organism), protein content (exudate >30 g/L; transu-

date <25 g/L), amylase (suggests pancreatitis), cytology for malignant cells and culture for infection.
- **Abdominal ultrasound** reveals liver size (e.g. cirrhosis), focal abnormalities (e.g. liver metastases), malignancy (e.g. ovarian, hepatoma), portal hypotension (e.g. splenomegaly) and vessel patency (i.e. thrombosis, Budd–Chiari syndrome).

Management

Treat the underlying cause. Initial management is medical (i.e. fluid/salt restriction, diuretics) and is most effective in 'transudative' ascites (e.g. cirrhosis) but less so in malignancy. Second-line therapeutic paracentesis is required for refractory ascites.

Transudative ascites management involves:
- **Fluid/salt restriction**: limit fluid intake to 1–1.5 L/day and dietary salt to <90 mmol/day (i.e. 5.2 g/salt/day). A 'no-added' salt diet is usually adequate.
- **Diuretics**: start spironolactone (100–400 mg/day), which increases sodium excretion and potassium reabsorption (hyperkalaemia may limits use). Then cautiously add loop diuretics (e.g. furosemide 40–160 mg/day; risks hyponatraemia).
- **Therapeutic paracentesis**: consider drainage in diuretic-resistant ascites or if side-effects (e.g. hyponatraemia) limit drug use. After large volume (i.e. >5 L) paracentesis, give 8 g albumin per litre ascites removed, for plasma expansion. *Transjugular intrahepatic portosystemic shunt* (TIPS) helps in refractory ascites requiring frequent paracentesis. It does not reduce mortality and may increase encephalopathy.

Exudative ascites may require treatment of:
- **Spontaneous bacterial peritonitis** in 10–30% of cases (mortality ~20%). Organisms (e.g. *E.coli*, enterococci) may not be detected, but start empirical antibiotics (e.g. cephalosporins) if the ascitic fluid WCC is >250/ml.
- **Underlying malignant ascites**: therapeutic paracentesis is required for symptomatic relief.

Critical Care Medicine at a Glance, Third Edition. Richard Leach. © 2014 John Wiley & Sons, Ltd. Published 2014 by John Wiley & Sons, Ltd.

59 Abdominal imaging

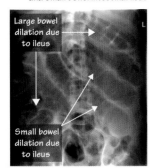

Figure 59a Abdominal X-ray showing large and small bowel intestinal ileus

Large bowel dilation due to ileus

Small bowel dilation due to ileus

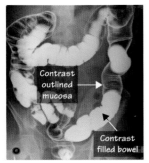

Figure 59b Normal barium enema

Contrast outlined mucosa

Contrast filled bowel

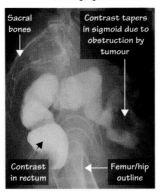

Figure 59c Barium enema (lateral view) showing sigmoid tumour

Sacral bones

Contrast tapers in sigmoid due to obstruction by tumour

Contrast in rectum

Femur/hip outline

Figure 59d Abdominal CT scan. Acute pancreatitis

Gallbladder — Swollen, contrast enhanced, inflamed pancreas — Necrotic tissue around pancreas

Liver — Spleen

Right kidney — Rib — Vertebra — Adrenal gland — Left kidney

Pearl of wisdom

Most gallstones are not radio-opaque (<10%) and cannot be seen on abdominal X-rays. In contrast ~80% of renal stones are visible

Figure 59e Typical radiation doses of common investigations

Diagnostic procedure	Radiation dose (mSv)	Equivalent number of CXRs	Equivalent period of background radiation
Chest (single PA film)	0.02	1	3 days
Abdominal X-ray	0.7	35	4 months
Barium swallow	1.5	75	8 months
Small bowel meal	3.0	150	13 years
Barium enema	7.2	360	3.2 years
Head CT scan	2	100	10 months
Chest CT scan	8	400	3.6 years
Abdominal or pelvic CT	10	500	4.5 years

The type of abdominal imaging selected depends on the clinical scenario, availability and benefit:risk ratio.

Plain abdominal radiograph (AXR) is often useful in patients with abdominal pain or distension but is of little value in haematemesis. Intestinal dilation (±fluid levels) is seen in paralytic ileus (e.g. post-operative) or bowel obstruction (e.g. ischaemia, volvulus). Obstructed small bowel is centrally located and 'ladder-like', whereas large bowel is peripheral (Figure 59a). Erect films may demonstrate air under the diaphragm after bowel perforation. Gallstones are rarely radiopaque whereas in renal colic ~80% of renal stones can be seen on large 'KUB' (kidney, ureter, bladder) films. Abnormal pancreatic calcification suggests chronic pancreatitis. Radiopaque foreign bodies and illicit drug packages (i.e. 'bodypackers') can be detected. A characteristic gas pattern suggests intussusception but AXR is unhelpful in appendicitis.

Contrast imaging (e.g. barium swallow, small/large bowel meal/enema): radio-opaque contrast is swallowed or infused into the small bowel or rectum by nasojejunal or rectal catheters respectively (Figures 59b and 59c). The contrast coats the lining of the oesophagus, small bowel or colon and images are acquired under fluoroscopic control. Introduction of air (e.g. into the colon) produces a double contrast view. These techniques detect tumours, oesophageal/bowel perforations, ulcers, diverticulae, intussusception and mucosal ulceration. Complications (e.g. perforation, barium impaction) are rare. Barium enemas are occasionally used therapeutically (e.g. to reduce large bowel volvulus, treat bleeding diverticulae). Contrast imaging is unpleasant and rarely used since the advent of endoscopy, ultrasound and CT scans.

Abdominal ultrasound scans (USS) do not use ionizing radiation, are non-invasive, widely available, painless and possibly the best technique for imaging soft tissues. Gallstones are highly echogenic and readily detected but they are common and often asymptomatic (i.e. not the cause of pain). Ultrasound delineates liver cysts and tumours, dilated bile ducts, head of the pancreas malignancy, pancreatitis (~25–50%) and abdominal aortic aneurysms. USS may determine bladder urine volume and detect urinary tract obstruction, renal stones, testicular disease (e.g. tumours) and, via the transrectal route, prostatic disease. In women, combined abdominal and transvaginal USS aids diagnosis of appendicitis, gynaecological problems and pelvic masses.

Abdominal CT scans are fast, non-invasive, painless and accurate. They generate detailed cross-sectional images of structures (e.g. blood vessels) and viscera (Figure 59d). CT scans often determine the cause of pain or abdominal/pelvic disease including infection (e.g. abscesses), inflammation (e.g. pancreatitis), malignancy, aneurysms or post-traumatic injuries. CT scans guide biopsies, drain abscesses and assess therapy. Disadvantages include cost and radiation doses (Figure 59e) with the associated risks (e.g. in pregnancy). Allergy may occur with contrast usage. For some conditions magnetic resonance imaging (MRI) may be preferable.

Endoscopy: Gastroscopy, cystoscopy and colonoscopy are widely available and the preferred 'first-line' investigation of hollow organs (e.g. oesophagus, stomach, colon, bladder). They are more accurate (i.e. the missed tumour rate in the 3 years after colonoscopy is ~2–6%, compared with ~20% after barium enema), preferred by patients and associated with fewer complications.

Critical Care Medicine at a Glance, Third Edition. Richard Leach. © 2014 John Wiley & Sons, Ltd. Published 2014 by John Wiley & Sons, Ltd.

60 Acute confusional state, coma and status epilepticus

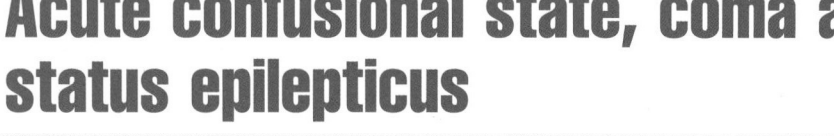

Figure 60a Causes of acute confusional states and coma

1. Metabolic Disorders
- Respiratory
  Hypoxia: P_aO_2 <5kPa
  Hypercapnia; P_aCO_2 >8kPa
- Renal and hepatic
  Na^+ <120 or >155 mmol/L
  Glucose <3 or <30 mmol/L
  Ca^{2+} <1.7 or <3.0 mmol/L
  Raised urea, ammonia
- Endocrine (e.g. thyrotoxicosis, myxoedema)
- Hypothermia / hyperthermia
- Alcohol withdrawal (2–5 days post admission)
- Nutritional deficiency (e.g. thiamine; Wernicke's encephalopathy)

2. Infection
- Sepsis, pneumonia, urine

3. Drug / Toxin ingestion
- Alcohol, LSD, sedatives

4. Neurological causes
- Epilepsy (i.e. ictal/post-ictal phase)
- Non-convulsive status epilepticus
- Infective (e.g. meningitis, encephalitis)
- Structural/traumatic (e.g. tumours, raised ICP, haematoma)
- Dementia (+superimposed illness)

5. Vascular causes
- Stroke (e.g. embolic in atrial fibrillation)
- Cardiac (e.g. myocardial infarction with hypotension)
- Hypertensive encephalopathy

Figure 60b Metabolic causes of acute confusional state

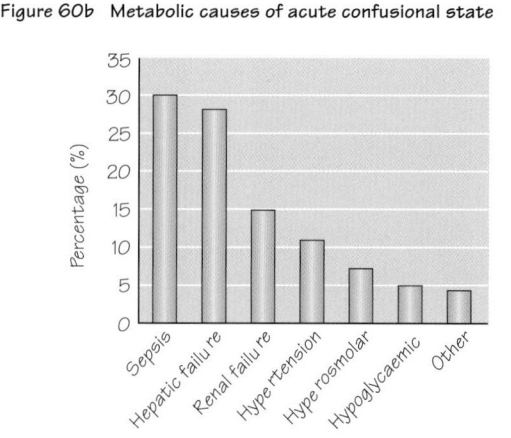

Figure 60c Potentially reversible causes of coma

Hypotension	Myxoedema (rare)
Hypoperfusion	Carbon monoxide
Hypoxaemia	Hypercalcaemia (rare)
Hypercapnia	Temperature disorders
Hypoglycaemia	Poisoning
Hypertension	CNS infections
Status epilepticus	CNS haemorrhage
Wernicke's encephalopathy (rare)	

Figure 60d Causes and complications of status epilepticus

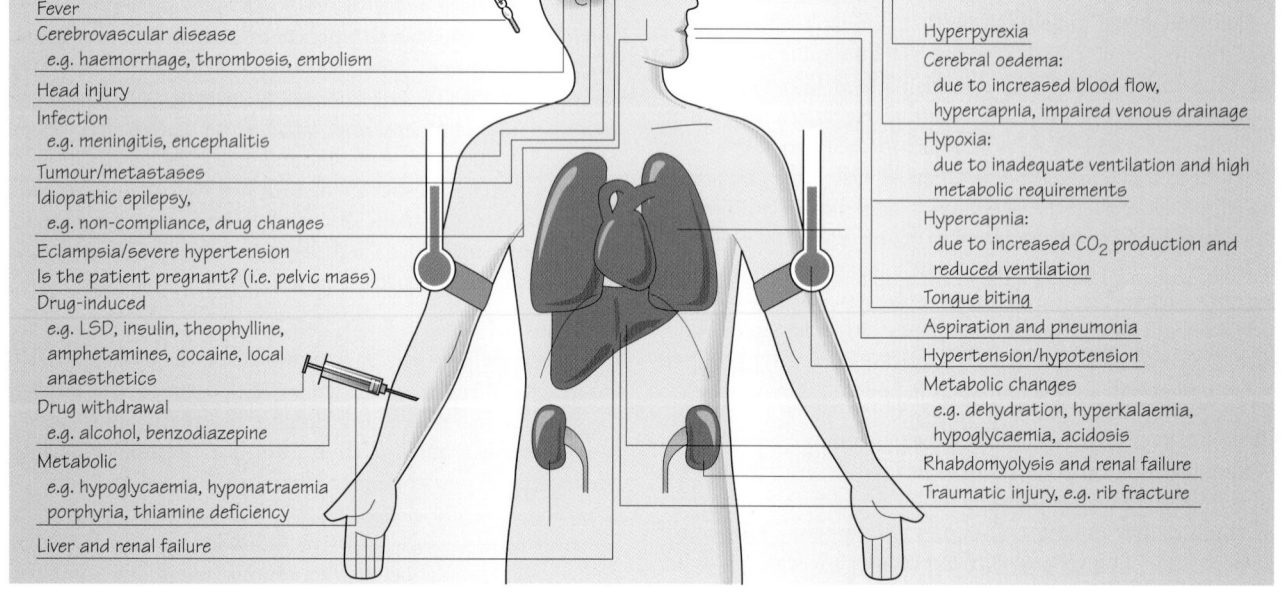

Causes of status epilepticus

Fever

Cerebrovascular disease
  e.g. haemorrhage, thrombosis, embolism

Head injury

Infection
  e.g. meningitis, encephalitis

Tumour/metastases

Idiopathic epilepsy,
  e.g. non-compliance, drug changes

Eclampsia/severe hypertension
Is the patient pregnant? (i.e. pelvic mass)

Drug-induced
  e.g. LSD, insulin, theophylline,
  amphetamines, cocaine, local
  anaesthetics

Drug withdrawal
  e.g. alcohol, benzodiazepine

Metabolic
  e.g. hypoglycaemia, hyponatraemia
  porphyria, thiamine deficiency

Liver and renal failure

Complications of status epilepticus

Hyperpyrexia

Cerebral oedema:
  due to increased blood flow,
  hypercapnia, impaired venous drainage

Hypoxia:
  due to inadequate ventilation and high
  metabolic requirements

Hypercapnia:
  due to increased CO_2 production and
  reduced ventilation

Tongue biting

Aspiration and pneumonia

Hypertension/hypotension

Metabolic changes
  e.g. dehydration, hyperkalaemia,
  hypoglycaemia, acidosis

Rhabdomyolysis and renal failure

Traumatic injury, e.g. rib fracture

Critical Care Medicine at a Glance, Third Edition. Richard Leach. © 2014 John Wiley & Sons, Ltd. Published 2014 by John Wiley & Sons, Ltd.

Acute confusional state (ACS)

ACS is common, affects ~10–15% of ward patients, especially older people, and increases mortality unless due to sedation. Characteristic features are impaired consciousness usually worse at night, disorientation in time and place, abnormal behaviour, altered perception particularly visual hallucinations, emotional lability (e.g. fear, anxiety) and memory loss. Figures 60a and 60b show common causes. Patients are nursed in quiet, gently lit rooms, with reassurance, orientation and constant observation. Treat the cause (e.g. infection). Cautious use of haloperidol and/or benzodiazepines may be required (Chapter 21).

Coma

Definition: a state of unconsciousness from which the patient cannot be aroused, often defined as a Glasgow Coma Score (GCS; Chapter 72) ≤8. ACS or gradual loss of consciousness may precede coma. **Cause** are listed inFigure 60a.

Immediate management

Assess airway, breathing and circulation. Give oxygen, support the circulation, treat seizures and protect the cervical spine as required. Consider intubation if the GCS is <8 to protect the airway or aid investigation (e.g. CT scan). Check the blood glucose (e.g. BM stix) and give intravenous dextrose if hypoglycaemia is suspected. Correct reversible causes of coma (Figure 60c). Naloxone and flumazenil temporarily reverse opiate- and benzodiazepine-induced coma respectively (Chapter 21). Give thiamine if alcohol abuse or Wernicke's encephalopathy is suspected. Subsequent management (e.g. antibiotics, anticoagulants, anticonvulsants, intracranial pressure [ICP] reduction) depends on the cause (Chapters 61–64, 72).

Assessment

1 Brief history (i.e. from family, witnesses) may establish the cause (e.g. overdose). An abrupt onset suggests a seizure or vascular event whereas a slower onset suggests a metabolic cause, tumour or extradural haematoma. Recent symptoms (e.g. headache), previous illness (e.g. diabetes, atrial fibrillation [AF]), travel and drug therapy direct ongoing investigation.

2 Examination: vital signs (e.g. blood pressure [BP]) aid diagnosis [Figure 60a]. Exclude trauma (e.g. haematoma, 'panda eyes') and immobilize the cervical spine if suspicious. Smell the breath (i.e. alcohol, ketones, hepatic foetor). Examine for stigmata of systemic disease (e.g. cirrhosis, uraemia), focal infection (e.g. pneumonia), venepuncture marks (i.e. illicit drug use) and neurological disease (e.g. meningitis). Incontinence and tongue lacerations indicate seizure. Neurological examination (mnemonic: SPERM) should include:

- **State of consciousness** (i.e. alert, lethargic [i.e. responds to command], stuporous [i.e. arousal to pain] or comatose [i.e. unrousable]). Record the GCS.
- **Pupillary reactions**: bilateral unreactive and pinpoint pupils suggest a brainstem lesion although many drugs affect pupillary response (e.g. morphine causes pinpoint pupils). Normal pupillary reactions during coma suggest a metabolic cause or a structural lesion above the midbrain.
- **Eye movements** are altered by frontal lobe, cortical or brainstem lesions. Loss of oculocephalic and oculovestibular reflexes (Chapter 29) suggests pontomedullary-midbrain damage.
- **Respiratory pattern**: tachypnoea is non-specific (e.g. acidosis). Ataxic breathing indicates severe brainstem dysfunction.
- **Motor function**: Record the best response (e.g. spontaneously moves all limbs, no response to pain). Pontine damage causes

decerebrate (i.e. extensor) posturing, whereas lesions above the pons cause decorticate (i.e. flexor) posturing.

Full neurological examination (+fundoscopy) localizes focal signs and identifies specific causes.

3 Investigations depend on the cause but include biochemistry, glucose, C-reactive protein (CRP), toxicology (±alcohol level), microbiology (±malaria), blood gases, carboxyhaemoglobin level, chest radiography (CXR), CT scan, electroencephalogram (EEG) and lumbar puncture (if ICP normal).

Prognosis deteriorates with duration of coma. It can be assessed from posture, pupillary and oculovestibular reflexes but only after drug, metabolic, cranial nerve and tympanic membrane defects have been excluded (Chapters 29, 72). Outcome can also be determined reproducibly from the GCS (Chapter 72). Patients with >3 days' postanoxic coma (i.e. cardiac arrest) rarely survive without severe disability. Poor prognostic features include decerebrate posturing and rigidity for >24 hours in non-trauma and >2 weeks in trauma patients, absent pupillary reflexes for >24 hours in postanoxic brain injury or >3 days in other patients, and absent oculovestibular reflexes for >24 hours.

Status epilepticus (SEp)

Definition: seizures lasting >30 min or repeated seizures without intervening consciousness. Prolonged seizures cause permanent brain damage due to hypoxia, hypotension, cerebral oedema and neuronal injury. Damage is proportional to seizure duration. Mortality is 15–30%.

Prognosis (Figure 60d): patients with epilepsy and metabolic disturbances have a good prognosis, whereas those with global hypoxia, structural damage or infective lesions have a poor prognosis.

Clinical features and complications (Figure 60d): severe lactic acidosis, metabolic imbalance, high fever, cerebral oedema and raised ICP may occur during SEp.

Investigations: immediately exclude (or treat) hypoglycaemia (i.e. bedside BM stix). After treatment has started, check biochemistry, toxicology, electrocardiogram (ECG) and anticonvulsant levels in known epileptics. In patients with new-onset seizures, CT imaging detects structural lesions (>50%) and EEG differentiates primary from secondary (focal) generalized seizures. In undiagnosed coma, the EEG occasionally reveals non-convulsive SEp.

Management

- **General**: maintain a patent airway (i.e. recovery position). Give oxygen (>60%) and thiamine if malnourished (i.e. alcoholics). Support the circulation but avoid hypotonic fluids that increase cerebral oedema. Correct pyrexia and electrolyte disturbances. Monitor EEG continuously in severe SEp.
- **Anticonvulsants**: rapid seizure control is often achieved with slow i.v. bolus or rectal benzodiazepines (e.g. diazepam). Continuous fitting may require a phenytoin or diazepam infusion. In resistant SEp, alternative therapies include sodium valproate, vigabatrin, barbiturates and i.v. anaesthetic agents (e.g. propofol).
- **Other therapies** include dexamethasone for tumours or vasculitis, surgery for space-occupying lesions (e.g. haematomas) and treatment for cerebral oedema (Chapter 72).

Pearl of wisdom
Over-sedation often aggravates acute confusional states in older patients

 # Stroke

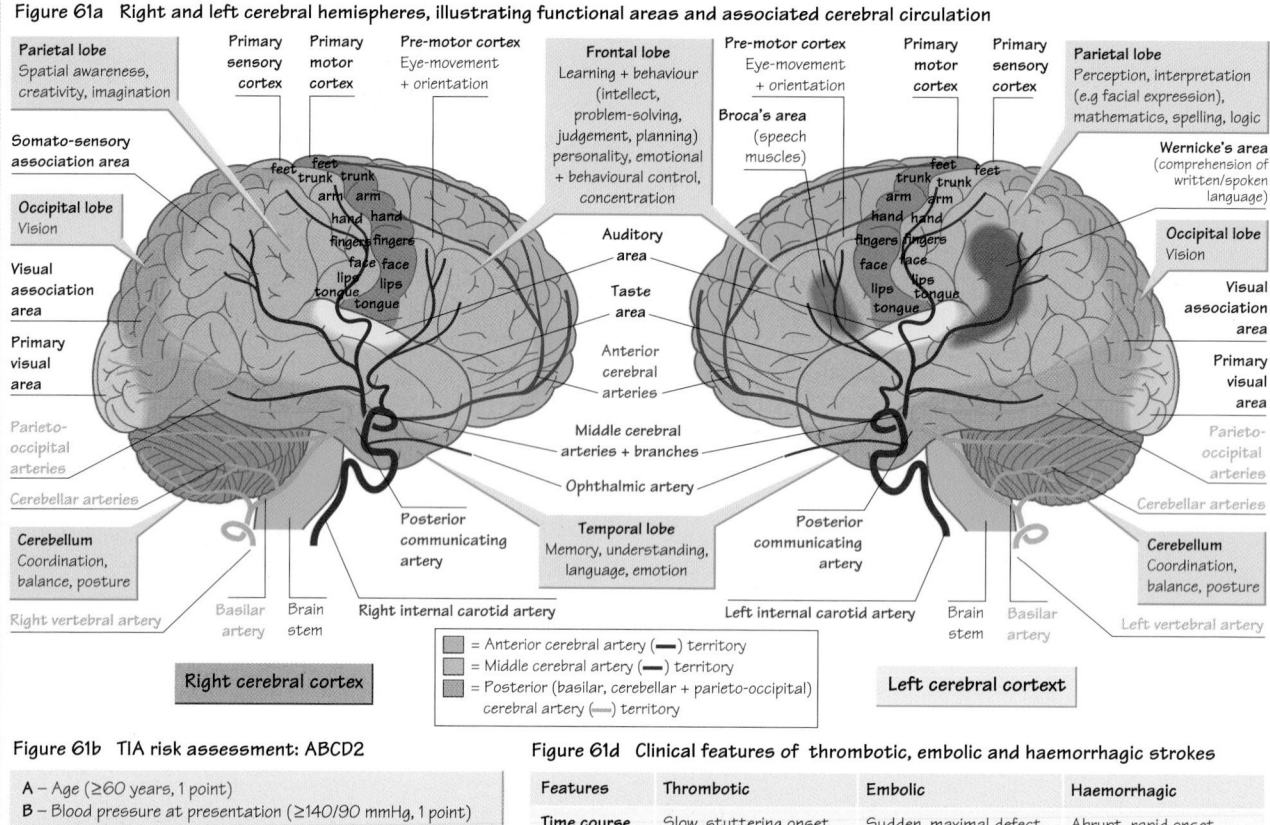

Figure 61a Right and left cerebral hemispheres, illustrating functional areas and associated cerebral circulation

= Anterior cerebral artery (——) territory
= Middle cerebral artery (——) territory
= Posterior (basilar, cerebellar + parieto-occipital) cerebral artery (——) territory

Right cerebral cortex

Left cerebral cortext

Figure 61b TIA risk assessment: ABCD2

A – Age (≥60 years, 1 point)
B – Blood pressure at presentation (≥140/90 mmHg, 1 point)
C – Clinical features (unilateral weakness, 2 points; speech disturbance without weakness, 1 point)
D – Symptom duration (>60 mins, 2 points; 10–59 mins, 1 point)
2 – Plus diabetes. Calculation of ABCD2 includes the presence of diabetes (1 point)
Total scores range from 0–3 (low risk) to 4–7 (high risk)

Figure 61c Risk factors for stroke

Risk factors for arterial disease
• Age, hypertension, male sex, smoking, diabetes
Genetic factors
• family history of vascular disease
Structural heart disease
• Myocardial infarction (1% have strokes post-MI)
• Atrial fibrillation (especially if >65 years old or CCF)
Excess alcohol
• Especially in young man
Hypercholesterolaemia
• Low cholesterol is important in secondary prevention
• High cholesterol is not a strong epidemiological risk factor
Thrombotic risk factors
• Polycythaemia, thrombophilia (e.g. factor V Leiden)
Intracerebral haemorrhage
• Main risk factors are hypertension, AVM, thrombolysis
Young stroke (additional risk factors in those <40 years old)
• Carotid/vertebral dissection (5–20% of stroke in young)
• Neurosyphilis (45% present as stroke)
• Vasculitis and antiphospholipid syndrome
• Drug induced e.g. cocaine
• Thrombophilia (e.g. protein C+S deficiency can cause venous sinus thrombosis)
• Structural extracranial abnormalities

AVM = arteriovenous malformation

Figure 61d Clinical features of thrombotic, embolic and haemorrhagic strokes

Features	Thrombotic	Embolic	Haemorrhagic
Time course	Slow, stuttering onset	Sudden, maximal defect	Abrupt, rapid onset
Location	Cortical infarcts Internal capsule	Cortical infarcts	Internal capsule, cortical, basal ganglia
Preceding history	TIA ± amaurosis fugax Retinal artery occlusion	Recent MI Arrhythmias (e.g. AF)	Anticoagulation Recent thrombolysis
Predisposing factors	DM, smoking, HT, hyperlipidaemia, heart disease	Endocarditis, ASD + PE, LV aneurysm + thrombus, air embolism, AF	HT, vascular malform[n], herald bleeds + headache cardiac catheterization
Treatment	Endarterectomy Aspirin (± thrombolysis?)	Aspirin anticoagulation	Surgical evacuation Correct coagulopathy

Figure 61e Stroke prognosis by circulation involved and size of stroke

	TAC	PAC	LAC	POC
30 day				
Independent	5	55	65	65
Dependent	55	40	30	30
Dead	40	5	5	5
1 year				
Independent	5	55	60	60
Dependent	35	30	30	20
Dead	60	15	10	20

TAC = total anterior circulation; PAC = partial anterior circulation; LAC = lacunar (internal capsule) infarct; POC = posterior circulation

Figure 61f Right-sided middle cerebral artery (MCA) infarction/stroke

Right-sided MCA infarct

Pearl of wisdom

Early, effective treatment of cardiovascular risk factors prevents strokes (±IHD) and always reflects the best medical management

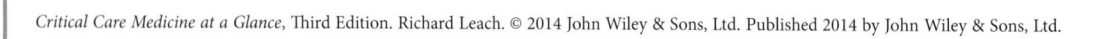

Transient ischaemic attacks (TIAs)

Definition: brief episodes of neurological dysfunction caused by focal brain or retinal ischaemia (without infarction) and clinical symptoms typically lasting <1 hour (maximum <24 hours). Onset is sudden and features focal, negative (e.g. arm weakness, blindness) and maximal at inception. Non-focal (e.g. syncope, incontinence) or positive (e.g. abnormal movement) signs indicate other causes (e.g. epilepsy, migraine). All vascular territories are affected with any pattern of neurological deficit (Figure 61a). Classically, *amaurosis fugax* causes brief unilateral blindness due to embolic ophthalmic artery occlusion.

Management: TIAs imply thrombosis on, or emboli from, atherogenic plaques. Early investigation reduces risk of disabling stroke, which is greatest in the first week. High-risk patients need specialist assessment within 24 hours; low-risk cases within a week (Figure 61b). Carotid artery ultrasonography (CUS) detects significant internal carotid artery (ICA) stenosis (i.e. 70–99% occlusion). Endarterectomy or radiological stenting within 2 weeks reduces subsequent stroke. Identify cardiac thrombosis, atrial fibrillation (AF) and other risk factors (Figure 61c). Give aspirin 300 mg immediately and then 75 mg daily. Start secondary prevention measures (e.g. reduce cholesterol, antihypertensives, antiarrhythmics). Cardiac emboli and AF may require anticoagulation.

Stroke

Definition: a clinical syndrome, characterized by rapid onset of a focal cerebral deficit lasting >24 hours due to a vascular cause (Figure 61a). *UK prevalence* is ~5/1000 population (100 000 new strokes/year). It is the most common cause of adult physical disability (i.e. limb disability [~30%], speech problems [~27%], cognitive impairment [~33%]). *Risk factors* are those predisposing to arterial disease, emboli and thrombosis/haemorrhage (Figure 61c).

Pathophysiology: strokes are thromboembolic (TE; ~80–90%) or haemorrhagic (~10–20%). Mortality rates are ~25% and >50% respectively.

- *'In-situ' thrombotic strokes* are due to atheroma, hypertension, vasculitis, oral contraceptives, alcohol excess or thrombophilia. They occur in small, internal capsule (IC) arteries as 'lacunar' infarcts (<1.5 cm^3) with large, often purely sensory or motor functional deficits. CT scans reveal hypodense (±later haemorrhagic) areas (Figure 61f).
- *Embolic strokes* are uncommon. Emboli occur from the heart (20%) or atheromatous plaques (80%). Arterial procedures, arrhythmias, endocarditis and cardiac defects increase the risk.
- *Haemorrhagic strokes* in the basal ganglia (~50 %) or pons (~5%) are due to hypertension, while cortical or cerebellar (~45%; Figure 62b; Chapter 62) bleeding is associated with arteriovenous malformations (AVM) and aneurysms. Risk factors are drug abuse (e.g. cocaine), anticoagulation and thrombolysis.

Clinical features are usually unheralded and occur suddenly. Occasionally, they present as 'stuttering' strokes. Stroke 'mimics' include migraine, hypoglycaemia, post-epileptic sequelae and haemorrhage into neoplasms. Size and location (cortex ~50%, basal ganglia ~25%, brainstem/cerebellum ~25%) characterize stroke (Figures 61a, 61d, 61e).

- *Anterior (i.e. carotid artery) strokes* present with hemiplegia. Language dysfunction occurs if the dominant, left hemisphere is affected. Left-sided neglect (±dyspraxia) occurs in non-dominant, right hemisphere strokes. Middle cerebral artery (MCA) occlusions cause hemianaesthesia, hemianopia and, if large, coma or death. IC strokes are similar but recover better because they are smaller.

- *Posterior (i.e. vertebrobasilar) strokes* affect the **brainstem** causing combinations of motor and sensory dysfunction (e.g. quadraparesis), gaze disturbance (e.g. pinpoint pupils, diplopia, nystagmus), dysarthria, dysphagia, locked-in syndrome and coma. *Cerebellar strokes* cause ataxia, unsteadiness and vomiting. **Ophthalmic strokes** impair vision. **Pontine strokes** cause catastrophic initial disability or death but, because the infarct is small, survival can be associated with good recovery.

Management (REACT)

- *Recognize* symptoms and signs early.
- *Evaluate risk factors and cause* (i.e. in-situ thrombosis, emboli).
- *Arrange prompt CT/MRI imaging*: to confirm diagnosis, site and cause (i.e. infarct/haemorrhage).
- *Co-ordinate management* (e.g. transfer to a hyperacute stroke unit [HASU] or neurosurgical unit).
- *Treat appropriately* (e.g. early thrombolysis, surgery).

Initially establish intravenous access, monitor and resuscitate. Prevent hypotension, even a 20% fall in blood pressure (BP) may be harmful. Avoid excessive, dextrose-containing fluids. Treat hypoxia, arrhythmias and seizures, and exclude hypoglycaemia. Keep the patient 'nil by mouth' until safe swallowing is confirmed. Admission to a HASU improves outcome and reduces mortality by ~25%. An *early CT scan* (<12–24h) identifies subtle signs of brain ischaemia (e.g. loss of grey–white differentiation, sulcal effacement). Consider MRI scanning in basal ganglia and brainstem strokes; CUS and echocardiography in TE strokes and angiography to exclude AVM/aneurysms in haemorrhagic strokes.

Primary therapy

- *Aspirin* (300 mg) improves outcome in TE strokes.
- *Thrombolysis*: tissue–type plasminogen activator (rtPA) is effective in selected ischaemic strokes within 3 hours of onset.
- *Anticoagulation* is contraindicated in hypertension and haemorrhagic or large strokes. Start 7–10 days after TE strokes due to AF. Consider therapy at 48 hours for intra-cardiac clot in small strokes.
- *Antihypertensives*: lower BP by ~15% if systolic pressure > 220 mmHg (or mean BP > 120 mmHg) in the first 24 hours post-stroke. Patients eligible for rtPA require a systolic BP < 185 mmHg and diastolic < 110 mmHg.
- *Blood sugar control*: hyperglycaemia (~30%) impairs outcome.
- *Surgery*: consider endarterectomy (±stenting) for ICA stenosis >70%. Surgical evacuation of posterior fossa bleeds with brainstem compression or cortical bleeds causing mass effects may improve outcome.

Secondary prevention strategies

- *Treat vascular risk factors* to reduce stroke recurrence (~10%/year). Lower BP (<140/85 mmHg), control diabetes, reduce cholesterol and give aspirin.
- *Prophylactic therapy* prevents deep venous thrombosis (~40%), pulmonary embolism (~5%) and peptic ulceration.
- *Nursing care* reduces pressure sores, malnutrition (20%) and incontinence (50%).
- *Swallowing assessment* detects dysfunction (~50%) and prevents aspiration.
- *Physiotherapy* reduces contractures and aids mobilization. Falls occur in ~35%.
- *Depression* (50%) may require antidepressants.
- *Post-stroke epilepsy* (5%) requires treatment.

Loss of independence persists in ~25–50% of first-stroke patients. They need nursing, rehabilitation, and financial and social support.

62 Other cerebral vascular disorders

Figure 62a
Dilated left pupil and carotid angiogram showing leaking aneurysm

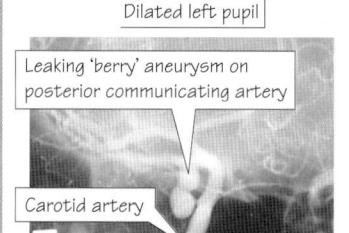

Dilated left pupil

Leaking 'berry' aneurysm on posterior communicating artery

Carotid artery

44-yr-old lady with headache and a dilated left pupil due to pressure of a posterior communicating aneurysm on the pupillary parasympathetic 'constrictor' fibres lying on the surface of the left third cranial nerve

Figure 62b
Haemorrhagic stroke on CT scan showing 'bright white' blood

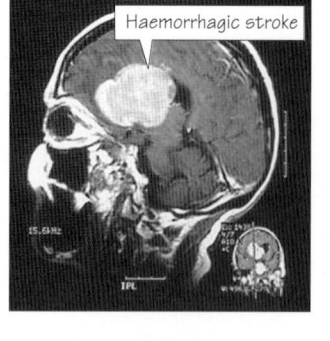

Haemorrhagic stroke

Pearl of wisdom
Suspect a subdural haematoma in a previously independent older patient who presents obtunded, confused or unexpectedly 'off their legs'

Figure 62c
Subdural haematoma on CT scan showing
① midline shift and
② ventricular compression

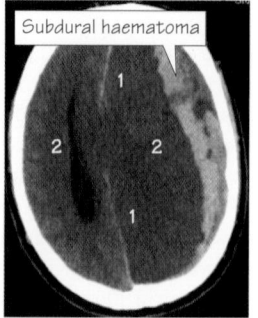

Subdural haematoma

Figure 62d
Brain linings, spaces and location of subdural haematoma

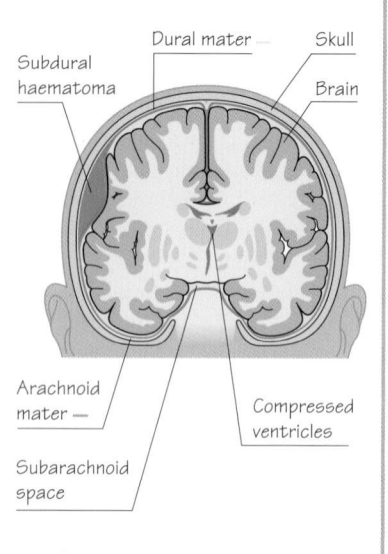

Dural mater — Skull
Subdural haematoma — Brain
Arachnoid mater —
Compressed ventricles
Subarachnoid space

Subarachnoid haemorrhage (SAH)

This follows spontaneous bleeding from ruptured intracranial 'berry' aneurysms (~85%; Figure 62a), arteriovenous malformations (AVM; ~15%) or, rarely, mycotic aneurysms in endocarditis. *UK prevalence* is 5/10000 population (~3000 cases/year). Risk factors are age >65 years, family history of SAH, connective tissue disease, polycystic disease and hypertension.

Clinical features include sudden onset 'thunderclap' headache, 'like a kick to the back of the head', with associated nausea, vomiting, confusion or coma. Occasionally, the headache is not severe. Neck stiffness and subhyaloid haemorrhage (~25%) are common. Infarction, haematoma, hydrocephalus and focal neurological signs, due to vasospasm or mass effect, may develop later. Other complications include arrhythmias and pulmonary oedema.

Investigation: a CT scan detects >95% of SAH (±complications) within 24 hours. Consider a lumbar puncture (LP) if CT is not diagnostic. This detects xanthochromia by spectrophotometry (i.e. yellow cerebral spinal fluid [CSF] discoloration due to bilirubin from haemoglobin breakdown) and/or uniform CSF blood staining. LP is only safe in the absence of focal deficits or if conscious level is normal. Angiography locates the aneurysm (~80% anterior cerebral circulation).

Management includes resuscitation, analgesia and anticonvulsants. Initially, maintain systolic blood pressure (BP) > 140 mmHg (i.e. fluid, inotropes). Long-term BP should be <145/85 mmHg. Nimodipine, a calcium channel blocker inhibits damaging cerebral artery vasospasm. Treat aneurysms by surgical clipping or radiological endovascular occlusion with 'Gugliemi' platinum coils.

Mortality is ~40% initially. Rebleeding affects ~25% of survivors with 60% mortality, if early surgical repair is not feasible. Severe neurological deficits affect ~30% of survivors.

Subdural haemorrhage/haematoma (SDH)

This is a venous bleed (Figures 62c and 62d) associated with 'brain atrophy' in dementia, old age and chronic alcoholism. It follows minor trauma that may not be remembered. Blood slowly oozes into the subdural space. Subsequently, osmotic breakdown products cause swelling and a gradually expanding 'space-occupying lesion'. Neurological impairment, with non-specific loss of mobility ('off-legs') and/or mental agility, occurs over weeks and is usually, but not always, associated with focal signs. CT scans are diagnostic. Surgical evacuation is often curative, even in very old people.

Extradural haematoma

This is due to middle meningeal artery rupture after head injury. A lucid period precedes rapid GCS deterioration. Prognosis is good after early surgical drainage if the initial GCS was high.

Cerebral venous sinus thrombosis (CVT)

This is rare, affecting mainly young women (e.g. peri/postpartum). Predisposing risk factors include oral contraception, dehydration, pregnancy, thrombophilia, inflammatory disease, ear infections, sinusitis, intracranial sepsis and, rarely, post-LP.

Clinical presentation mimics stroke, tumours, encephalitis, abscess or benign intracranial hypertension. Features depend on the occluded vein but include acute or subacute headache, seizures, papilloedema, proptosis, ophthalmoplegia, reduced consciousness and focal features.

Diagnosis: magnetic resonance imaging with contrast angiography detects thrombus, haemorrhage (~40%) and infarcts.

Treatment: heparin improves prognosis but consider local thrombolysis for those who deteriorate. Correct the underlying cause and reduce intracranial pressure with mannitol if necessary.

Critical Care Medicine at a Glance, Third Edition. Richard Leach. © 2014 John Wiley & Sons, Ltd. Published 2014 by John Wiley & Sons, Ltd.

63 Infective neurological emergencies

Critical Care Medicine at a Glance, Third Edition. Richard Leach. © 2014 John Wiley & Sons, Ltd. Published 2014 by John Wiley & Sons, Ltd.

Figure 63a Bacterial causes of meningitis

Organism	Special clinical features	Microbiology and antibiotic
Community acquired		
Pneumococcus (*Streptococcus pneumoniae*)	Affects older adults + neonates Spreads from infected ears, sinuses, pneumonia, endocarditis. Develops rapidly (hrs) Mortality ~25%	Gram +ve diplococci in CSF and often in blood. Benzyl-penicillin (± vancomycin if penicillin resistance is common)
Meningococcus (*Neisseria meningitidis*)	Affects children and adolescents Occurs in closed communities (e.g. barracks). Part of septicaemia (±shock). Purpuric rash common	Gram -ve diplococci in CSF and occasionally blood. Benzylpenicillin. Rifampicin for contacts
Haemophilus influenzae	Affects children under 6 years old	Gram -ve bacilli. Ceftriaxone, cefotaxime
Hospital acquired		
Staphylococcus (*S. aureus* or *S. epidermidis*)	Post neurosurgery, endocarditis, immunocompromised	Gram +ve cocci. Flucloxacillin (± vancomycin if MRSA)
Enteric Gram -ve rods (e.g. *E. coli*)	Neonates, immunocompromised, postoperative	Gram -ve bacilli. Cefotaxime (± aminoglycoside)

Figure 63b Clinical features and associated conditions* in meningitis

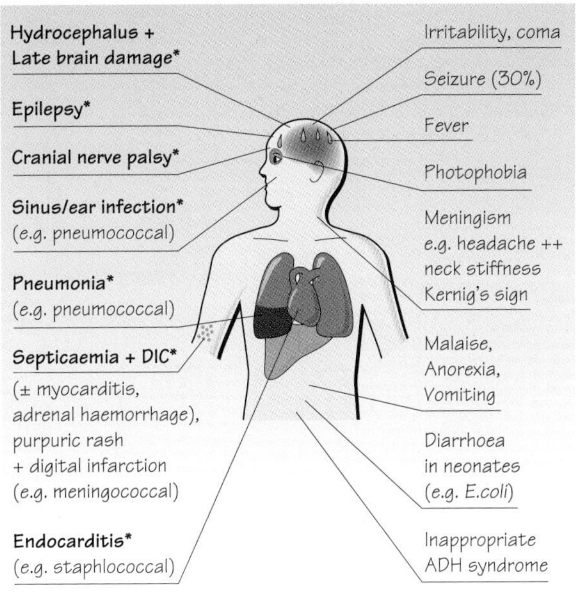

Hydrocephalus + Late brain damage*

Epilepsy*

Cranial nerve palsy*

Sinus/ear infection* (e.g. pneumococcal)

Pneumonia* (e.g. pneumococcal)

Septicaemia + DIC* (± myocarditis, adrenal haemorrhage), purpuric rash + digital infarction (e.g. meningococcal)

Endocarditis* (e.g. staphlococcal)

Irritability, coma

Seizure (30%)

Fever

Photophobia

Meningism e.g. headache ++ neck stiffness Kernig's sign

Malaise, Anorexia, Vomiting

Diarrhoea in neonates (e.g. *E.coli*)

Inappropriate ADH syndrome

DIC = disseminated intravascular coagulation; ADH = antidiuretic hormone

Meningitis (Chapters 65, 66, 67, 68)

Bacterial meningitis presents with fever, headache, neck stiffness and photophobia but should be suspected in any patient with fever and confusion, because 'meningism' is not always present. It is often associated with rapidly progressive, life-threatening sepsis (±disseminated intravascular coagulation [DIC]). Early recognition and treatment is life-saving. Viral meningitis is rarely severe.

Causes: bacteria are listed in Figure 63a. Viruses, *Mycobacterium tuberculosis* (tuberculosis [TB]) and leptospirosis (Weil's disease) present less acutely. *Listeria monocytogenes* and *Cryptococcus neoformans* meningitis affect immunocompromised patients (e.g. AIDS).

Clinical features (e.g. sepsis, meningism) are illustrated in Figure 63b. Precipitating causes must be excluded (e.g. pneumococcal meningitis is often secondary to chest, ear or sinus infection). Chronic TB meningitis is easily missed. Subarachnoid haemorrhage, malignancy and abscess may present with meningism. **Complications** (Figure 63b) include seizures, digital infarctions, cerebral oedema and obstructive hydrocephalus.

Investigation: a CT scan is performed before lumbar puncture if there are focal central nervous system (CNS) deficits, papilloedema, trauma or suspected mass lesions. In bacterial infections, cerebrospinal fluid (CSF) reveals raised polymorphs ($>500\,\text{mm}^3$), increased protein ($0.5–3\,\text{g/L}$), low CSF:blood sugar (BS) ratio (CSF/BS < 40%) and bacteria on stain or culture. Blood cultures may be positive. In viral meningitis, CSF reveals raised lymphocytes ($<500\,\text{mm}^3$) and protein ($0.5–1\,\text{g/L}$), but normal CSF/BS ratio (~60%). Viral culture and immunology of CSF, throat swabs or faeces are diagnostic. In TB meningitis, CSF shows raised lymphocytes ($<500\,\text{mm}^3$), protein ($1–5\,\text{g/L}$) and a low CSF/BS ratio (<40%). Staining or culture of acid-fast bacilli confirms TB. India ink stains detect *Cryptococcus*.

Treatment (Figure 63a): benzylpenicillin is effective against most pneumococcal and meningococcal meningitis. Cefotaxime or ceftriaxone treats *H. influenzae*. Until an organism has been isolated, treat with empirical cefotaxime (±penicillin) and await cultures. Aminoglycosides and antistaphylococcal agents are required in hospital-acquired meningitis. TB meningitis is treated with standard quadruple therapy. Steroids improve outcome and reduce complications in bacterial and TB meningitis. Rifampicin is given to close contacts of meningococcal and *H. influenzae* meningitis.

Encephalitis (Chapter 66)

This is an acute, usually viral, brain infection (e.g. herpes simplex). It is a rare complication of common viral diseases (e.g. mumps). Immunocompromised patients are at greatest risk. Initial features include drowsiness, irritability, fever, meningism and occasionally focal neurological signs. Severe cases progress to seizures, coma and death. CSF reveals lymphocytosis and raised protein. Viral serology may identify the cause. Management is supportive but aciclovir treats herpes simplex and ganciclovir, cytomegalovirus (CMV) infections. Prognosis varies but mortality is high with some viruses (e.g. Japanese B).

Other neurological infections

- **Tetanus** (Chapter 65): a toxin-mediated disease caused by *Clostridium tetani* infection of necrotic wounds. Generalized muscle rigidity, spasms and respiratory failure require sedation, paralysis and mechanical ventilation. Cardiovascular instability is controlled with magnesium infusions. Antibiotics, surgical debridement and immune globulin treat the infection and toxin.
- **Poliomyelitis, botulism and rabies** cause paralytic infections.
- **Others**: cerebral abscesses, cerebral malaria, prion disease.

64 Neuromuscular conditions

Figure 64a Symptoms and signs of Guillain-Barré syndrome

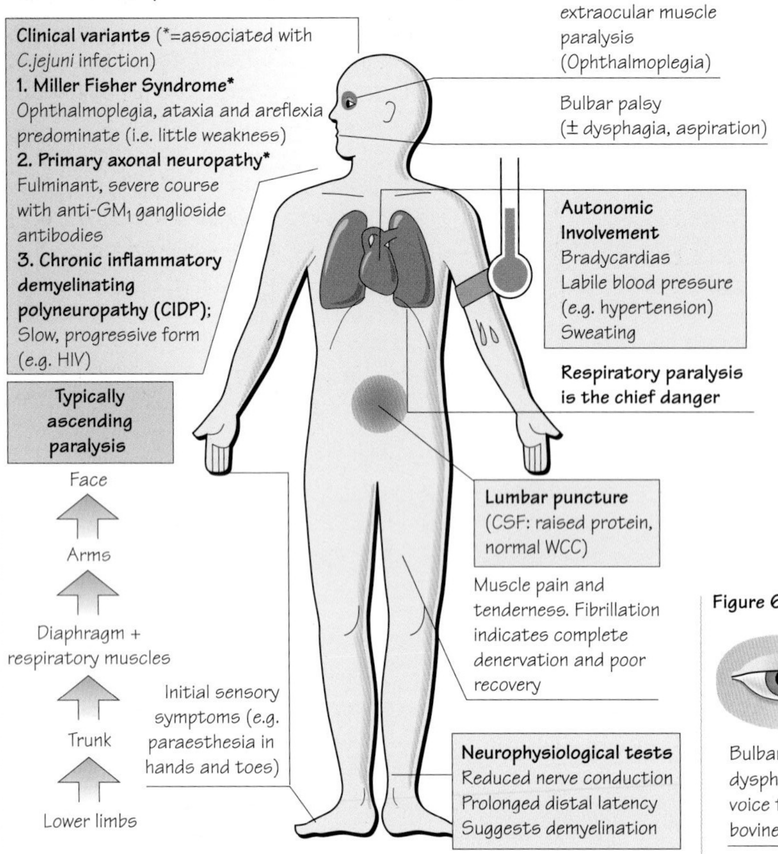

Clinical variants (*=associated with *C.jejuni* infection)
1. Miller Fisher Syndrome*
Ophthalmoplegia, ataxia and areflexia predominate (i.e. little weakness)
2. Primary axonal neuropathy*
Fulminant, severe course with anti-GM_1 ganglioside antibodies
3. Chronic inflammatory demyelinating polyneuropathy (CIDP);
Slow, progressive form (e.g. HIV)

Typically ascending paralysis

Face
↑
Arms
↑
Diaphragm + respiratory muscles
↑
Trunk
↑
Lower limbs

Initial sensory symptoms (e.g. paraesthesia in hands and toes)

Double vision due to extraocular muscle paralysis (Ophthalmoplegia)

Bulbar palsy (± dysphagia, aspiration)

Autonomic Involvement
Bradycardias
Labile blood pressure (e.g. hypertension)
Sweating

Respiratory paralysis is the chief danger

Lumbar puncture
(CSF: raised protein, normal WCC)

Muscle pain and tenderness. Fibrillation indicates complete denervation and poor recovery

Neurophysiological tests
Reduced nerve conduction
Prolonged distal latency
Suggests demyelination

Figure 64b Differential diagnosis and investigation of acute neuromuscular diseases

Differential diagnosis	Investigations
Toxic (e.g. heavy metal)	Blood tests: haematology, biochemistry (e.g. K^+), serology, toxicology, ACR assays, autoimmune screen (e.g. ANA)
Biochemical (e.g. hypokalaemia)	
Metabolic (e.g. porphyria)	
Nutritional (e.g. neurotoxic fish)	Urine tests (e.g. porphyrins)
Connective tissue disease (e.g. SLE)	Microbiology/virology
Systemic disease (e.g. lymphoma)	CXR (e.g. lung cancer)
Infective (e.g. polio, tetanus, diphtheria, botulism, HIV)	CSF fluid examination
	Edrophonium test (e.g. myasthenia gravis)
Neuromuscular diseases (e.g. myasthenia gravis)	Electromyography (e.g. nerve conduction studies)
Malignancy related Lambert-Eaton myasthenic syndrome (i.e. small cell lung cancer)	Nerve biopsies

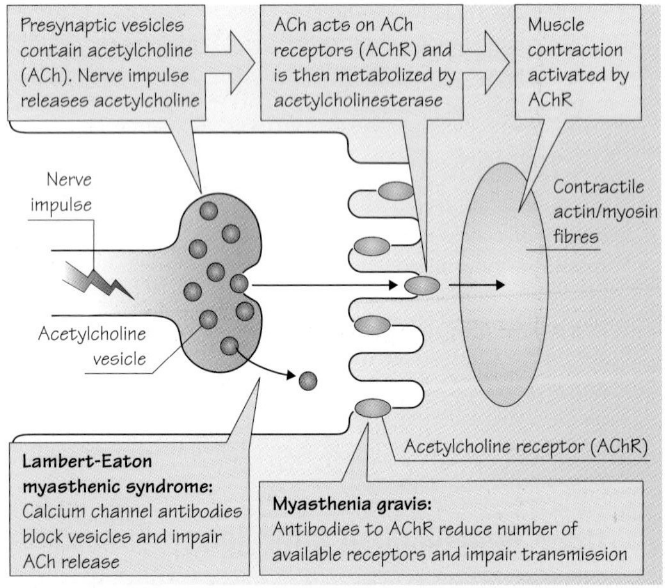

Figure 64d Symptoms and signs of myasthenia gravis

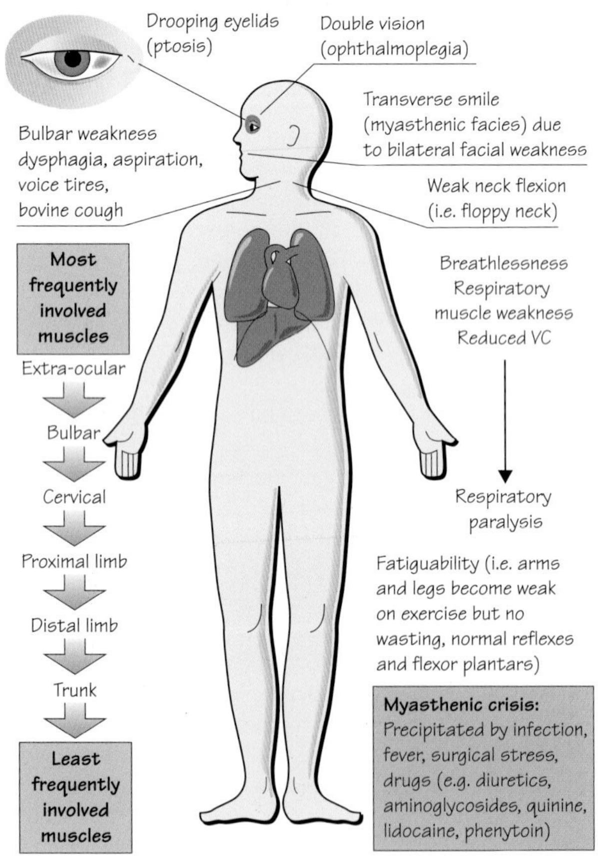

Drooping eyelids (ptosis)
Double vision (ophthalmoplegia)
Transverse smile (myasthenic facies) due to bilateral facial weakness
Weak neck flexion (i.e. floppy neck)

Bulbar weakness dysphagia, aspiration, voice tires, bovine cough

Most frequently involved muscles

Extra-ocular
⇓
Bulbar
⇓
Cervical
⇓
Proximal limb
⇓
Distal limb
⇓
Trunk
⇓
Least frequently involved muscles

Breathlessness Respiratory muscle weakness Reduced VC

Respiratory paralysis

Fatiguability (i.e. arms and legs become weak on exercise but no wasting, normal reflexes and flexor plantars)

Myasthenic crisis:
Precipitated by infection, fever, surgical stress, drugs (e.g. diuretics, aminoglycosides, quinine, lidocaine, phenytoin)

Figure 64c Pathophysiology of myasthenia gravis

Presynaptic vesicles contain acetylcholine (ACh). Nerve impulse releases acetylcholine → ACh acts on ACh receptors (AChR) and is then metabolized by acetylcholinesterase → Muscle contraction activated by AChR

Nerve impulse

Acetylcholine vesicle

Contractile actin/myosin fibres

Lambert-Eaton myasthenic syndrome:
Calcium channel antibodies block vesicles and impair ACh release

Acetylcholine receptor (AChR)

Myasthenia gravis:
Antibodies to AChR reduce number of available receptors and impair transmission

Guillain–Barré syndrome (GBS)

Incidence: the most common cause of acute generalized flaccid paralysis. It affects $\sim$1.7/10^5/population/year.

Pathophysiology: an acute, inflammatory, demyelinating polyradiculoneuropathy, that occurs a few weeks after surgery, flu vaccination or minor respiratory (45%) or gastrointestinal (20%) infections. Implicated organisms include *Campylobacter jejuni* (20–45%), cytomegalovirus (CMV) (10–20%), Epstein–Barr virus and mycoplasma. Cross-reactivity between the immune response to an organism and peripheral nerves is the likely mechanism. Figure 64b lists other acute neuropathies.

Clinical features (Figure 64a): initial symptoms are often sensory (e.g. distal paraesthesia 50–75%). Subsequent ascending weakness (i.e. lower limbs to face), areflexia and paralysis can be surprisingly rapid. In severe cases, bulbar (e.g. ophthalmoplegia) and autonomic involvement (e.g. bradycardia) occur. Respiratory paralysis is the chief danger. **Clinical variants** (Figure 64a) include: (i) **Miller Fisher syndrome**: mainly ophthalmoplegia, ataxia and areflexia; (ii) **primary axonal neuropathy**: fulminant, severe illness with poor prognosis; and (iii) **chronic inflammatory demyelinating polyneuropathy** (CIDP): prolonged illness with stepwise deterioration.

Prognosis: flaccid quadriparesis and respiratory paralysis can occur within 24–72 hours. About 30% require mechanical ventilation (MV) for a few days to >1 year. Neurological deficit peaks at $\sim$14–21 days, followed by recovery over weeks or months. Mortality is <10% but $\sim$10% of survivors have residual neurological deficits. Outcome is worse in older people and those with rapid onset or axonal damage.

Investigation (Figure 64b): excludes other causes of weakness (e.g. hypokalaemia). **Electrophysiology** may suggest demyelination (i.e. $\downarrow$ nerve conduction velocity, $\uparrow$ distal latency). **Cerebrospinal fluid (CSF) analysis** reveals raised protein (>0.5 g/L) and a normal white cell count.

Management: monitor respiratory reserve (i.e. vital capacity [VC] 1–4 hourly) because respiratory distress and arterial blood gas (ABG) deterioration are late features of respiratory failure (RF). Intubation is indicated if VC is <15 ml/kg ($\sim$1 L) or pharyngeal paralysis impairs secretion clearance. Respiratory function usually recovers within 2–3 weeks but consider a tracheostomy if paralysis persists. Chest physiotherapy and microbiological monitoring reduce respiratory infections. Minimize autonomic dysfunction (e.g. hypotension, arrhythmia, ileus) with fluid resuscitation and sedation. Profound bradycardia occasionally requires a temporary pacemaker. **General measures** include skin care, nutrition, analgesia (e.g. neuropathic pain), thromboembolic prophylaxis and physiotherapy to prevent joint contractures. **Specific measures** include high-dose (i.v.) immunoglobulin therapy and plasma exchange (plasmapheresis). Both speed recovery if used early (<7 days). Steroids are of no benefit except for radicular (root) pain and in CIDP.

Myasthenia gravis (MG)

An autoimmune disorder characterized by skeletal muscle fatigability and weakness. Antibodies to postsynaptic, acetylcholine receptors (AChR) are detected in 90%. AChR loss reduces transmission across neuromuscular junctions (Figure 64c). It affects 5/10^5 population (1 : 2 M : F ratio). Women are affected earlier (<50 years) and men later (>50 years) in life. The thymus gland is abnormal in 75%; mainly thymic hyperplasia in young women and benign thymoma ($\sim$10%) in older males. MG is associated with autoimmune disorders (e.g. hyperthyroidism, SLE), drugs (e.g. penicillamine) and thymic tumours.

Clinical features (Figure 64d) usually develop insidiously over weeks. Typically, muscle weakness increases with repetitive use and recovers with rest. Extraocular muscles are most frequently involved, trunk muscles least (Figure 64d). Ptosis and diplopia are the most common presenting features. MG is confined to the extraocular muscles in 20%. Bulbar muscle involvement causes dysphagia, aspiration and a snarling smile (myaesthenic facies). **Myaesthenic crisis,** a life-threatening deterioration, is precipitated by infection, fever, surgery or drugs (e.g. aminoglycosides). RF requires intubation and MV.

Investigations include blood for AChR antibodies. Chest radiography (CXR)/CT scans exclude thymoma. **Electromyography** shows declining muscle action potentials on repetitive stimulation. The **edrophonium (Tensilon) test** is diagnostic. Edrophonium prevents breakdown of acetylcholine (ACh) by acetylcholinesterase. Increased ACh temporarily restores neuromuscular transmission, abolishing weakness, ptosis and diplopia. However, AChR stimulation causes autonomic side-effects (e.g. sweating, bradycardia) requiring treatment with atropine. Inject a test dose of edrophonium (2 mg), followed by a further 8 mg if side-effects are not excessive. Improved strength lasting several minutes supports the diagnosis. Facilities for intubation must be available because excess ACh inhibits neuromuscular transmission and may precipitate a **cholinergic crisis** (e.g. apnoea, paralysis, bulbar palsy, excess secretions, colic).

Management: monitor respiratory function in patients with dyspnoea or difficulty swallowing. Consider intubation if VC is <15 ml/kg ($\sim$1 L) or secretion clearance is inadequate. MV is required in $\sim$10%. Assess swallowing in dysphagic patients and start thromboembolic prophylaxis.

Specific treatments include: (i) **anticholinesterase drugs** (e.g. pyridostigmine). Slowly increase the dose to achieve symptom relief. Excessive therapy, in an attempt to abolish all weakness, may result in cholinergic crisis. Give anticholinergics to control muscarinic side-effects (e.g. salivation, colic, diarrhoea). (ii) **Immunosuppressive therapy**: steroids may benefit patients with isolated ocular MG or a poor response to anticholinesterases. Improvement after several weeks follows initial deterioration. Consider azathioprine in severe MG. (iii) **Plasma exchange** produces short-lived ($\sim$4 weeks) but marked improvements during myaesthenic crisis or ventilator weaning. (iv) **Thymectomy** improves $\sim$80% of MG, hastening remission and reducing mortality compared with medical therapy alone.

Other neuromuscular disorders

Many neuromuscular diseases (e.g. muscular dystrophy, poliomyelitis) require MV following RF or surgery. Weaning can be difficult.

Critical illness polyneuropathy occurs after sepsis or high-dose steroids particularly if combined with prolonged paralysis. Axonal degeneration of the motor ($\pm$sensory) peripheral nerves leads to weakness, wasting, weaning failure and loss of reflexes. Nerve conduction studies confirm axonal loss. Treatment is symptomatic and recovery may take months.

Pearl of wisdom

Recent onset of a bizarre gait should raise the possibility of Guillain–Barré syndrome (GBS)

65 Specific bacterial infections

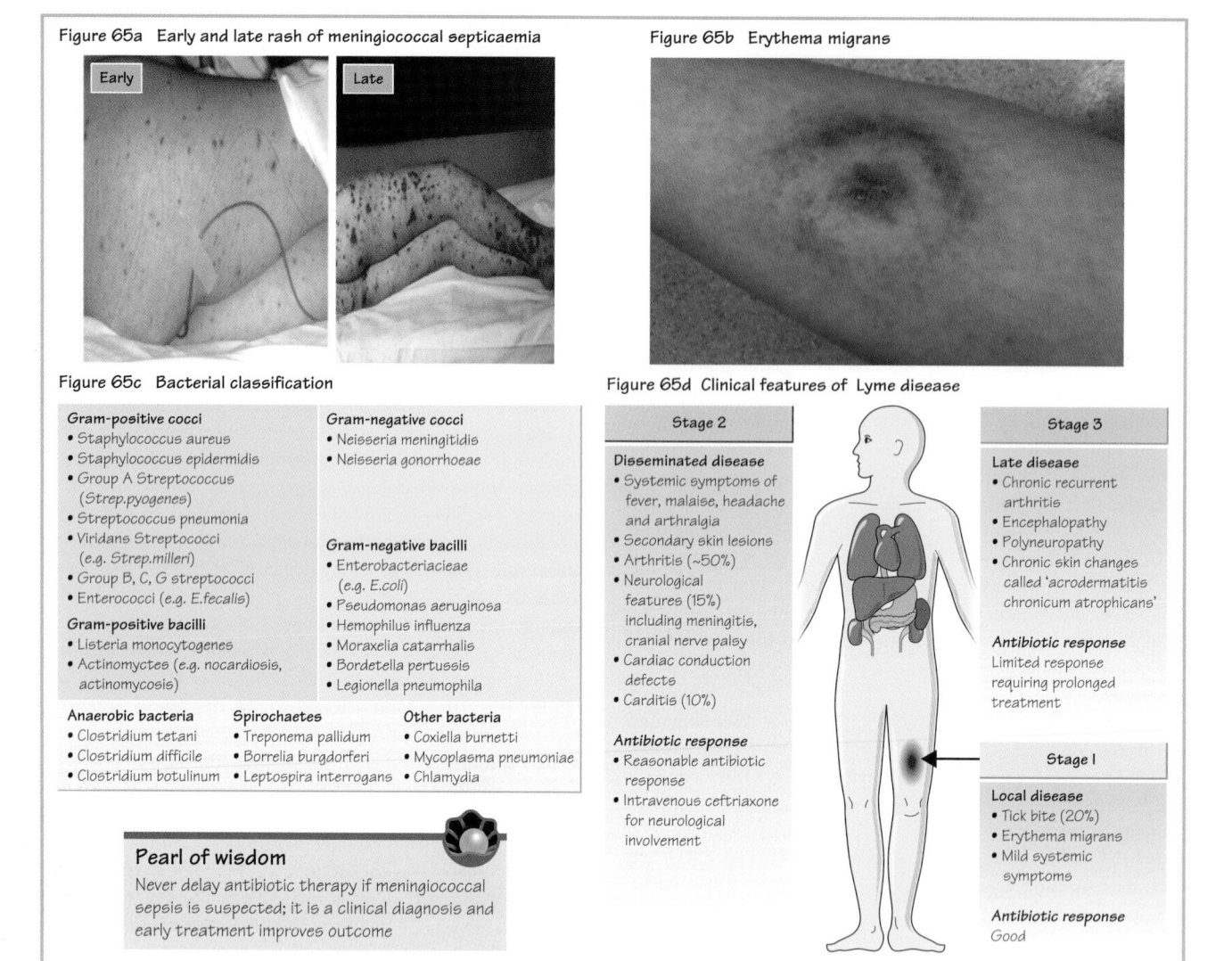

Figure 65a Early and late rash of meningiococcal septicaemia

Early

Late

Figure 65b Erythema migrans

Figure 65c Bacterial classification

Gram-positive cocci
- Staphylococcus aureus
- Staphylococcus epidermidis
- Group A Streptococcus (Strep.pyogenes)
- Streptococcus pneumonia
- Viridans Streptococci (e.g. Strep.milleri)
- Group B, C, G streptococci
- Enterococci (e.g. E.fecalis)

Gram-positive bacilli
- Listeria monocytogenes
- Actinomyctes (e.g. nocardiosis, actinomycosis)

Gram-negative cocci
- Neisseria meningitidis
- Neisseria gonorrhoeae

Gram-negative bacilli
- Enterobacteriacieae (e.g. E.coli)
- Pseudomonas aeruginosa
- Hemophilus influenza
- Moraxelia catarrhalis
- Bordetella pertussis
- Legionella pneumophila

Anaerobic bacteria
- Clostridium tetani
- Clostridium difficile
- Clostridium botulinum

Spirochaetes
- Treponema pallidum
- Borrelia burgdorferi
- Leptospira interrogans

Other bacteria
- Coxiella burnetti
- Mycoplasma pneumoniae
- Chlamydia

Pearl of wisdom
Never delay antibiotic therapy if meningiococcal sepsis is suspected; it is a clinical diagnosis and early treatment improves outcome

Figure 65d Clinical features of Lyme disease

Stage 2

Disseminated disease
- Systemic symptoms of fever, malaise, headache and arthralgia
- Secondary skin lesions
- Arthritis (~50%)
- Neurological features (15%) including meningitis, cranial nerve palsy
- Cardiac conduction defects
- Carditis (10%)

Antibiotic response
- Reasonable antibiotic response
- Intravenous ceftriaxone for neurological involvement

Stage 3

Late disease
- Chronic recurrent arthritis
- Encephalopathy
- Polyneuropathy
- Chronic skin changes called 'acrodermatitis chronicum atrophicans'

Antibiotic response
Limited response requiring prolonged treatment

Stage 1

Local disease
- Tick bite (20%)
- Erythema migrans
- Mild systemic symptoms

Antibiotic response
Good

Bacteria are classified by morphological appearance (i.e. cocci, bacilli), staining (Gram-positive dark purple, Gram-negative light pink) and oxygen requirements (i.e. aerobic, anaerobic). Initial antibiotic therapy is guided by Gram-stains and morphology and adjusted when culture and antibiotic sensitivities are available. Figure 65c classifies common bacteria, many of which are discussed in specific chapters.

Meningococcal sepsis

Acute meningococcaemia is a medical emergency. It is a common cause of community-acquired septicaemia , due to Neisseria meningitides, and can occur in the absence of meningitis. Fever, myalgia, malaise and a non-blanching purpuric rash on the extremities (Figure 65a) evolves to septic shock, coagulopathy, organ failure, coma and death, often within hours. Many cases present with meningitis, headache, photobobia and neck stiffness

(Chapter 63). Coagulopathy is due to disseminated intravascular coagulation (DIC) and microvascular thromboses can progress to gangrene of extremities. Rarely, chronic meningiococcaemia presents over days or weeks with fever, arthralgia and a rash that is maculopapular or pustular rather than petechial.

Neisseria meningitides: a Gram-negative diplococci with many serotypes (A, B, C, W, Y135), is part of the normal oropharyngeal flora in asymptomatic carriers (5–15%). Transmission is respiratory in infected droplets especially in overcrowded or closed communities. The young (15–19 years old) and children (<5 years old) are most susceptible. In the UK, serotypes B and C are most common and cause epidemic outbreaks in schools or barracks. Serotype A causes dry season epidemics on the 'meningitis belt' of sub-Saharan Africa. Meningiococci are isolated from blood cultures (~50%) or skin lesions (~70%). Cerebrospinal fluid from lumbar puncture is often diagnostic and throat swabs detect car-

Critical Care Medicine at a Glance, Third Edition. Richard Leach. © 2014 John Wiley & Sons, Ltd. Published 2014 by John Wiley & Sons, Ltd.

riage. Investigation and specimen collection should never delay treatment. Immediate high-dose intravenous penicillin or ceftriaxone (chloramphenicol if penicillin allergic) are standard. Give oral rifampicin prophylaxis to close contacts. Vaccination is available for serotype C but not other serotypes.

Tetanus

Clostridium tetani is an anaerobic, spore-forming, Gram-positive bacillus found in soil. It infects necrotic 'anaerobic' wounds and produces tetanospasmin toxin. The toxin prevents inhibitory central nervous system (CNS) neurons releasing pre-synaptic transmitter, and this causes the characteristic muscular rigidity. The incubation period (IP) is 1–21 days. Generalized tetanus presents with spasm of the masseter muscles causing trismus (lockjaw) and 'risus sardonicus' (characteristic 'sardonic' grin due to facial muscle spasm) followed by widespread, painful muscle spasms that may be precipitated by noise or touch. Autonomic instability with arrhythmias and labile blood pressure occur. Neonatal tetanus, common in the developing world, is usually due to infection of the umbilical stump. The diagnosis is clinical and human tetanus toxin is given to neutralize circulating toxin. Initially, debride the infected wound and eliminate the organism with metronidazole or penicillin. Benzodiazepams reduce spasms but mechanical ventilation may be required. Treat autonomic instability with α- or β-blockade and/or inotropes. Primary *immunization* with tetanus toxoid prevents tetanus. Mortality, due to respiratory failure or autonomic instability, is ~20%.

Lyme disease

The spirochaete *Borrelia burgdorferi* causes Lyme disease. It is transmitted to humans by a painless bite from *Ixodes sp.* ticks from host mice or deer. In the UK, tick exposure occurs in late spring (early summer) in the New Forest, Exmoor, Lake District and Scottish Highlands. It causes 2–3000 cases annually. Regions of East Coast USA, Europe, Russia and China are also affected.
• **Localized (stage 1) disease** (3–30 days) presents with a well-demarcated, erythematous annular lesion with central clearing (erythema migrans) at the site of the bite (Figures 65b and 65d).
• **Disseminated (stage 2) disease** follows blood spread. Fluctuating systemic symptoms (e.g. fever, malaise, myalgia, headache), monoarticular, large joint arthritis (60%), meningitis, cranial nerve defects, myelitis (15%), myocarditis and conduction defects (10%) resolve spontaneously after several weeks.
• **Late (stage 3) disease** develops months later if the initial infection is untreated. Features include chronic arthritis (probably autoimmune), chronic skin disease, encephalopathy and polyneuropathy.
Serology confirms clinical diagnosis because organisms are rarely isolated. Treat early disease with oral doxycycline (or amoxicillin). Late disease requires longer antibiotic courses (>3 weeks) or ceftriaxone (i.v.) in patients with neurological involvement.

Toxic shock syndrome

Toxins produced during *Staph. aureus* (e.g. infected tampons) or *Strep. pyogenes* (e.g. deep tissue infections like necrotising fasciitis) infection cause toxic shock syndrome. It presents abruptly with fever, myalgia, vomiting and diarrhoea, followed by severe hypotension, conjunctival injection, a deep red ('sun-burn') erythematous rash and multi-organ failure (e.g. acute kidney injury [AKI],

acute respiratory distress syndrome [ARDS], confusion). Subsequent desquamation affects mainly the soles and palms. Treatment is supportive with fluid resuscitation and antibiotics. Mortality is high.

Listeriosis

Listeria monocytogenes, a Gram-positive bacillus, usually acquired from food (e.g. cold meats, pate, soft cheese) causes disease in pregnant women, neonates and immunocompromised patients. In pregnancy, bacteraemia produces a flu-like illness and, rarely, meningitis, but it can lead to abortion, stillbirth or neonatal sepsis. Meningioencephalitis occurs in the late neonatal period and in immunocompromised and older patients. In systemic disease, blood cultures may be positive. In neurological syndromes, a few organisms may be present in cerebrospinal fluid (CSF) but cultures are usually positive. Treatment is with high-dose ampicillin and gentamicin.

Syphilis

Treponema pallidum, a sexually transmitted spirochaete, causes syphilis. Incidence has increased in developed countries recently. Blood dissemination follows entry through epithelial breaches in a sexual partner.
• **Primary syphilis** (IP ~3 weeks) is associated with a painless, ulcerated papule ('primary chancre) at the site of inoculation on the penis, labia or cervix, and inguinal lymphadenopathy. It heals spontaneously within weeks.
• **Secondary syphilis** occurs 6–8 weeks later with fever, sore throat, headache, generalized maculopapular rash (affects palms and soles), lymphadenopathy (~50%) and highly infective condylomata (moist plaques in intertriginous areas).
• **Tertiary syphilis** with widespread, hard, granulomatous lesions (gummata) occurs after 3–10 years. Neurosyphilitic features include meningovascular disease (~5 years), general paresis of the insane (~15 years) and tabes dorsalis (~20 years). Dark ground microscopy detects *Treponema pallidum* in primary or secondary syphilitic lesions. Penicillin is the drug of choice. In late syphilis, steroids are required to prevent anaphylaxsis to dead spirochaetes (Jarisch–Herxheimer reaction). Contacts should be traced and treated.

Gonorrhoea

Neisseria gonorrhoeae causes sexually transmitted genitourinary tract infections with associated urethritis, cervicitis, proctitis and asymptomatic throat infections. In <1% it causes bacteraemia. Disseminated disease causes septic monoarthritis, polyarthritis (i.e. knees, ankles, wrists), fever, pustular skin rash, tenosynovitis and hepatitis (due to local spread). Urethral swabs and blood or urethral cultures detect Gram-negative intracellular-diplococci and determine antibiotic sensitivities. Single-dose intramuscular ceftriaxone treats most cases. Alternative therapies include ciprofloxacin or ofloxacin.

Pearl of wisdom
Never delay antibiotic therapy if meningococcal sepsis is suspected; it is a clinical diagnosis and early treatment improves outcome

66 Common adult viral infections

Figure 66a Varicella-zoster infection

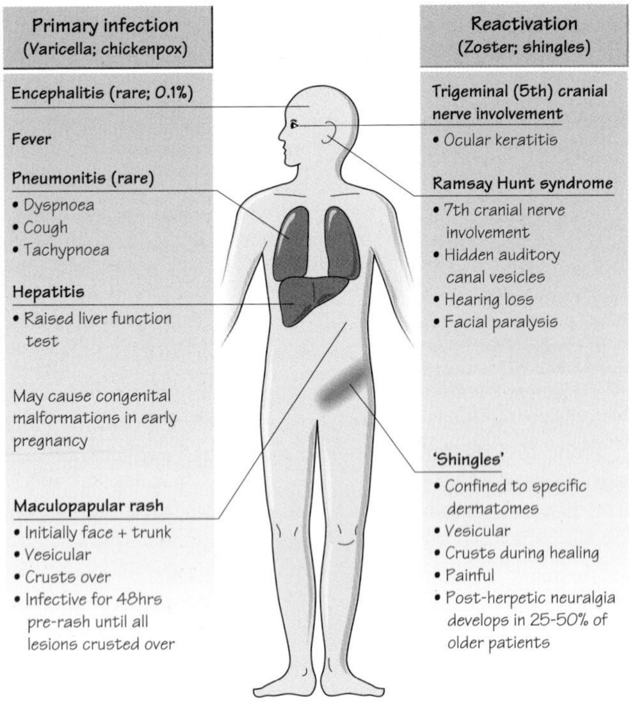

Primary infection (Varicella; chickenpox)	Reactivation (Zoster; shingles)

Primary infection (Varicella; chickenpox)

Encephalitis (rare; 0.1%)

Fever

Pneumonitis (rare)
- Dyspnoea
- Cough
- Tachypnoea

Hepatitis
- Raised liver function test

May cause congenital malformations in early pregnancy

Maculopapular rash
- Initially face + trunk
- Vesicular
- Crusts over
- Infective for 48hrs pre-rash until all lesions crusted over

Reactivation (Zoster; shingles)

Trigeminal (5th) cranial nerve involvement
- Ocular keratitis

Ramsay Hunt syndrome
- 7th cranial nerve involvement
- Hidden auditory canal vesicles
- Hearing loss
- Facial paralysis

'Shingles'
- Confined to specific dermatomes
- Vesicular
- Crusts during healing
- Painful
- Post-herpetic neuralgia develops in 25-50% of older patients

Figure 66b Herpes zoster (shingles rash)

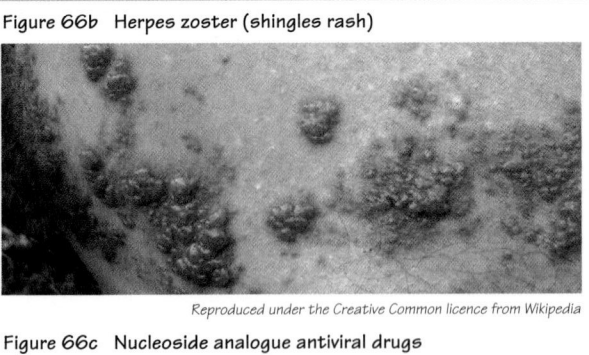

Reproduced under the Creative Common licence from Wikipedia

Figure 66c Nucleoside analogue antiviral drugs
(interfere with viral polymerases and replication)

Drug	HSV	VZV	CMV	Comments
Aciclovir (iv, o) Valaciclovir	+++	++	-	Short half life requiring frequent dosing orally
Famciclovir	+++	++	-	
Foscarnet	++	++	++	Nephrotoxic but useful in resistant HSV or CMV
Ganciclovir (iv) Valganciclovir (o)	+	+	+++	Myelotoxic

Pearl of wisdom

Annual flu vaccination saves lives and is essential in old peolple with co-morbid disease or any patient with significant respiratory impairment

Figure 66d Other common childhood viruses

Virus	Incubation period	Clinical features	Diagnosis and treatment
Measles	8–12 days	Fever, cough, pharyngitis and conjunctivitis over days 3–4, followed by a maculopapular rash initially affecting the face and then spreading to the trunk, hands and feet over 2–3 days. White plaques (Koplik's spots) on the buccal mucosa are pathognomonic. Worldwide, 1 million children die annually but mass vaccination has reduced mortality in the developed world. Complications are more serious in adults including pneumonitis, otitis media and meningioencephalitis (0.1%).	Serology confirms diagnosis. Management is supportive but immune globulin can be given to susceptible pregnant women and the immunocompromised. Measles, mumps and rubella (MMR) vaccination is effective and safe
Mumps	17–19 days	Fever, headache, pharyngitis, myalgia and tender, enlarged parotid glands resolves over 1–2 weeks. Adolescents may present with unilateral epididymo-orchitis (sterility is uncommon) or meningitis (without parotid enlargement). Pancreatitis, oophoritis, deafness and arthitis can occur	Treatment is symptomatic with analgesia for orchitis which can be severe MMR vaccination is safe and effective
Rubella or German measles	16–18 days	Often subclinical in children. Adults develop fever, pharyngitis, headache, myalgia and post auricular lymphadenopathy. A facial rose-pink maculopapular rash spreads distally and lasts 3 days. Polyarthralgia may persist for weeks. Non-immune pregnant women risk congenital rubella syndrome (i.e. microcephaly, cataracts, deafness and diabetes) during early gestation. Rubella is infectious 5 days before and after the rash	Treatment is symptomatic Serology confirms the diagnosis Consider termination in early pregnancy MMR vaccination is effective
Parvovirus B19	13–18 days	Erythematous cheek rash (slapped cheek syndrome) that extends over 2 weeks. Fever is absent, arthragia of the hands, ankles and wrists in adults. Transient aplastic anaemia may occur in sickle cell disease	No specific treatment May cause fetal death in pregnancy
Enteroviruses (e.g. Cosackie, echoviruses)	2–10 days	Causes meningitis, pericarditis and myocarditis in adults. Coxsackie B causes fever, pharyngitis and intercostal myalgia (Bornholm disease). Coxsackie A causes herpangina (small painful oropharyngeal vesicles) in infants. Coxsackie A16 causes hand, foot and mouth disease with associated painful vesicles in childhood	Highly contagious, faecal oral transmission Diagnosis confirmed by serology No specific treatment
Hepatitis viruses A–E	7–21 days	Fever and prodromal constitutional symptoms in hepatitis A but the fever resolves before jaundice develops	Serological diagnosis and symptomatic treatment

Viral infections are common and usually self-limiting. The common cold, characterized by fever, sore throat, sneezing and nasal congestion is often caused by rhinoviruses, but also adenoviruses, respiratory syncytial virus, parainfluenza and coronaviruses. In developing countries, measles, mumps and rubella (MMR) cause major morbidity and a million children <5 years old die from measles annually. Mass vaccination in developed regions has reduced MMR incidence, which only occurs in those who were not fully vaccinated, in childhood.

Influenza

Influenza, an orthomyxovirus (incubation period [IP] 1–3 days), occurs as two strains.

- **Influenza A** infects many species but birds are nature's main reservoir. It is highly infectious causing worldwide pandemics by respiratory droplet spread. The virus has two surface antigens: haemaglutinin (H) and neuraminidase (N). Major antigenic 'shifts' cause pandemics every 10–30 years (e.g. 'Spanish' flu (H1N1) caused 20 million deaths worldwide in 1918). Minor antigenic 'drift' causes regional epidemics every 1–3 years. The latest pandemic in 2009, 'swine flu' (H1N1), originated in Mexico.
- **Influenza B** causes less severe epidemic infections.

Presentation is with fever (>38°C), pharyngitis, headache, rigors, myalgia and malaise. Secondary bacterial pneumonia is common whereas viral pneumonia with chest radiograph (CXR) infiltrates is rare and potentially fatal. Throat swab polymerase chain reaction (PCR) establishes the diagnosis. Management is usually symptomatic and most patients recover spontaneously. Mortality is high in older patients and those with chronic respiratory disease. In these cases, oseltamivir may be effective against both A and B strains if started within 48 hours of infection. Annual vaccination is recommended in those at risk.

Varicella–zoster virus (VZV)

Varicella (chicken-pox), the primary infection, and herpes zoster (shingles), the recurrent infection (Figure 66a), are caused by VZV (IP 10–21 days).
- **Varicella**, a benign childhood disease transmitted by respiratory droplets, affects 90% of children. Fever and malaise precede a maculopapular rash, initially on the face and trunk, which becomes vesicular before crusting over. Patients are infectious until every vesicle has scabbed over (~5 days). In adults, it is a serious illness (15-fold rise in mortality) associated with pneumonitis (0.25%); encephalitis (0.1%, fatal in 20%) and hepatitis. VZV causes congenital malformations in early pregnancy and disseminated infection in the immunocompromised.
- **Herpes zoster** occurs in older people after reactivation of latent VZV infection in dorsal root ganglia. Pain or itching precedes a unilateral 'varicella-like' rash (i.e. maculopapular, vesicular) with a dermatomal distribution (Figure 66b). Trigeminal nerve involvement may cause sight-threatening keratitis. Ramsay Hunt syndrome (i.e. 'hidden' auditory canal vesicles, deafness, facial nerve palsy, taste loss) follows geniculate ganglion VZV reactivation. Paralysis due to anterior horn cell involvement, transverse myelitis or encephalitis also occurs. Post-herpetic neuralgia occurs in 25–50% of >50 years olds.
Diagnosis is confirmed by electron or immunofluorescence microscopy of vesicular scrapping. Early oral acyclovir therapy reduces severity in adults with chickenpox or shingles. Intravenous therapy is needed in pneumonitis, encephalitis and the immunocompromised. Give prophylactic immunoglobulin in pregnant and immunocompromised patients exposed to infection.

Herpes simplex virus (HSV)

HSV is common and affects mainly mucocutaneous sites. It is transmitted by oral or sexual contact. Two types occur, HSV1 and HSV2, with different clinical and epidemiological presentations (but some overlap). HSV1 infection usually occurs in childhood, whereas HSV2 is due to sexual contact. Recurrent infection, due to 'latency' in sensory nerve ganglions, is precipitated by stress, viral infections, trauma or sunlight.
- **Oral mucocutaneous HSV** with recurrent 'cold sores', usually follows asymptomatic HSV1 primary infection or mild febrile pharyngitis. 'Tingling' over the lip edge precedes painful vesicles, which 'crust' before healing.
- **Genital HSV** is due to HSV2 (~80%). Painful vesicles affect the penis, vulva, perineum or vagina, 2–7 days after the primary contact (but may be asymptomatic). Fever, dysuria, malaise and tender inguinal lymphadenopathy may occur. Vesicular ulceration can persist for weeks and often recurs. Asymptomatic viral shedding infects sexual partners.
- **Other HSV conditions** include primary eye infections (dendritic ulcers), atopic dermatitis infection (eczema herpeticum), encephalitis and herpetic finger whitlows.
Acyclovir is required in systemic illness (e.g. encephalitis) or primary/recurrent genital HSV. Early use of acyclovir cream may prevent or reduce severity of 'cold sores'.

Epstein–Barr virus (EBV)

EBV, a herpes virus, causes glandular fever (IP 2–6 weeks). Infection follows contact with infected saliva ('kissing disease'). It affects 90% of people before adulthood. Asymptomatic infection affects 50% of children <5 years old in developed countries.
Clinical disease occurs in adolescence and later life. A prodrome of fever, headache, myalgia and malaise is followed by sore throat due to exudative tonsillitis, lymphadenopathy, splenomegally (50%) and palatial petechiae. A maculopapular rash often follow treatment with amoxicillin/ampicillin (~90%). Haemolytic anaemia, hepatitis, myocarditis and meningoencephalitis are rare complications. Lymphoproliferative disorders may develop in transplant and HIV patients. Recovery occurs in 2–3 weeks but may be followed by chronic fatigue. Differential diagnosis includes streptococcal tonsillitis, cytomegalovirus (CMV) and toxoplasma infection.
Investigation: lymphocytosis with >10% atypical lymphocytes, thrombocytopaenia and raised serum transaminase occur. Heterophil antibodies (e.g. antibodies to sheep red blood cells) are rapidly detected (e.g. Paul Bunnell, Monospot) but are non-specific tests. EBV serology is diagnostic.
Treatment is non-specific (i.e. symptomatic). Steroids prevent airways obstruction, thrombocytopaenia or haemolytic anaemia.

Cytomegalovirus

CMV is a herpes virus transmitted by intimate contact with body fluids (e.g. saliva). Although most adults are infected, it rarely causes clinical disease except in the immunocompromised (e.g. transmission in transplanted tissue).
- Symptomatic primary CMV infection causes a mild illness like glandular fever with mononucleosis and trivial hepatitis that rapidly resolves, although fever may persist for weeks. Congenital infection follows primary infection during pregnancy.
- Immunocompromised post-transplant patients may develop pneumonitis, hepatitis, retinitis or diarrhoea within 3 months of transplantation. Colitis, encephalitis and sight-threatening retinitis occur in advanced human immunodeficiency virus (HIV) infection. Treat with i.v. ganciclovir or oral valganciclovir. Immunoglobulin is used to treat pneumonitis.

Gastro-intestinal viral infections

Norovirus (small round or Norwalk-like virus) causes 'Winter vomiting' disease. It is the most common cause of gastroenteritis in developed countries. The IP is 12–48 hours and transmission is by the faecal–oral route. Outbreaks occur in 'enclosed' environments (e.g. ships, hospital wards). Management includes isolation, barrier nursing and re-hydration. Recovery takes 1–2 days.
Rotovirus is the most common cause of gastroenteritis in infants. Figure 66d lists less common and childhood viral infections.

67 Common fungal and protozoal infections

Figure 67a Pathogenic fungal infections

Fungus	Clinical features, diagnosis and treatment
Histoplasmosis	Due to inhalation of soil particles contaminated by *histoplasma capsulatum* in bird and bat faeces. Most cases are asymptomatic or cause mild respiratory tract infection with hilar adenopathy and patchy CXR shadows. Chronic lung infection occurs in emphysema with low grade fever, productive cough, weight loss and upper lobe cavitation on CXR. Disseminated infection occurs in the immunocompromised (e.g. HIV) with fever, lymphadenopathy, hepatosplenomegaly, skin lesions, meningitis and weight loss. It may be chronic or rapidly fatal. Serology is diagnostic, as are cultures, but may take weeks. Immunocompetent patients may not need treatment but give itraconazole if symptomatic. Amphotericin B is given for serious infections in the immunocompromised
Pneumocystis jiroveci	Causes a potentially fatal pneumonia in immunosuppressed patients especially those with HIV (see chapter 68)
Blastomycosis	Causes acute and chronic infections of the lungs, skin or bones following exposure to infected dust with *Blastomyces dermatitidis*
Coccidiodomycosis	Usually a self-limiting pneumonic illness following inhalation of dust contaminated by *Coccidioides immitis* in desert climates. Disseminated infection can cause meningitis
Paracoccidiodomycosis	Caused by infection with paracoccidiodes brasiliensis in central and south American agricultural workers. An acute form in young adults presents with fever, lymphadenopathy and weight loss. Chronic disease occurs in older adults with pulmonary and mucocutaneous disease

Figure 67b Oral candida infection

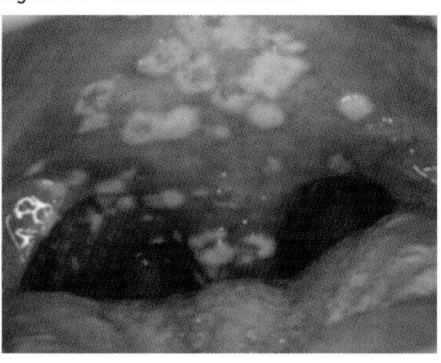

Figure 67c Aspergillus infection

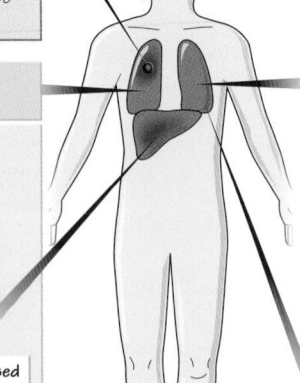

Aspergilloma
- Fungal ball in pre-existing cavity
- Fever, cough, dyspnoea
- CXR shows air-crescent sign
- Associated haemoptysis can be severe

Acute invasive pulmonary aspergillosis
- Fever
- Dyspnoea, cough, tachypnoea
- Haemoptysis
- Chest pain

CXR: Nodular infiltrates + multiple small cavities

Spread occurs to the brain, spleen and liver

Affects the immunosuppressed
- Steroid therapy
- Advanced AIDS
- Profound neutropaenia (e.g. acute leukaemia)
- Organ transplantation
- Prolonged antibiotic therapy

Invasive sino-orbital disease
(acute leukaemia/BMT)
- Fever, headache
- Infected sinuses
- Periorbital swelling (extension from infected sinuses)

Allergic bronchopulmonary aspergillosis (APBA)
- Wheeze, dyspnoea, cough
- Expectoration of dark mucous plugs
- Often chronic asthmatics
- Bronchoconstriction, airways inflammation and bronchiectasis
- ↑IgE, blood eosinophilia
- CXR: flitting lung infiltrates

Chronic necrotising pulmonary aspergillosis
- Progressive cavitation and aspergilloma formation in alcoholics, diabetics, COPD
- Fever, weight loss, cough
- Haemoptysis

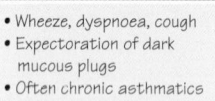

Figure 67d Lung biopsy in invasive aspergillus infection

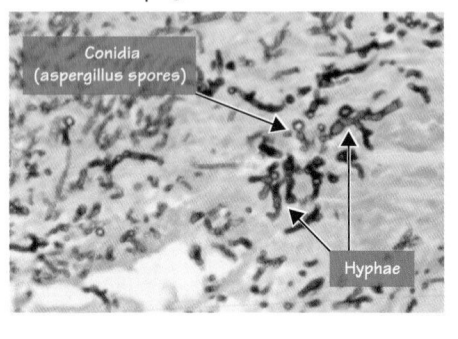

Conidia (aspergillus spores)

Hyphae

Figure 67e CXR and CT scan of allergic bronchopulmonary aspergillosis

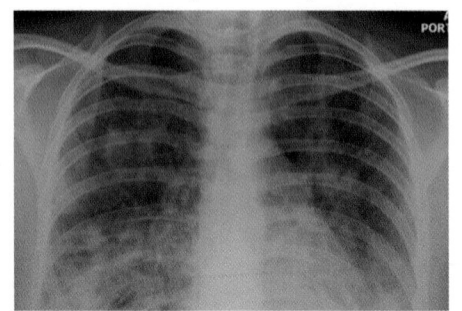

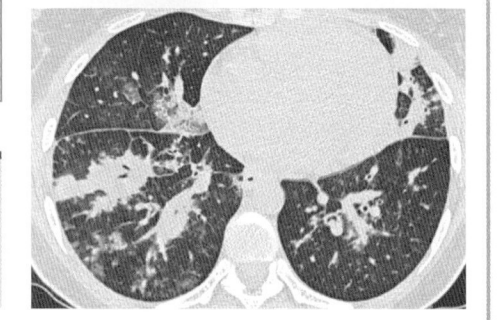

Pearl of wisdom

If sepsis fails to respond to antibiotic therapy, consider opportunistic fungal infections. They are more common than generally realized, account for ~5% of sepsis and are often missed. Candidaemia is the fourth most common nosocomial blood stream infection. Delayed therapy increases mortality

Critical Care Medicine at a Glance, Third Edition. Richard Leach. © 2014 John Wiley & Sons, Ltd. Published 2014 by John Wiley & Sons, Ltd.

Normal adult fungal infections are relatively innocuous. However, 'opportunistic' fungi can cause life-threatening disease in the immunocompromised and are important in modern medicine. Pathogenic fungi cause systemic 'granulomatous' infections but are relatively rare (Figure 67a).

Candida species

Candida is ubiquitous and a normal commensal in the respiratory, gastrointestinal and genitourinary tracts.

• **Local, mucocutaneous infection** (i.e. oral, skin, vaginal) is common and caused by *Candida albicans*. Diabetics and human immunodeficiency virus (HIV) patients are most susceptible. Oral candida infection is characterized by creamy white 'curd-like' patches on the tongue and mucosa (Figure 67b). In immunosuppressed hosts (e.g. HIV), oesophageal candida may cause dysphagia and retrosternal chest pain. Intertrigo (i.e. infection of warm, damp skinfolds with associated inflammation, 'maceration' and 'satellite' lesions) and pruritic vaginal infections are common, especially in diabetics. Treat oral and vaginal infections with topical therapy or short-term systemic therapy (e.g. oral fluconazole). Oesophageal or serious mucocutaneous disease requires prolonged systemic therapy.

• **Disseminated (invasive) candidiasis** occurs in immunosuppressed (e.g. HIV, steroid therapy) or neutropaenia patients (e.g. acute leukaemia), after prolonged antibiotic therapy or infected intravenous (i.v.) or urinary catheters. Less common *Candida* species (e.g. *C. tropicalis*) may be responsible. Candidaemia may present as septic shock with fever, but can be asymptomatic. Blood cultures are positive in ~50%. Micro-abscesses occur in the liver, spleen and brain. Eye lesions occur in 10% and patients with candidaemia (or two or more local infection sites) require examination by an ophthalmologist to exclude endopthalmitis. *Candida* spp. may be detected in the urine. Treat disseminated candidiasis with i.v. azoles (e.g. fluconazole), echinocandins (e.g. caspofungin) or amphotericin. Fluconazole resistance occurs in patients on fluconazole prophylaxis (e.g. bone marrow transplant recipients). Remove potentially infected lines.

Aspergillus species

Aspergillus is common in soil, dust (e.g. demolition) and decaying vegetation (e.g. hay). Human disease (Figure 67c) follows spore inhalation and causes:

• **Allergic bronchopulmonary aspergillosis** (ABPA): allergy to *Aspegillus fumigatus* that causes bronchoconstriction, airways inflammation and bronchiectasis. Chronic asthma patients present with increasing wheeze, dyspnoea, cough and expectoration of dark mucous plugs. Diagnostic features include raised IgE, blood eosinophilia and flitting lung infiltrates (±central bronchiectasis) on chest radiograph (CXR) and CT scan (Figure 67e). Treat acute episodes with prolonged high-dose steroids (±itraconazole).

• **Aspergilloma**: a fungal ball (with an air-crescent sign on a CXR) results from heavy aspergillus colonization of pre-existing (e.g. tuberculous) lung cavities. Erosion of the cavity wall causes minor haemoptysis (75%) but occasionally life-threatening bleeding requires surgical resection. Antifungals are not beneficial.

• **Chronic necrotising pulmonary aspergillosis**: a semi-invasive infection occurring in the mildly immunosuppressed (e.g. diabetes, alcoholism) or chronic lung disease. It causes slowly progressive cavitation and aspergilloma formation presenting with fever, weight loss, cough and haemoptysis.

• **Invasive infection** affects the immunocompromised (e.g. steroid therapy, advanced AIDS), those with profound neutropaenia or organ transplants and patients on prolonged antibiotics. It causes:

• **Invasive sino-orbital disease** with fever, headache and periorbital swelling follows extension from infected sinuses especially in acute leukaemia or bone marrow transplant recipients. Surgical debridement is required in addition to antifungal agents.

• **Acute invasive pulmonary aspergillosis** presents with fever, cough, haemoptysis and chest pain. Early blood spread occurs to the brain, spleen and liver. Nodular infiltrates with multiple small cavities are seen on CXR. A halo sign (i.e. pulmonary nodule surrounded by ground-glass opacification) suggests 'angio-invasive' disease on the CT scan. Diagnosis requires lung biopsy because cultures are rarely helpful (Figure 67d). Early therapy with i.v. amphotericin, voraconazole or caspofungin is effective. Mortality is high: >20%.

Cryptococcal species

Cryptococcus neoformans causes cryptococcosis and is acquired by inhalation from pigeon droppings or soil. Pulmonary disease affects normal and immunosuppressed adults. Meningitis only affects the immunocompromised and presents with slowly progressive headache, confusion and occasionally cranial nerve lesions or papilloedema. Neck stiffness is often absent. In advanced AIDS (CD4 count <100 cells/mm^3), it is the most common cause of meningitis. Disseminated disease with pulmonary and skin (~10%) infections occurs occasionally. Diagnosis is confirmed by direct visualization of India ink-stained cryptococci, culture and lymphocytosis, low glucose and high protein in cerebrospinal fluid (CSF). Serum cryptococcal antigen is present in 85% of meningitis cases. Treat meningitis with i.v. amphotericin and oral flucytosine followed by prolonged prophylaxis with oral fluconazole in advanced AIDS. Repeated CSF fluid removal may be required for raised intracranial pressure to prevent blindness and coma.

Mucormycosis

Mucormycosis infects patients with uncontrolled diabetes, immunosuppression, iron overload states and previous deferoxamine or steroid therapy. Rhinocerebral mucormycois follows spore inhalation. Rapidly progressive, invasive sinusitis involves the orbits and skull base with a characteristic black eschar on the hard palate and associated proptosis, orbital cellulitis, double vision and cranial nerve palsies. Local spread causes cerebral abscesses and cavernous sinus or carotid artery thrombosis. Treatment requires surgical debridement and i.v. amphotericin. Fulminant lung and disseminated infection also occur.

Toxoplasmosis

Toxolasma gondii, a common protozoan parasite spread in cat faeces, can survive for months in damp soil. Infection follows ingestion of contaminated water or foods (e.g. raw meats).

• In immunocompetent cases, 10–20% of primary infections are symptomatic. Enlarged lymph nodes, often cervical, may be the only finding but malaise, sore throat, sweats and low-grade fever can occur. Symptoms and lymphadenopathy may persist for months.

• In immunocompromised patients (e.g. HIV), toxoplasma infection is serious, causing encephalitis, pneumonitis and hepatitis.

• Congenital toxoplasmosis is acquired *in utero* due to infection during pregnancy. It causes hydrocephalus, mental retardation and chorioretinitis. Treat with spiramycin as soon as possible.

Serology is usually diagnostic but toxoplasma can be isolated in tissue biopsy samples. The immunocompetent rarely need treatment, but pyrimethamine and sulfadiazine are used in the immunosuppressed. Steroids reduce oedema in cerebral toxoplasmosis.

68 The immune compromised patient

Figure 68a Clinical features of AIDS and causes of critical illness

Clinical features and diseases that are indicators of AIDS

Cerebral
HIV encephalopathy, dementia
Cerebral toxoplasmosis
Cryptococcus neoformans
Primary brain lymphoma

General
Weight loss, fatigue
Lymphadenopathy
CMV retinitis

Respiratory
Pneumocystis carinii
   pneumonia
Mycobacterium avium
   intracellulare
Mycobacterium tuberculosis
Pneumonia
(e.g. S.pneumoniae)

Gastrointestinal
Diarrhoea
Cytomegalovirus colitis
Oral and oesophageal candida
Small bowel lymphoma

Skin
Herpes simplex
Kaposi's sarcoma
Dermatitis

Malignancy
Non-Hodgkin's lymphoma
Burkitt's lymphoma

Blood
Lymphopenia
Bacteraemia

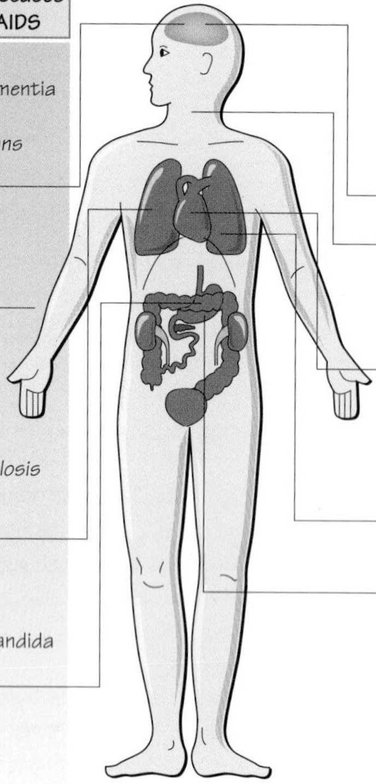

Causes of critical illness *commonest

Neurological emergencies*
Seizures
Meningitis
Encephalitis
Infection

Upper airways obstruction

Hypotension*
Sepsis (e.g. candida)
Adrenal insufficiency
Cardiac arrhythmias

Respiratory failure*
Pneumocystis jiroveci
   pneumonia
Tuberculosis
Interstitial pneumonitis

Gastrointestinal
GI bleeding

Malignancy
Side effects of therapy
Secondary infection
Drug toxicity

Other
Drug toxicity
Self harm

Figure 68b Cerebral CT scan illustrating cerebral toxoplasmosis with ring enhancement following contrast

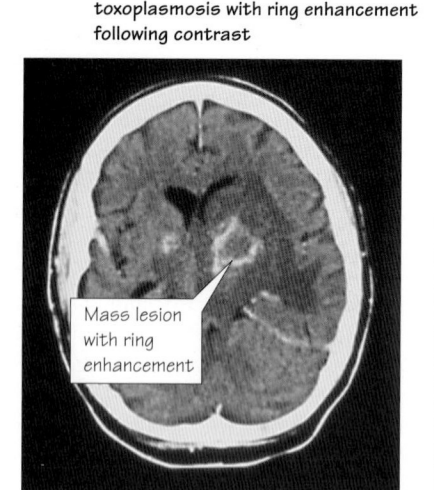

Mass lesion with ring enhancement

Figure 68c Causes of new pulmonary infiltrates

Infectious
• Bacterial pneumonia
• Fungal pneumonia (e.g. aspergillosis)
• Opportunistic pneumonia (e.g. PCP)
• Viral pneumonia

Non-infectious
• Pulmonary oedema, ARDS
• Radiation pneumonitis
• Drug induced e.g. amiodarone, busulfan
• Malignant infiltration
• Pulmonary haemorrhage
• Non-specific interstitial pneumonitis

Figure 68d Pneumocystis jiroveci pneumonia showing bilateral diffuse infiltrates

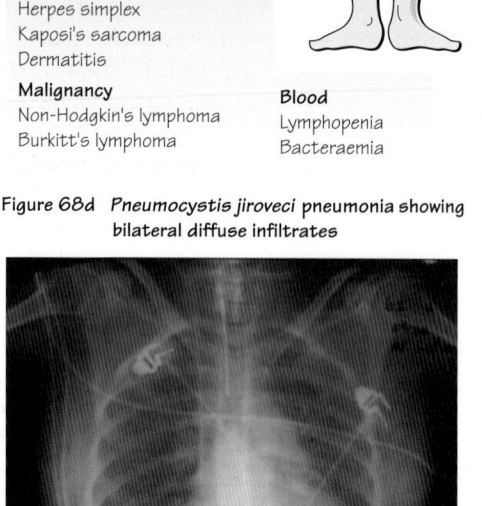
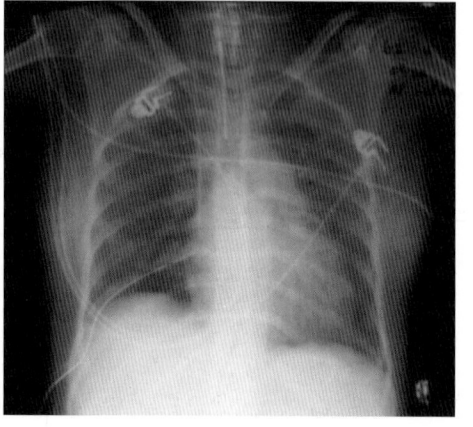

Figure 68e Causes of immunosuppression

Pathogenesis	Condition	Comments
Physiological	Elderly	Pneumonia
	Pregnancy	Listeriosis
Acquired	Diabetes	Septicaemia
	Malnutrition	Septicaemia
	Malignancy	Opportunistic infection
	Radiation	T-cell suppression
	Drugs (e.g. steroids)	Varying effects
Congenital	B-lymphocyte	e.g. IgA deficiency
	T-lymphocyte	e.g. Thymic aplasia (DiGeorge syndrome)
		• fungal infections
	T+B-lymphocytes	e.g. Wiskott-Aldrich syndrome
		• increased bacterial infections
	Granulocyte	e.g. chronic granulomatous disease
		• staphylococcal infection
	Complement	e.g. C2, C3
		• septicaemia
Others	Cystic fibrosis	Viscid sputum
		• pneumonia

Critical Care Medicine at a Glance, Third Edition. Richard Leach. © 2014 John Wiley & Sons, Ltd. Published 2014 by John Wiley & Sons, Ltd.

General factors

Malnutrition, disease (e.g. diabetes, acquired immunodeficiency syndrome [AIDS]) and medical interventions (e.g. chemotherapy) impair the immune system and risk critical illness due to **infection** or **non-infectious** (e.g. neoplasia, drug reactions, graft vs. host disease) causes (Figures 68a, 68e). Primary failure of **T-lymphocyte** (cell-mediated) function predisposes to viral or fungal infections and neoplasia. **B-lymphocyte** (antibody-mediated; 'humoral') disorders and **granulocytopenia** promote bacterial infections.

Fever in profoundly neutropenic (<1000 granulocytes/mm^3) patients is an emergency, particularly if due to infection, and survival depends on rapid diagnosis and treatment. Unfortunately, infection with commensal organisms (e.g. *Pneumocystis*) and an absence of local inflammation often makes diagnosis difficult. Primary bacteraemia and soft tissue infections are characteristic although any site can be involved. **Pulmonary infiltrates** may not indicate infection because non-infective causes are common (Figure 68c). Establishing the diagnosis may require invasive investigation (e.g. bronchoscopy) with the associated risks.

General management

Survival of febrile neutropenic patients depends on **early effective empirical antibiotic ($\pm$antifungal) therapy**. Potential infecting organisms (Chapters 65, 66, 67) include gram-negative rods (e.g. *Pseudomonas*), staphylococci and fungi (e.g. *Aspergillus*). Impaired cell-mediated immunity predisposes to *Pneumocystis* and *Candida* infection. Obtain cultures of blood, urine, sputum and skin lesions before starting broad-spectrum antibiotics including extended-spectrum penicillins, third-generation cephalosporins, aminoglycosides and, in some cases, cover against methicillin-resistant *Staphylococcus aureus* (MRSA) infections. Consider the addition of antifungal therapy (e.g. amphotericin) if fever persists for >72 hours after starting antibiotics.

Specific causes

Acquired immunodeficiency syndrome

AIDS is caused by human immunodeficiency virus (HIV), which infects, replicates within, impairs and eventually depletes CD4 T-lymphocytes. HIV is transmitted by sexual contact, in blood products, during pregnancy from mother to child and through breast milk. Over 40 million people are infected worldwide. AIDS is defined by the presence of indicator diseases (Figure 68a) in HIV-infected individuals with a blood CD4 count <200/ml (or a CD4 count $<14\%$ of all lymphocytes).

Clinical features, diseases and critical illnesses that indicate AIDS (Figure 68a) include:
- *Pneumocystis (carinii) jiroveci* **pneumonia (PCP)** with respiratory failure. Although common, incidence has decreased with prophylactic Septrin therapy.
  - **Clinical features** include fever, dry cough and dyspnoea. Pneumothorax occurs in ~2% cases.
  - **Investigations** reveal generalized alveolitis with impaired diffusion on lung function tests and exercise desaturation. Chest radiography (CXR) typically shows bilateral interstitial infiltrates (Figure 68d) but may be normal or focally consolidated. Giemsa, silver and immunofluorescent stains of sputum, particularly if induced with nebulized 2.7% saline, detects pneumocystis in >70% cases. Bronchoscopic washings detect >90% of cases but transbronchial lung biopsies are most reliable.

- **Treatment** is with oxygen ($\pm$continuous positive airways pressure [CPAP]) and high-dose intravenous co-trimoxazole, which can cause severe skin rashes (~30%), vomiting, colitis and hepatitis. The alternative therapy, pentamidine, also causes side-effects. High-dose steroids reduce alveolitis, respiratory failure and mortality.
- **Other opportunistic infections** include mycobacteria, toxoplasmosis (Figure 68b), candidiasis, *Cryptococcus neoformans*, cytomegalovirus (CMV) and herpes simplex. Consider tuberculosis ($\pm$isolation) in HIV patients with undiagnosed respiratory illness.

Hospital precautions: assume all patients are HIV-positive and take appropriate precautions (e.g. gloves, masks). The infection risk following HIV-contaminated needlestick injury is ~0.4%. After cleansing, seek expert advice ($\pm$start prophylactic therapy).

Other specific causes

1 **Malignant diseases** are increasingly associated with improved outcomes, especially haematological and lymphoproliferative disorders. Patients admitted to hospital for treatment (e.g. chemotherapy) or management of life-threatening effects of the tumour (e.g. hypercalcaemia) are susceptible to infection due to profound leucopenia (i.e. 10–14 days after chemotherapy or bone marrow transplantation), disease-mediated immunosuppression and invasive procedures (e.g. line insertion). In general, mortality rates are high ($>70\%$) when patients with malignant disease develop acute illness but prolonged survival may justify aggressive management in some cases.

2 **Post-splenectomy**: infection, typically with encapsulated bacteria (e.g. pneumococci, *Haemophilus*), may be fatal because loss of splenic phagocytic function allows rapid bacterial proliferation and spread. Prophylactic antibiotics (e.g. penicillin) and vaccination against influenza, pneumococcus, *H. influenza* and meningococcus are recommended.

3 **Systemic disease** can increase infection risk (e.g. diabetes). **Cirrhosis** impairs hepatic phagocytic function. **Connective tissue diseases** (e.g. SLE) are immunosuppressive due to associated leucopenia and the effects of therapy (e.g. steroids). **Primary immunodeficiency disorders** (e.g. DiGeorge syndrome) occasionally cause infection.

4 **Transplant surgery** requires post-operative immunosuppressive therapy (e.g. ciclosporin, steroids) to prevent graft vs. host organ rejection. Ciclosporin acts primarily on T-cells, is less immunosuppressive and prevents rejection better than azathioprine. This has reduced secondary infections and increased graft survival. Rejection risk is greatest for 6–12 weeks post-transplant, after which tolerance develops to the graft and the ciclosporin dose can be reduced. During this period of intense T-cell suppression, transplant recipients are prone to CMV, cryptococcus, PCP, herpes simplex and *Aspergillus* infections. The long-term risk of opportunistic infections and, to a lesser extent, malignancy (e.g. lymphoma) is also increased.

5 **Immunosuppressive therapy** is used in many diseases (e.g. Crohn's, rheumatoid arthritis). These drugs (e.g. steroids, cyclophosphamide, methotrexate) and therapies (e.g. radiotherapy) are immunosuppressive and increase the risk of infection.

Pearl of wisdom
Beware occult malignancies in patients with immunosuppressive disease or on long-term immunosuppressive therapy

69 Coagulation disorders and transfusion

Figure 69a Initial (previous extrinsic pathway) and amplification (previous intrinsic pathway) phases of the clotting cascade and causes of prolonged PT (vitamin K dependent factors) and APPT (measures amplification phase)

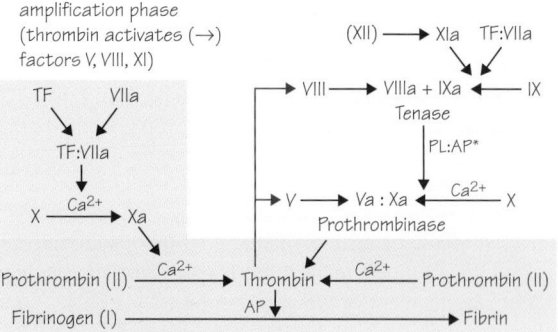

(i) Initial phase produces relatively little thrombin but activates the amplification phase (thrombin activates (→) factors V, VIII, XI)

(ii) Amplification phase produces >90% of thrombin produced (measured by APPT)

*As IXa and Xa only work when tethered to AP via PL, clotting is confined to the platelet plug

TF=tissue factor (thromboplastin)
PL=phospholipid, AP=activated platelets
PT= prothrombin time, APPT= activated partial thromboplastin time
INR=international normalized ratio
DIC=disseminated intravascular coagulation

PT prolonged by:
Liver disease + DIC
Warfarin
Vitamin K deficiency
Salicylate poisoning
Circulating anticoagulants
Excessive heparin
Circulating anticoagulants
PT is expressed as the INR, the ratio of the PT to a standardized reference sample. INR is normally 1

APPT prolonged by:
Haemophilia
Heparin
Von Willebrand's Disease
Under-filled blood bottle
(e.g. spurious result)
Delay in assay performance
Circulating anticoagulants

Figure 69b Causes of thrombocytopenia

Decreased Platelet Production
- Leukaemias, marrow depression
- Infiltration by malignancy
- Drugs e.g. chlorpropamide, thiazides, gold, penicillin, methyldopa, quinine, TB therapy, chloroquine, chloramphenicol

Increased Platelet Consumption
- Sepsis (most important)
- Shock
- Disseminated intravascular coagulation
- Splenomegaly with hypersplenism
- Idiopathic thrombocytopenic purpura (ITP) due to anti-platelet IgG autoantibodies
- Thrombotic thrombocytopenic purpura (TTP)
- Haemolytic uraemic syndrome (HUS)
- Heparin-induced thrombocytopenia (HIT)

Extracorporeal Platelet Loss
- Cardiopulmonary bypass
- Renal replacement therapy

Figure 69c Factors contributing to coagulation failure in acute illness

- Vessel trauma
  e.g. surgical, traumatic
- Acquired factor deficiencies
  e.g. trauma, transfusion, liver failure, DIC, extracorporeal circuits
- Anticoagulants
  e.g. heparin, thrombolytics
- Thrombocytopenia
  e.g. heparin-induced, idiopathic thrombocytopenic purpura (ITP), sepsis
- Hereditary factors
  e.g. haemophilia
- Hypothermia

Figure 69d Conditions predisposing to disseminated intravascular coagulation (DIC)

- Sepsis e.g. E. coli, malaria, viral
- Surgery e.g. cardiac bypass
- Liver failure
- Malignancy
  e.g. promyelocytic leukaemia
- Incompatible transfusions
- Intravascular haemolysis
- Shock e.g. burns, trauma
- Poisoning e.g. snake venom
- Autoimmune disease
- Pregnancy-related
  e.g. eclampsia, puerperal sepsis, amniotic fluid embolism etc.

Figure 69e Management of bleeding, transfusion reactions and effects of massive transfusion

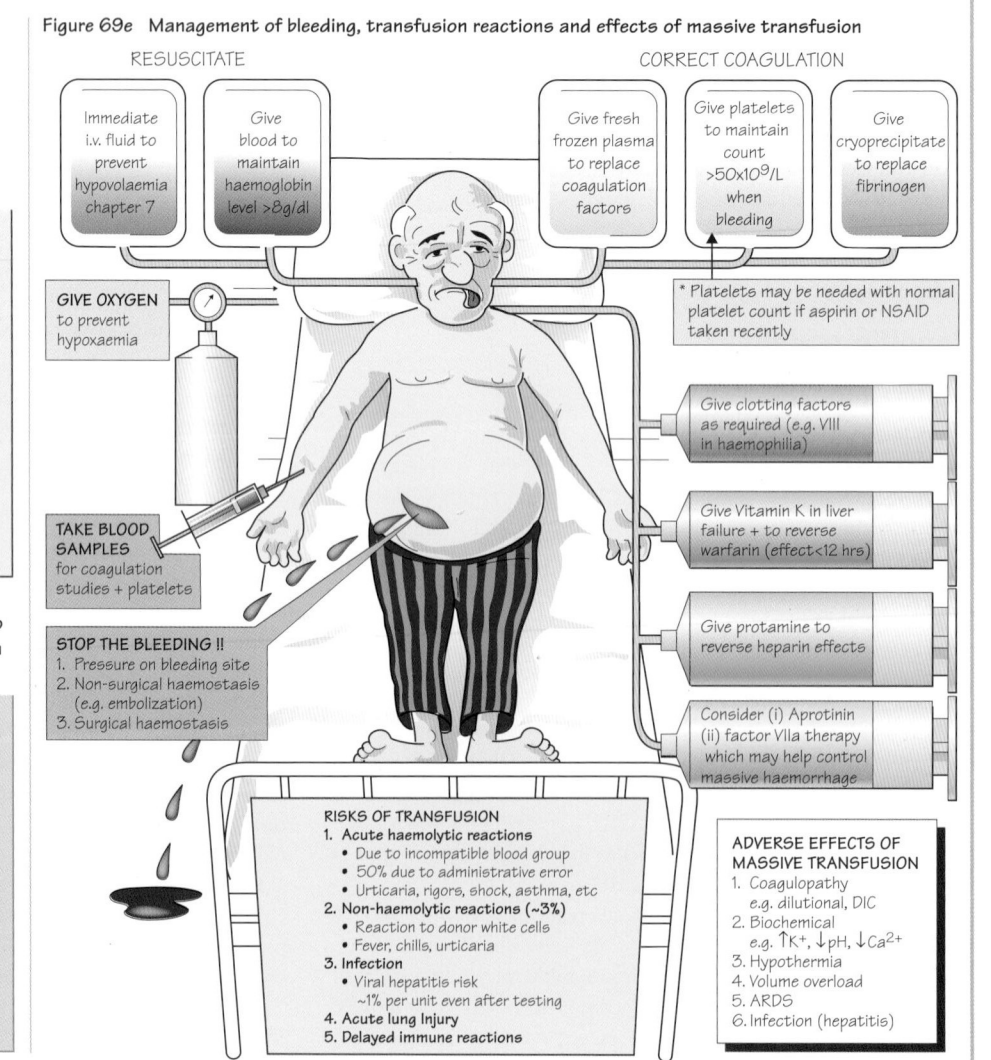

RESUSCITATE

Immediate i.v. fluid to prevent hypovolaemia chapter 7

Give blood to maintain haemoglobin level >8g/dl

CORRECT COAGULATION

Give fresh frozen plasma to replace coagulation factors

Give platelets to maintain count >50x10⁹/L when bleeding

Give cryoprecipitate to replace fibrinogen

GIVE OXYGEN to prevent hypoxaemia

* Platelets may be needed with normal platelet count if aspirin or NSAID taken recently

Give clotting factors as required (e.g. VIII in haemophilia)

Give Vitamin K in liver failure + to reverse warfarin (effect<12 hrs)

Give protamine to reverse heparin effects

Consider (i) Aprotinin (ii) factor VIIa therapy which may help control massive haemorrhage

TAKE BLOOD SAMPLES for coagulation studies + platelets

STOP THE BLEEDING !!
1. Pressure on bleeding site
2. Non-surgical haemostasis (e.g. embolization)
3. Surgical haemostasis

RISKS OF TRANSFUSION
1. **Acute haemolytic reactions**
   - Due to incompatible blood group
   - 50% due to administrative error
   - Urticaria, rigors, shock, asthma, etc
2. **Non-haemolytic reactions (~3%)**
   - Reaction to donor white cells
   - Fever, chills, urticaria
3. **Infection**
   - Viral hepatitis risk ~1% per unit even after testing
4. **Acute lung Injury**
5. **Delayed immune reactions**

ADVERSE EFFECTS OF MASSIVE TRANSFUSION
1. Coagulopathy e.g. dilutional, DIC
2. Biochemical e.g. ↑K⁺, ↓pH, ↓Ca²⁺
3. Hypothermia
4. Volume overload
5. ARDS
6. Infection (hepatitis)

Critical Care Medicine at a Glance, Third Edition. Richard Leach. © 2014 John Wiley & Sons, Ltd. Published 2014 by John Wiley & Sons, Ltd.

Blood and blood components

Blood is expensive; before transfusion it must be cross-matched because it is antigenic and screened for human immunodeficiency virus, hepatitis, human lymphocytic virus 1, syphilis and cytomegalovirus to reduce infection risk. Donated **whole blood** is collected into citrate, phosphate, dextrose-adenine (CPD-A) anticoagulant; 1 unit is ~430 ml. Subdivision of blood (i.e. red cells, platelets) aids storage (i.e. shelf-life) and targets use at specific needs. Red cells, separated by centrifugation, are resuspended in SAG-M (sodium chloride, adenine, glucose; mannitol prevents haemolysis) as **packed red cells** with a haemocrit of ~0.65 and a shelf-life of ~42 days. The platelet-rich plasma fraction (~250 ml) is divided into platelets and plasma. **Platelets** have a short shelf-life of ~7 days and 1 unit increases serum platelet count by ~4–9 × 10^9/L. **Fresh frozen plasma** (FFP) contains the clotting factors but ≥4 units are required for useful increases in serum levels. Storage time is ~12 months. FFP can be further separated into **cryoprecipitate** (factor VIII, fibrinogen) and supernatant (albumin). **Fresh whole blood** is rich in clotting factors and platelets but transfusion reactions are common. It is only used to reduce clotting factor dilution during massive transfusions. **Stored blood** is metabolically active; pH, 2,3 diphosphoglycerate (DPG), adenosine triphosphate (ATP), platelets and clotting factors decrease, K^+ increases (cell rupture) and microaggregates form.

Coagulation disorders

Coagulation disorders occur when the haemostatic balance between **vascular endothelium**, **platelets** and the **clotting–fibrinolytic system** is disrupted. In severe illness the cause is often multifactorial (Figure 69c), whereas hereditary disorders stem from a single soluble factor deficiency. **Bleeding disorders** are easily identified because clinical features are obvious and laboratory monitoring widely available. By contrast, **hypercoagulability** and microvascular thrombosis is less obvious.

Coagulation tests

Figure 69a illustrates the clotting cascade. **Prothrombin time** (PT) is the time to clot formation following addition of tissue factor (TF) and Ca^{2+} to plasma; normally 12–14 secs. It measures the initial phase and vitamin K dependent clotting factor (II, VII, X) activity (e.g. warfarin control). Causes of prolonged PT are listed in Figure 69a. **Activated partial thromboplastin time** (APTT) is the time to clot formation after adding kaolin (surface activator), phospholipid and Ca^{2+} to plasma; normally ~40 secs. It measures the amplification phase factor activities (but not factor VII). Figure 69a lists causes of prolonged APTT. **Platelet counts** < 20 × 10^9/L (<50 × 10^9/L with co-existing platelet dysfunction) increase the risk of spontaneous bleeding. **Bleeding time** tests platelet function: after a standard skin incision, bleeding should stop within 9 min. **Activated clotting time**, a bedside test of heparin action, examines clotting in whole blood but is prolonged by thrombocytopenia, hypothermia and fibrinolysis. **Factor assays** (e.g. fibrinogen, VII) are available. **Fibrinogen degradation products** (FDPs) and **d-dimers** are products of fibrinolysis and increase during DIC, sepsis, trauma and venous thromboembolism (VTE). FDP assays are widely available. D-dimers are sensitive but not specific for VTE; a negative result reliably excludes VTE (Chapter 36). A detailed history, medication review (e.g. aspirin) and PT, APTT and platelet count detect most acquired bleeding disorders.

Bleeding disorders

- **Genetic coagulopathies**: haemophilias A and B are sex-linked, recessive diseases causing spontaneous bleeding in affected males.

Haemophilia A is due to factor VIII deficiency. **Haemophilia B** (Christmas disease) is less common and due to factor IX deficiency. Treatment is with factors VIII and IX respectively. **Von Willebrand's disease**, an autosomal dominant trait, is the most common hereditary coagulation disorder. It decreases factor VIII activity and reduces platelet adherence to vascular injury sites. Treatment with desmopressin acetate or arginine vasopressin (DDAVP) augments factor VIII and reduces the bleeding risk. Cryoprecipitate and FFP correct the deficit.

- **Liver disease, malnutrition and antibiotics** cause vitamin K-dependent coagulation factor deficiency. Vitamin K therapy is rapidly effective except in severe liver damage.
- **Anticoagulants**: oral agents deplete vitamin K-dependent clotting factors. FFP transiently reverses and vitamin K corrects warfarin-induced anticoagulation. **Heparin** potentiates antithrombin III, which blocks the action of thrombin (±factors IX, X), inhibiting coagulation and prolonging APTT. Protamine sulphate reverses its effects. Antibodies to heparin can cross-react with platelet antigens causing heparin-induced thrombocytopenia (HIT; ~10%) and thrombosis. **Antiplatelet agents** (e.g. aspirin) irreversibly inhibit platelet function for ~10 days. **Thrombolysis** may cause haemorrhage (e.g. gastrointestinal tract). Intracranial bleeds occur in <0.5–2%. FFP and platelets stop bleeding. **Circulating anticoagulants** develop with some drugs (e.g. penicillin) and diseases (e.g. SLE).
- **Disseminated intravascular coagulation (DIC)** follows extensive activation of coagulation and fibrinolysis (e.g. sepsis) with simultaneous bleeding, often the presenting feature, and thrombosis. Platelets and fibrinogen levels fall and PT, APTT and FDP increase. Red cell fragmentation may occur. Figure 69d lists the causes of DIC. Treat the cause, supplement clotting factors (±platelets) and start low-dose heparin.
- **Thrombocytopenia** is due to decreased production, increased consumption or extracorporeal loss of platelets (Figure 69b). Treat the cause (e.g. steroids/immune globulin in immune thrombocytopaenia [ITP], FFP/plasma exchange in thrombotic thrombocytopaenia [TTP]).

Transfusion and management of bleeding

Full cross-matching takes ~45 min but ABO type can be determined in ≤10 min. Give O-negative blood (universal donor) if blood is needed immediately. It may provoke minor transfusion reactions. Type-specific (ABO-, rhesus-compatible) blood is preferred if time permits. After ~5 units of blood, dilutional clotting disorders and biochemical abnormalities (e.g. hypocalcaemia) develop and may require correction. Use blood filters during large transfusions. Management of bleeding and the consequences of transfusions are illustrated in Figure 69e.

Hypercoagulable disorders

Thromboembolism (Chapter 36) is due to a predisposing genetic disorder in ~20% of cases (e.g. antithrombin III deficiency, protein C and S deficiency, lupus anticoagulant). A family history of, or repeated thromboses, unusual sites (e.g. arms) and recurrent spontaneous abortions are suggestive.

Pearl of wisdom
Dilution of clotting factors and platelets may potentiate bleeding after massive transfusion unless actively supplemented with fresh frozen plasma (FFP) and platelet transfusions

70 Drug overdose and poisoning

Figure 70a Clinical features assisting drug identification

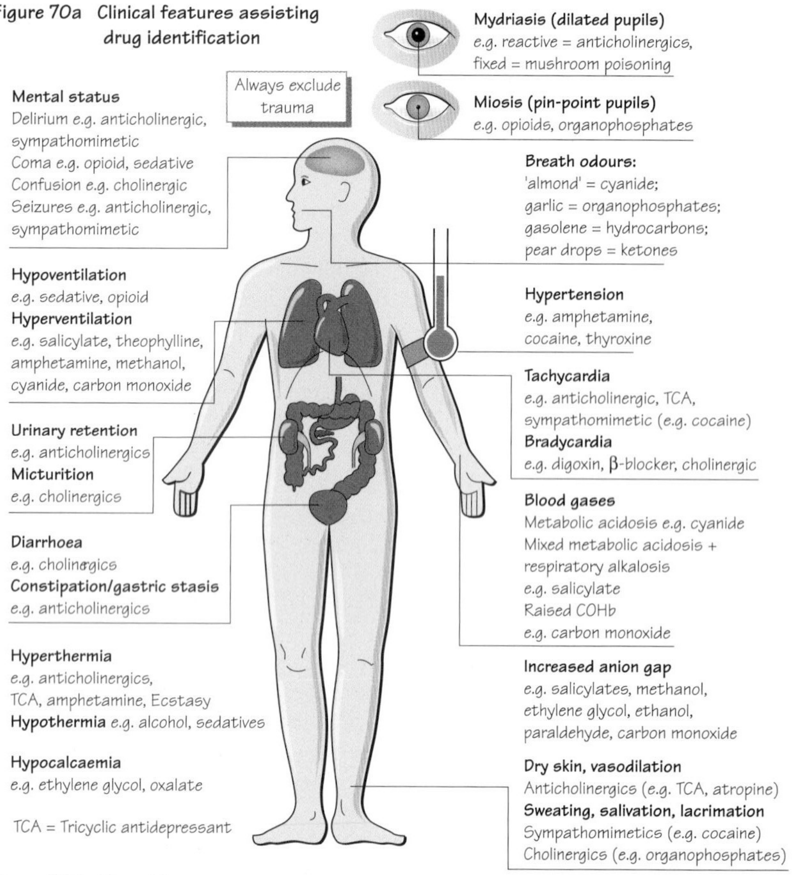

Always exclude trauma

Mental status
Delirium e.g. anticholinergic, sympathomimetic
Coma e.g. opioid, sedative
Confusion e.g. cholinergic
Seizures e.g. anticholinergic, sympathomimetic

Hypoventilation
e.g. sedative, opioid
Hyperventilation
e.g. salicylate, theophylline, amphetamine, methanol, cyanide, carbon monoxide

Urinary retention
e.g. anticholinergics
Micturition
e.g. cholinergics

Diarrhoea
e.g. cholinergics
Constipation/gastric stasis
e.g. anticholinergics

Hyperthermia
e.g. anticholinergics, TCA, amphetamine, Ecstasy
Hypothermia e.g. alcohol, sedatives

Hypocalcaemia
e.g. ethylene glycol, oxalate

TCA = Tricyclic antidepressant

Mydriasis (dilated pupils)
e.g. reactive = anticholinergics, fixed = mushroom poisoning

Miosis (pin-point pupils)
e.g. opioids, organophosphates

Breath odours:
'almond' = cyanide;
garlic = organophosphates;
gasolene = hydrocarbons;
pear drops = ketones

Hypertension
e.g. amphetamine, cocaine, thyroxine

Tachycardia
e.g. anticholinergic, TCA, sympathomimetic (e.g. cocaine)
Bradycardia
e.g. digoxin, β-blocker, cholinergic

Blood gases
Metabolic acidosis e.g. cyanide
Mixed metabolic acidosis + respiratory alkalosis
e.g. salicylate
Raised COHb
e.g. carbon monoxide

Increased anion gap
e.g. salicylates, methanol, ethylene glycol, ethanol, paraldehyde, carbon monoxide

Dry skin, vasodilation
Anticholinergics (e.g. TCA, atropine)
Sweating, salivation, lacrimation
Sympathomimetics (e.g. cocaine)
Cholinergics (e.g. organophosphates)

Figure 70b ECG features in overdose

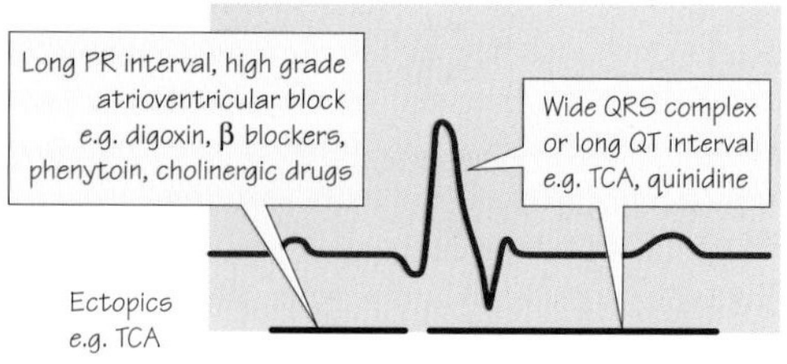

Long PR interval, high grade atrioventricular block e.g. digoxin, β blockers, phenytoin, cholinergic drugs

Wide QRS complex or long QT interval e.g. TCA, quinidine

Ectopics e.g. TCA

Figure 70c Paracetamol overdose treatment lines

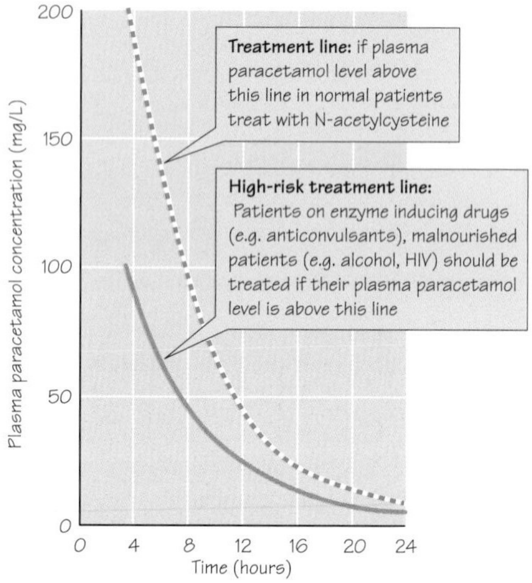

Treatment line: if plasma paracetamol level above this line in normal patients treat with N-acetylcysteine

High-risk treatment line: Patients on enzyme inducing drugs (e.g. anticonvulsants), malnourished patients (e.g. alcohol, HIV) should be treated if their plasma paracetamol level is above this line

(Graph: Plasma paracetamol concentration (mg/L) vs Time (hours); y-axis 0–200, x-axis 0–24)

Figure 70d Clinical features and therapy of common overdoses

Drug	Clinical features	Specific therapy and antidotes
Paracetamol (see text)	Initially few; later hepatotoxicity monitored by liver function tests and prothrombin time	Antidote: N-acetylcysteine
Tricyclics (see text)	Anticholinergic features (e.g. hyperthermia, fixed dilated pupils, dry skin etc.), seizures and arrhythmias	Diazepam for agitation. Dialysis of no value
Aspirin	Nausea, vomiting, tinnitus, agitation, sweating and rarely hyperthermia and seizures. Initially CNS stimulation causes hyperventilation and a respiratory alkalosis followed by a metabolic acidosis, if severe, due to inhibition of oxidative phosphorylation and glucose metabolism. Pulmonary oedema occurs with large doses. Absorption may be delayed and blood concentrations misleadingly low	GL and AC may be effective up to 4h after ingestion. If plasma salicylate is >500 mg/L or pH <7.0 forced diuresis (± iv sodium bicarbonate) enhances urine excretion. Severe overdose (>750 mg/L) requires haemodialysis
Anticholinergics • Belladonna alkaloids, atropine, phenothiazines (e.g. chlorpromazine)	Anticholinergic features: hyperthermia, fixed dilated pupils, dry skin, CNS symptoms (e.g. agitation, ataxia, fits, coma), labile BP, arrhythmia, urine retention and ileus	No specific antidote. Diazepam for agitation. Physostigmine, an anticholinesterase, may be useful in severe cases. Dialysis is of no value
Sedatives/Hypnotics • Benzodiazepines • Opiates • Barbiturates	Sedatives cause drowsiness, coma, low BP + hypoventilation. Opioids associated with pinpoint pupils, sweating, needle tract marks + complications (e.g. rhabdomyolysis, endocarditis, infection). Barbiturates cause dilated pupils, and red wheals on bony prominences	Ventilation is rarely required in sedative overdoses. Naloxone is a short-acting, iv antagonist for opioids and flumazenil for benzodiazepines. Dialysis is of little value
Stimulants: amphetamines + Ecstasy (MDMA)+Cocaine	Sympathomimetic features: arrhythmias, hypertension, seizures, coma, hyperthermia, rhabdomyolysis, hyponatraemia + strokes. Cocaine's vasoconstrictor effects can cause MI without IHD	No specific antidotes. Fluid resuscitation and supportive therapy (e.g. AC, cooling, anxiolytics) are required
Alcohols • Ethanol • Methanol • Ethylene glycol	CNS depression ± aspiration, high anion gap metabolic acidosis. Ethanol depresses gluconeogenesis causing hypoglycaemia. After a latent period (~2–12 h) methanol metabolites (e.g. formaldehyde) cause GI symptoms (e.g. vomiting), eye signs (blurring, blindness), metabolic acidosis and hyperosmolality. Ethylene glycol metabolites (e.g. glycoaldehyde) cause metabolic acidosis, hyperosmolality, oxalate crystaluria, hyperthermia, hypoglycaemia and hypocalcaemia	Ethanol is an antidote for methanol and ethylene glycol acting as a competitive inhibitor. Haemodialysis is indicated in severe cases with renal failure, visual disturbance and acidosis that does not respond to bicarbonate
Organophosphates and carbamates (e.g. pesticides)	Inhibit acetylcholinesterase causing cholinergic overactivity (e.g. mnemonic DUMBELS = diarrhoea, urination, miosis, bronchospasm, emesis, lacrimation and salivation; sweating and abdominal pain also occur). Symptoms develop within 0.5–2 h. Delay follows cutaneous absorption	Atropine given for 24 h blocks cholinergic symptoms. Pralidoxime, a specific cholinesterase reactivator, is effective if given within 24 h. Skin decontamination
Theophylline	Tremors, gastrointestinal upset, arrhythmias and seizures at serum levels >40 mg/L	AC, dialysis, haemoperfusion
Lithium	Initally polyuria, thirst, vomiting, diarrhoea and agitation. Then coma, seizures + NDI	Haemodialysis for severe toxicity
Digoxin	Nausea, vomiting, confusion, bradycardia and paroxysmal atrial tachycardia	Supportive (± Digibind)
Mushroom poisoning	Nausea, vomiting and diarrhoea followed by hepatorenal failure	Forced diuresis, activated charcoal, haemodialysis

BP = blood pressure, GL = gastric lavage, AC = activated charcoal, MI = myocardial infarction, IHD = ischaemic heart disease, GI = gastrointestinal, NDI = nephrogenic diabetes insipidus

Critical Care Medicine at a Glance, Third Edition. Richard Leach. © 2014 John Wiley & Sons, Ltd. Published 2014 by John Wiley & Sons, Ltd.

Overdoses (ODs) and poisonings cause ~10% of hospital admissions. In-hospital mortality is <1% because most deaths occur before admission due to arrhythmia or respiratory arrest. A few drugs (i.e. paracetamol, tricyclic antidepressants) account for ~90–95% of self-administered OD. Most cases are 'a cry for help' rather than genuine suicide attempts and occur in young people (<35 years old; M : F 1 : 1.5) with a history of similar episodes. Fatal overdoses are more likely in patients >45 years old with serious suicidal intent. In children, poisoning is usually accidental due to ingestion of a single agent.

In general, supportive care and prevention of absorption are more important than active measures to hasten drug elimination. Be guided by poisons information services. A practical approach to OD management entails:

1 Resuscitation, including airways protection, respiratory support, fluid replacement and acid–base balance. Prolonged unconsciousness is associated with hypothermia, aspiration, rhabdomyolysis and compartment syndrome. Drug-induced hyperthermia (e.g. anticholinergics) is uncommon (Chapter 23).

2 Substance identification: although **history** is unreliable, important information includes *drugs taken* (±time taken, dosage, route); *past history* (i.e. previous OD); *circumstances* (e.g. witnesses, empty containers, syringes) and *associated trauma*.
- **Examination** (Figure 70a) detects diagnostic clues.
- **Investigations** (Figures 70a, 70b) include drug identification (e.g. blood, urine, gastric aspirates); paracetamol, aspirin and alcohol levels; blood tests including liver function, coagulation and serum osmolality (e.g. ethylene glycol); blood gases and anion gap (Chapter 20); chest radiography (CXR) (e.g. pulmonary oedema with salicylates); and electrocardiogram (ECG) (e.g. myocardial ischaemia with cocaine).

3 Prevention of absorption is best achieved with:
- **Activated charcoal (AC)**: an effective adsorbent that promotes drug elimination (e.g. salicylates) and is first-line therapy for most poisonings. It is best given within 1 hour of drug ingestion (later if drug delays gastric emptying), after gastric lavage (GL) and at 4-hourly intervals with specific drugs (e.g. theophylline). AC does not bind iron, lithium, alcohols, acids, alkalis, cyanide or pesticides. It causes constipation and is given with a cathartic (e.g. sorbitol) as an aqueous slurry.
- **GL** is not recommended unless performed within 1 hour of drug ingestion, is harmful after intake of caustic or petroleum products and ineffective after alcohol. Perform lavage in the left lateral position using a large bore (~38 Fr) orogastric tube to facilitate removal of pill fragments. Intubate obtunded patients to reduce the risk of gastric aspiration. Oropharyngeal trauma and oesophageal perforation also occur.
- **Additional measures** include: (i) **cathartics**, which promote diarrhoea and reduce drug absorption but risk fluid and electrolyte loss; (ii) **skin decontamination** for transdermally absorbed toxins (e.g. organophosphates); and (iii) **endoscopy/surgery** (e.g. body packers). Induced vomiting is not recommended because it is ineffective, limits AC use and risks aspiration (±oesophageal tears).

4 Enhanced drug elimination is only indicated in life-threatening poisoning because some techniques have risks.
- **Gut dialysis** uses repeated doses of AC to bind drugs with an enterohepatic circulation that are excreted in bile (e.g. theophylline, digoxin, carbamazepine).
- **Forced diuresis** enhances drug excretion by increasing urine production to 2–5 ml/kg/h with intravenous fluid (±diuretic)

but risks fluid overload. Alkalinization with sodium bicarbonate promotes salicylate, tricyclic antidepressant and barbiturate excretion but is only used in severe cases.
- **Haemodialysis** removes low molecular weight, water soluble molecules, with a small volume of distribution and low protein binding (e.g. salicylates, methanol, theophylline).
- **Haemoperfusion** using charcoal or resin columns is useful for lipid soluble drugs (e.g. theophylline, barbiturates) but may cause hypocalcaemia and coagulopathy.

5 Lipid emulsion therapy is considered for severe poisoning with a lipophilic drug that has not responded to other measures.

Specific management

Figure 70d summarizes the clinical features and management of OD and poisonings. Paracetamol and tricyclic antidepressants are most common, often in combination with alcohol.
- **Paracetamol overdose** (POD) causes 200 deaths/year in the UK (>12 g (150 mg/kg) can be lethal). It depletes hepatic glutathione stores, with accumulation of a hydroxylamine metabolite that causes liver and renal damage. Malnourished patients (e.g. alcoholics) and those taking anticonvulsants are at most risk of hepatotoxicity. Initially there are few symptoms apart from nausea, vomiting and abdominal pain. Signs and biochemical evidence of hepatocellular necrosis present after 24 hours and peak at 3–4 days. The recovery phase lasts ~8 days. Management during the initial 4 hours includes GL and AC. If paracetamol levels at 4 hours are above the treatment line (Figure 70c) or if >10 g has been ingested, treatment with intravenous *N*-acetylcysteine (NAC) for 24 hours (or more in severe liver injury) raises glutathione levels and improves outcome. It is most effective if given within 12 hours of POD. Later administration may not prevent liver damage but it improves recovery. Rapid administration can cause bronchospasm, urticaria and anaphylaxis. Methionine is an oral alternative to NAC. Consider early referral to a liver unit if liver failure develops because liver transplantation may be indicated.
- **Tricyclic antidepressants** (TCA) cause most OD fatalities (~300 deaths/year in the UK) but hospital mortality is <1%. Toxicity is due to anticholinergic effects that cause fixed dilated pupils, dry red skin, hyperthermia, tachycardia, urine retention and central nervous system (CNS) hyper-reactivity (e.g. psychosis, hallucinations). Hypotension, arrhythmias, respiratory depression, fits and coma occur in severe intoxication. There is no specific antidote. GL and AC are essential due to associated ileus, delayed gastric emptying and enterohepatic circulation. The ECG signals cardiac and CNS toxicity when the QRS complex is >0.12 secs. Life-threatening arrhythmias respond to correction of hypoxia, acidosis and cardioversion but are resistant to antiarrhythmic agents. Lidocaine is the most beneficial antiarrhythmic; avoid type 1a drugs (e.g. quinidine), which further impair conduction. Increasing arterial pH to >7.45 reduces free drug availability and toxicity. Mild hyperventilation and sodium bicarbonate (8.4%) in 50 ml aliquots improves outcome, especially in those with prolonged QRS, arrhythmias, hypotension or metabolic acidosis. Recovery occurs in ~24 hours due to rapid metabolism.

Pearl of wisdom

Patients with tricyclic antidepressant toxicity exhibit anticholinergic features and appear as 'hot as a hare, blind as a bat, dry as a bone and mad as a hatter'

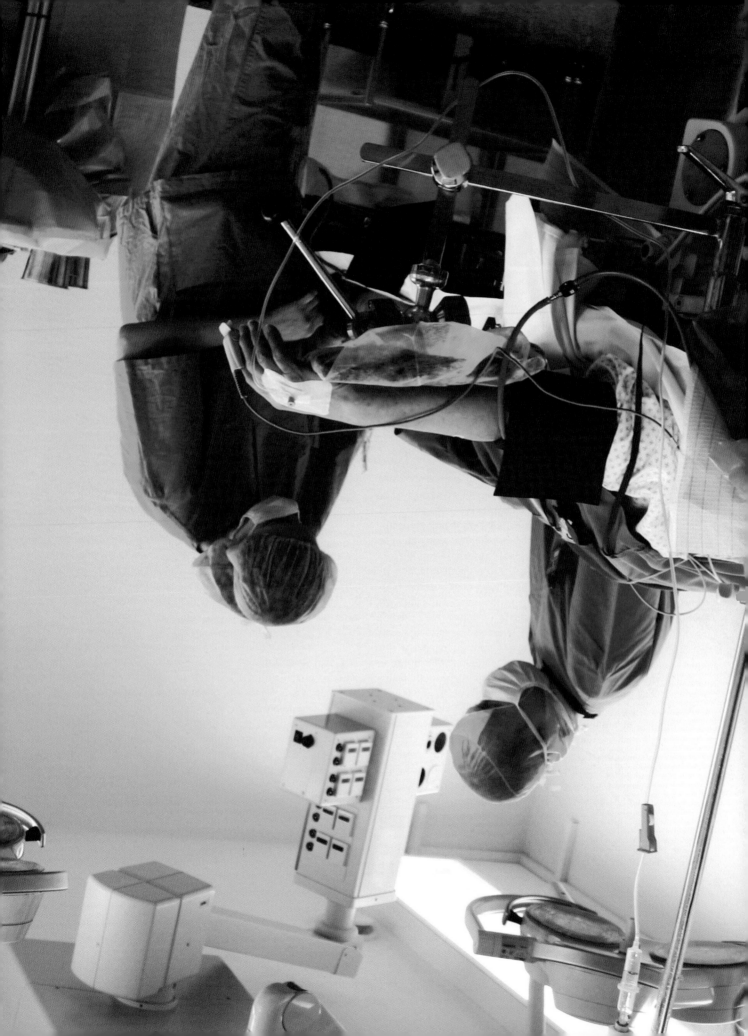

Surgical

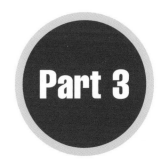

Part 3

Chapters

71 Trauma

Figure 71a   Manual in-line immobilization

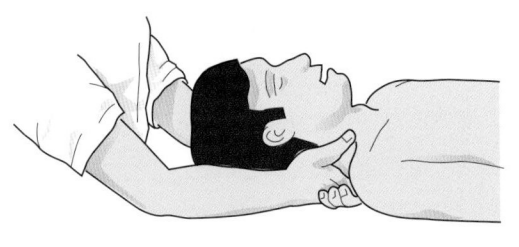

Figure 71b   C2 hangman's fracture and C2 on C3 facet joint fracture dislocation (arrow) causing loss of alignment, bony contour and lordosis with interspinous opening

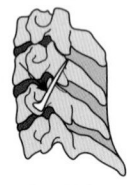

Figure 71c   Classification of haemorrhage severity

Class	Circulating volume loss	Approx volume loss (70kg man)	Clinical signs
Class 1	<15%	<750 mL	Minimal signs
Class 2	15–30%	<1500 mL	↑HR + ↓BP; sweating ↓pulse pressure
Class 3	30–40%	<2000 mL	Agitated, sweating, oliguria, ↑HR (>120 /min) ↓BP (systolic ~90 mmHg)
Class 4	>40%	>2000 mL	Preterminal, drowsy ↓BP (systolic <90 mmHg)

Figure 71d   Examining the cervical X-ray and examples of cervicle fracture (#)

Cervical X-rays compromise 3 views AP, lateral and open mouth. The lateral must clearly visualize the occiput to the C7/T1 junction
Check the following on the 3 views to assess the presence of injury

1. Alignment (see figure)
The following indicate injury a. loss of lordosis b. ↑ anterior soft tissue shadows >4 mm at C4, >15 mm at C6
c. ↑ interspinous distance
d. malaligned spinous processes
e. cortical discontinuity

2. Bony abnormality

3. Contours (+ cartilages)
Check vertebral bodies and spinous processes. Look for avulsion, burst and wedge fractures (i.e. >3 mm height difference between front and back of the body)

4. Disc spaces and soft tissues
e.g. distance from C3 to the back of the pharynx (>4 mm = haematoma)

5. Odontoid peg
Open mouth and lateral views. Distance between the anterior arch of C1 and the peg should be <3 mm

Normal alignment

RP →
RT →
1 2 3 4

1. Anterior vertebral line
2. Posterior vertebral line
3. Spinolaminar line
4. Spinous process line
5. RP= retropharyngeal Soft tissue space C4 <4 mm
6. RT=retrotracheal space C6 <15 mm

Odontoid process fracture
(a) AP view through mouth
(b) Lateral view in extension.
Usually an unstable injury, that requires stabilization. Rarely associated with cord injury, as injury to the cord at this level leads to sudden death

(a)   (b)
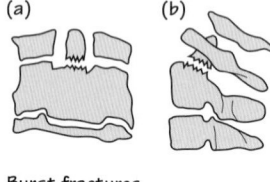

Burst fractures
A compression injury tends to be stable unless significant displacement of bony fragments posteriorly causes cord damage

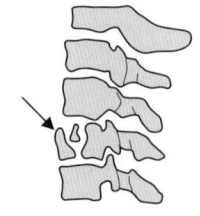
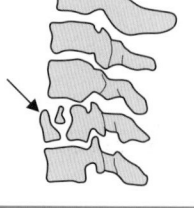

Extension injuries
These injuries occur commonly in the elderly, are associated with central cord neurological deficit and are usually stable and may be treated expectantly. The role for surgical decompression is equivocal

Fracture dislocations (distraction) injuries
Very unstable injuries with both anterior and posterior ligamentous and bony disruption with a high association of cord damage. Usually requires surgical correction and fixation to stabilize the spine

Trauma is the leading cause of death in young people (<40 years old). **Advanced trauma life support (ATLS) programmes** recommend a **structured approach** to severe and multiple trauma management, by a well-organized **trauma team**. Assessment, diagnosis and therapy should be concurrent and lack of a definitive diagnosis must not delay appropriate therapy. Treat the greatest risk to life first, recognizing that **airways obstruction** is more rapidly fatal than **inadequate ventilation**, which is more serious than **loss of circulating volume**, followed by expanding **intracranial mass lesions** (i.e. ABC system).

Although early resuscitation improves outcome, **pre-hospital treatment** is limited to ensuring adequate oxygenation, ventilation and spinal immobilization. Fluid resuscitation should not delay transfer to hospital. The sequence of trauma management is as follows.

Primary survey/initial resuscitation

Assess and treat:

1 Airway and cervical spine: ensure a patent upper airway and start oxygen therapy. Immobilize the spine with manual in-line cervical stabilization (MILS; Figure 71a) or a hard cervical collar, sandbags and tape. If the airway is at risk, intubate using rapid sequence induction with MILS and cricoid pressure (Chapter 17). Profound hypotension may occur during anaesthestic induction due to hypovolaemia.

2 Breathing: treat life-threatening chest injuries (e.g. flail segment, haemothorax) and anticipate pneumothorax, especially during mechanical ventilation (MV). Consider early MV in head-injured patients at risk of hypoxia, hypercapnia and blood pressure fluctuations (Chapters 72, 73).

3 Circulation: control external haemorrhage with direct pressure, establish intravenous access, institute electrocardiogram (ECG) monitoring and cross-match blood. Shock is usually hypovolaemic due to blood loss, but other causes include sepsis, tension pneumothorax, neurogenic shock and myocardial contusion or tamponade (secondary survey). Clinical signs indicate haemorrhage severity (Figure 71c) but hypotension (±shock) may not be apparent until loss of >30% circulating volume in young patients. Early fluid replacement prevents tissue ischaemia and subsequent organ dysfunction (Chapters 5, 6, 7). Fluid is warmed as hypothermia increases bleeding. Give blood if haemocrit is <0.3 or haemoglobin <10 g/dl. **Immediate surgery** may be required to control bleeding.

4 Neurological status: record pupillary responses and Glasgow Coma Score (GCS) (Chapters 60, 72). Record blood alcohol levels.

5 General management: undress the patient to aid examination but avoid hypothermia. Catheterize to monitor urine output after excluding urethral injury. In basal skull fractures, nasogastric tubes may cause meningeal infection. The oro-gastric route is preferred.

Secondary survey/definitive therapy

Detailed clinical examination and referral for specialist treatment follow resuscitation.

• **Head and face**: inspect for lacerations, haematomas, depressed fractures, eye and orbit injury and mobile mid-face or mandible segments. Clinical features of basal skull fracture include racoon eyes, bruising over the mastoids (Battle's sign), subhyaloid haemorrhage, haemotympanum and cerebrospinal fluid rhinorrhoea or otorrhoea. See head injury (Chapter 72).

• **Chest**: treat life-threatening tracheobronchial injuries, pulmonary or cardiac contusions and aortic, oesophageal or diaphragmatic ruptures (Chapter 73).

• **Abdomen**: suspect concealed intra-abdominal bleeding or viscus perforation if shock persists despite fluid replacement. Examine for associated abdominal bruising, tenderness and distention. Rectal examination may reveal bleeding after bowel injury, a high prostate suggests urethral injury and reduced perianal sensation and sphincter tone indicate spinal injury. Abdominal ultrasound, CT scan, diagnostic peritoneal lavage and, rarely, laparotomy are required if examination is unreliable in unconscious, ventilated or persistently hypotensive patients.

• **Peripheral trauma**: occult haemorrhage and neurovascular injuries must be identified and treated after long-bone fractures. Crush injuries cause compartment syndromes requiring decompressive fasciotomy. Associated rhabdomyolysis causes hypovolaemia, hyperkalaemia and renal failure unless preventative measures are instituted (Chapters 45, 46).

• **Spinal injury** occurs in ~3% of major trauma victims (Figure 71b, 71d). Most injuries are cervical (~50%). The most common sites are $C_{5/6}$, $C_{6/7}$ and T_{12}/L_1.

Examination: carefully log-roll the patient to allow palpation of the spine for tenderness and 'step-off' deformity. Neurological assessment is vital, particularly motor and sensory function below suspected cord lesions, which has prognostic implications.

Investigations: cervical (i.e. lateral, anteroposterior [AP] and open mouth views), thoracic and lumbar spine X-rays are required although injury may occur *without radiographic abnormality*. CT scans assess regions not clearly seen on X-ray. MRI scans detect ligament and cord damage.

Management aims to prevent secondary cord damage by immobilization and spinal cord ischaemia with resuscitation.

• **Spinal stability**: disruption of the posterior ligamentous complex produces an unstable spine. Many specialist units advocate early referral for fixation. Potentially unstable cervical fractures (Figure 71d) may require stabilization with a halo frame.

• **Respiration**: cord lesions above C_4 inhibit diaphragmatic function and always require ventilatory support. Intercostal muscles are innervated by T_2–T_{12}; patients with lesions above this depend on diaphragmatic breathing which impairs tidal volumes and cough.

• **Circulation**: following initial hyperstimulation and hypertension, loss of sympathetic control in cord lesions above T_{1-6} limits cardiovascular responses causing bradycardia, peripheral vasodilation, hypotension and neurogenic shock (Chapter 7). Unopposed vagal activity (e.g. during bronchial suctioning) can cause profound bradycardia.

• **Neurology**: spinal shock is the muscle flaccidity and areflexia that follows spinal injury. It lasts for 2–70 days. Muscle contractures and spasms follow resolution. Autonomic dysreflexia occurs with cord injuries above T_7 (~65%); stimulation below the lesion (e.g. bladder distension) causes a sympathetic reflex (i.e. flushing, sweating, hypertension, bradycardia) that can precipitate seizures or strokes. Early steroids may improve neurological outcome.

• **General factors** include hypothermia due to vasodilation, paralytic ileus and bladder atony requiring catheterization. Meticulous nursing avoids pressure sores.

72 Head injury

Figure 72a Cerebral herniation due to raised ICP

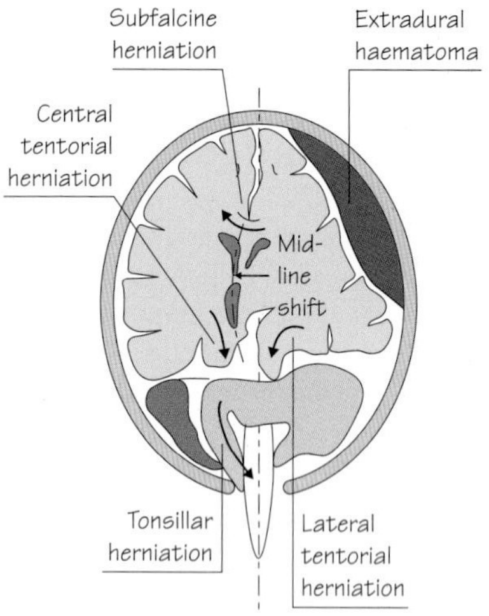

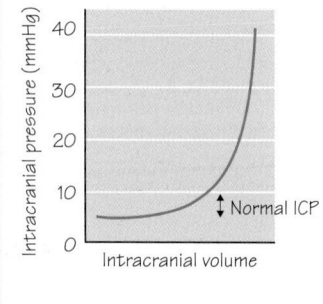

- Subfalcine herniation
- Extradural haematoma
- Central tentorial herniation
- Mid-line shift
- Tonsillar herniation
- Lateral tentorial herniation

Figure 72b CT scan: Head injury after road traffic accident

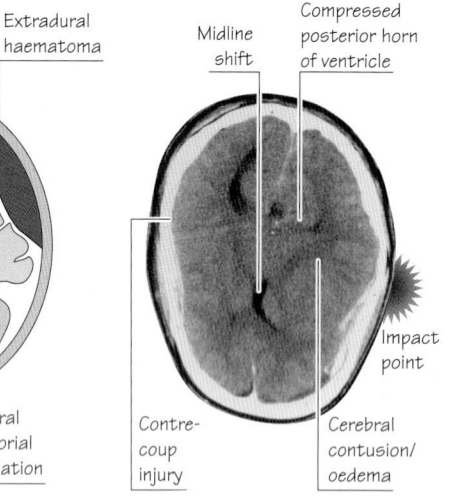

- Midline shift
- Compressed posterior horn of ventricle
- Contre-coup injury
- Impact point
- Cerebral contusion/oedema

Figure 72c The Glasgow Coma Scale

Eyes	Open	Spontaneously	4
		To verbal command	3
		To pain	2
		No response	1
Best motor response	To verbal commands	Obeys	6
	To painful stimuli	Localizes pain	5
		Flexion - withdrawal	4
		Flexion - decorticate	3
		Extension - decerebrate	2
		No response	1
Best verbal response		Orientated converses	5
		Disorientated converses	4
		Inappropriate words	3
		Incomprehensible sounds	2
		No response	1
		Total	3–15

Figure 72d Effect of cerebral oedema on ICP

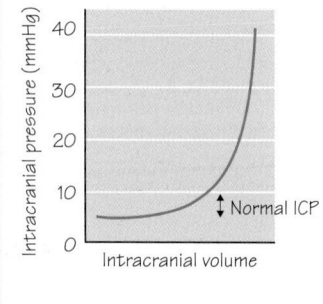

Intracranial pressure (mmHg) vs Intracranial volume

Normal ICP

Figure 72e Factors influencing cerebral blood flow

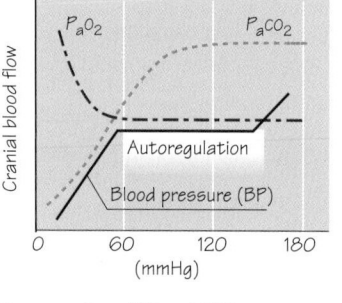

Cranial blood flow

P_aO_2 P_aCO_2

Autoregulation

Blood pressure (BP)

0   60   120   180 (mmHg)

Figure 72g Complications associated with severe head injury

Pulmonary
- Neurogenic pulmonary oedema; catecholamine-induced venoconstriction
- Autonomic induced hypoxaemia due to V/Q mismatching
- Acute respiratory distress syndrome
- Atelectasis due to restricted physiotherapy

Neuroendocrine
- Hypothalamic injury reduces ADH secretion causing diabetes insipidus
- Pituitary damage with reduced ACTH, GH, etc.

Neurological
- Meningitis
- Obstructive hydrocephalus

Haematological
- DIC (~ 25%) and coagulation disorders due to brain thromboplastin release
- Deep venous thrombosis

Skin
- Decubitus pressure sores

ADH, antidiuretic hormone; GH, growth hormone

Figure 72f The effect of hyperventilation and hypocapnia on ICP and CPP

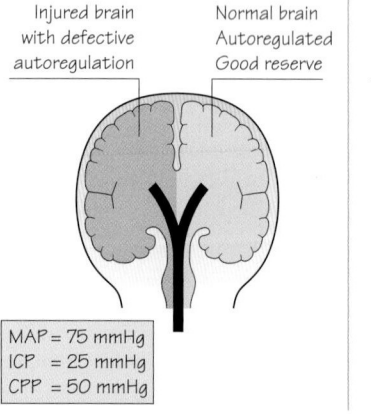

Normal P_aCO_2 = 45mmHg

- Injured brain with defective autoregulation
- Normal brain Autoregulated Good reserve

MAP = 75 mmHg
ICP = 25 mmHg
CPP = 50 mmHg

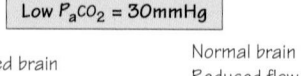

Low P_aCO_2 = 30mmHg

- Injured brain Better perfused Not autoregulated
- Normal brain Reduced flow (Fig 72e) but not compromised due to a good reserve Shrinks = ↓ICP
- Reduced flow due to vasoconstriction i.e. autoregulated

MAP = 75 mmHg
ICP = 10 mmHg
CPP = 65 mmHg

Critical Care Medicine at a Glance, Third Edition. Richard Leach. © 2014 John Wiley & Sons, Ltd. Published 2014 by John Wiley & Sons, Ltd.

Head injury causes ~33% of trauma deaths. Most serious head injuries are due to road traffic accidents, falls, assaults and gunshot wounds. Two mechanisms cause neural tissue damage:

1 Primary injury sustained during trauma includes brain lacerations, contusions and diffuse axonal injury due to shear forces during acceleration or deceleration. It is irreversible.

2 Secondary injury (Figures 72a, 72b) due to raised intracranial pressure (ICP) and poor cerebral perfusion. It accounts for ~50% of deaths. Preventive therapy may improve outcome. Causes are:

- **Intracranial**, including cerebral oedema, hydrocephalus, space occupying lesions (SOLs; e.g. extradural haemorrhage), cerebral ischaemia (e.g. seizures) and inflammation.
- **Systemic**, including hypotension, hypoxia, anaemia, hyper-/hypoglycaemia, hyper-/hypocapnia and hyperthermia.

Pathophysiology

The skull is a fixed volume containing brain, blood and cerebrospinal fluid (CSF). Initially, cerebral oedema (±SOL) displaces blood and CSF with little effect on the ICP (~5–10 mmHg). Further swelling rapidly raises ICP (Figure 72d). After trauma, ICP peaks at ~72 hours and may cause cerebral herniation (Figure 72a). Increased ICP (e.g. >25 mmHg) reflects the severity of brain injury but reduced **cerebral perfusion pressure** (CPP: the difference between mean arterial pressure [MAP] and ICP) is more important because this impairs cerebral blood flow (CBF) causing ischaemia. Therapy aims to maintain a normal CPP (>60 mmHg) because neuronal failure and death occur at <40 and <20 mmHg respectively.

Normally CBF is independent of blood pressure (BP) (i.e. autoregulated) but sensitive to P_aO_2 and P_aCO_2 (Figure 72e). In injured brain, autoregulation fails and perfusion directly parallels CPP.

- **Hypoxia or hypercapnia** dilates normal vessels and diverts blood flow away from damaged cerebral tissue. The associated increase in cerebral blood volume (CBV) raises ICP, reduces CPP and CBF, and further aggravates ischaemia in damaged brain.
- **Hypocapnia** (Figure 72f) constricts normal vessels, reducing CBV and ICP. This increases CPP and CBF. Also, vasoconstriction in normal tissue and failure of autoregulation in damaged tissue diverts blood flow to injured brain relieving ischaemia. Unfortunately, raised CPP increases oedema and ICP in damaged brain and, with vasoconstriction, may cause ischaemia in normal tissue. Consequently, a low–normal P_aCO_2 (~35–40 mmHg) is currently recommended.

Immediate management

(i) **Prompt resuscitation**: oxygen therapy corrects hypoxaemia, ventilatory support prevents hypercapnia and fluid resuscitation and antiarrhythmics maintain haemodynamic stability and CPP. (ii) **Spinal immobilization**: assume all head-injured patients have spinal injuries. (iii) **Airways protection**: cervical stabilization is required during intubation (Chapter 71). (iv) **General review**: ~50% have serious thoracic or abdominal injuries. (v) **Sedation** (±**paralysis**) reduces ICP and spinal injury in agitated patients.

Assessment

The **Glasgow Coma Score** (GCS) is a prognostic, reproducible method of assessing patient responsiveness (Figure 72c). Severe head injury is defined as GCS ≤8; post-resuscitation GCS ≤8 within 48 hours of injury; or any intracranial contusion, haematoma or laceration.

- **Physical examination** detects head wounds and spinal cord damage. CSF rhinorrhoea, blood behind the tympanic membrane,

'racoon eyes' or bruising behind the ears (Battle's sign) occur in basilar skull fractures. Papilloedema indicates raised ICP. Neurological examination is essential.

- **Radiographic evaluation** includes skull radiographs and/or CT scan (Figure 72b). Indications for immediate CT scan are coma, deteriorating consciousness, GCS ≤8, GCS 9–13 with skull fractures or planned surgery. Intracranial haematoma is 10 times as common with skull fractures.
- **Monitoring**: GCS is often adequate, but severe injuries may require **ICP monitoring** using extradural, subarachnoid or brain (e.g. Camino bolt) pressure transducers. Infection risks and inaccuracy limit use. **Cerebral oxygen saturation** (S_jO_2) is measured using a jugular venous bulb fibreoptic catheter. S_jO_2 <55% suggests inadequate CBF. Monitor **blood sugar** (BS) and occasionally **electroencephalogram (EEG)**.

Management

The aim is to prevent secondary cerebral damage.

- **General measures**: optimize CBF (i.e. MAP >70 mmHg, ICP <15–20 mmHg, CPP >60 mmHg) and oxygenation (i.e. P_aO_2 > 90%, S_jO_2 >55%).
- **Reduce ICP**: treatment options are: (i) **hyperventilation** (P_aCO_2 25–30 mmHg); rapidly (~30 secs) reduces ICP (~25%) but is not recommended routinely (ii) **Loop diuretics** (e.g. furosemide) **and osmotic agents** (e.g. mannitol) transiently (~6–8 hours) but effectively reduce ICP, which may prevent cerebral herniation. Mannitol increases intravascular osmotic pressure, reducing brain cell volume and ICP. (iii) **Optimise venous drainage**. Hard collars, neck flexion and tracheostomy ties can impede venous drainage, increasing ICP. Drainage is improved by midline head position and 15–30° elevation. Suctioning, physiotherapy and PEEP increase venous pressure. Consider (iv) **ventriculostomy drainage/decompressive surgery** if other methods fail. CSF drainage is useful in obstructive hydrocephalus. **Steroids** do not reduce ICP or improve outcome.
- **Reduce cerebral metabolism**: options include: (i) **tight glycaemic control** (BS 4–7 mmol/L). Reduced cerebral lactate production improves outcome. (ii) **Prophylactic anticonvulsants** prevent seizures that complicate ~10–40% of severe head injuries. (iii) **Sedation and paralysis** decrease agitation and metabolism. Propofol may be neuroprotective. Barbiturates reduce cerebral metabolism but cause haemodynamic instability. Benzodiazepines are a good alternative. (iv) **Antipyretics and cooling** prevent hyperthermia, which damages injured brain. Moderate hypothermia (33–34 °C) may be neuro-protective.
- **Treat complications** (Figure 72g). Avoid nasogastric tubes in basilar skull fractures and treat signs of meningitis with antibiotics.

Prognosis

Road safety measures (e.g. seat belts, helmets, drink-driving legislation) have reduced head injury related deaths. Nevertheless, in the USA, ~50,000 severely head-injured patients (GCS ≤8) die before reaching hospital and ~50,000 after hospital admission. Of survivors with an initial GSC ≤8, ~33% never regain independent function, whereas ~66% are largely self-reliant.

Pearl of wisdom
Assume all head-injured patients have spinal injuries and immobilize the spine until clearance is obtained

73 Chest trauma

Figure 73a Kerbstone fractures

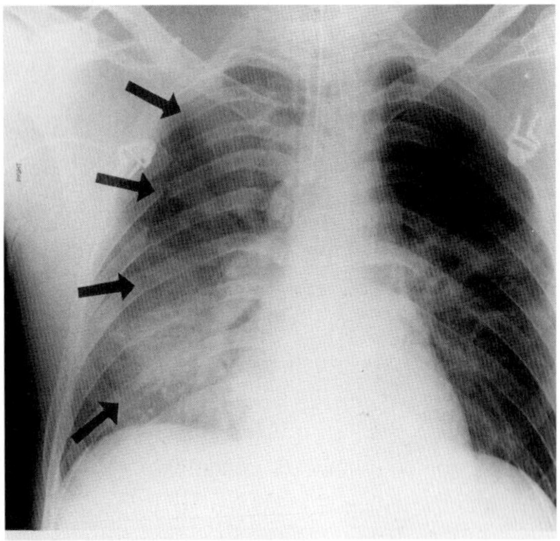

Figure 73b Rib fracture complications

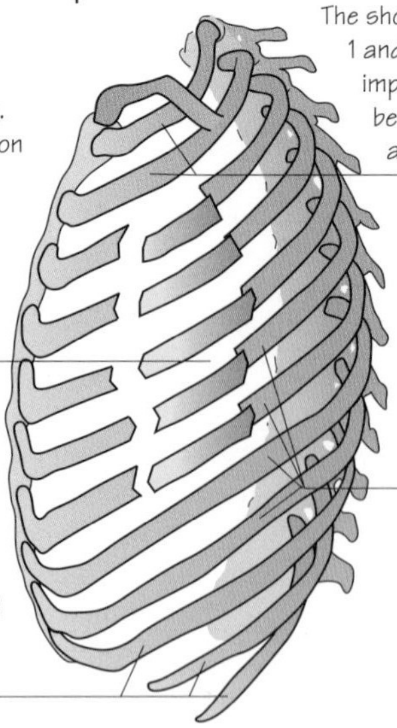

Rib fractures damage underlying lung. Pneumothorax is common

Flail segment causes respiratory failure and atelectasis

The shoulder girdle protects ribs 1 and 2. Fracture of these ribs implies a forceful blow and may be associated with airways and great vessel damage

Ribs fracture at the site of maximum curvature on the posterior axillary line: 'kerbstone fractures'

Fractures of ribs 10-12 may damage the liver, spleen and kidneys

Figure 73c Chest injuries

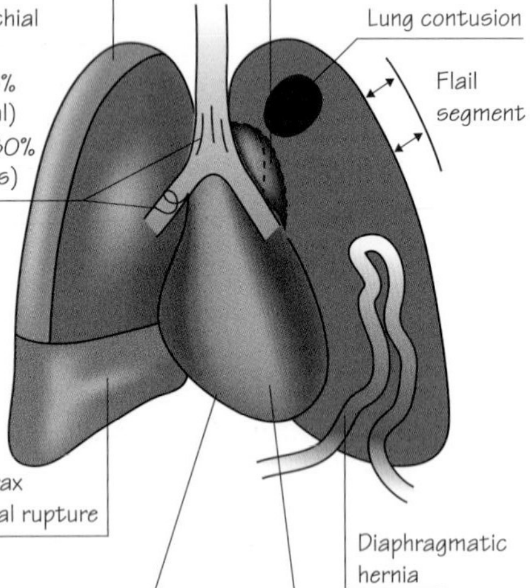

Pneumothorax

Tracheobronchial tears
• Tracheal 15% (longitudinal)
• Bronchial 80% (spiral tears)

Aortic rupture

Lung contusion

Flail segment

Pleural effusion
Haemothorax
Oesophageal rupture

Diaphragmatic hernia

Pericardial tamponade

Cardiac
• Contusion
• Traumatic damage (valve and papillary muscle rupture)

Figure 73d Aortic damage

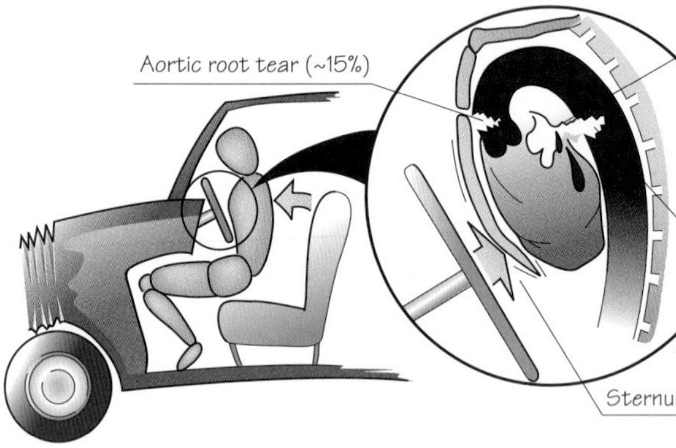

Aortic root tear (~15%)

Ligamentum arteriosum (LA)

Aorta tears just distal to LA (~80%)

Sternum

Figure 73f Radiographic features of aortic rupture

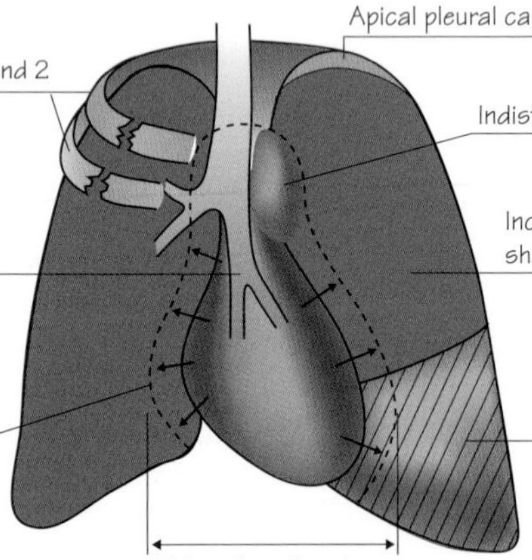

Fracture of ribs 1 and 2

Apical pleural capping

Indistinct aortic arch

Depression of left main bronchus

Increased left-sided shadowing

Occasional pericardial tamponade

Pleural effusion

Widened mediastinum

Figure 73e Specific injury mortality in chest trauma

Chest Injury	Mortality
Bilateral contusion and haemothorax	54%
Three fractured ribs bilaterally	41%
Unilateral lung contusion	25%
Three fractured ribs unilaterally	17%

Chest trauma may be penetrating or blunt. It is often associated with multiple trauma (Chapters 71, 72). Treatment of associated hypoxaemia, hypercapnia and hypotension prevents secondary organ damage (Chapters 7, 14). Ongoing management anticipates complications and detects missed injuries.

Penetrating chest trauma

- **Stab (e.g. knife) and low-velocity gunshot wounds** cause haemopneumothorax. Simple chest drainage is effective in most cases. Indications for thoracotomy include transmediastinal injury, cardiac tamponade, initial chest drain blood loss >1.5–2 L or >200–250 ml drainage/h indicating ongoing bleeding.
- **High-velocity gunshot wounds** cause extensive cavitation and tissue injury. Early surgery is needed to control haemorrhage and air leaks, evacuate blood clots and remove damaged lung. Consider air embolism if neurological (e.g. cerebrovascular accident) or cardiac (e.g. arrhythmia) complications develop. Although air embolism can complicate any parenchymal lung damage, it is more common in high-velocity gunshot wounds and during mechanical ventilation (MV).

Blunt chest trauma

Non-penetrating blunt chest trauma is relatively common. There may be few external clinical signs apart from bruising. A high index of suspicion is required to avoid delayed diagnosis of serious internal injury (Figure 73c, 73e).

Three mechanisms cause intrathoracic injury:

1 Rib fractures (Figures 73a and 73b) damage underlying structures (e.g. pneumothorax, haemothorax, lung contusion) and cause severe pain with splinting, hypoventilation and atelectasis. Older patients are most frequently affected. In young patients, chest wall flexibility causes intrathoracic damage without rib fractures. Treatment involves chest drainage, physiotherapy, nerve blocks and potent opioid (±epidural) analgesia.

2 Increased intrathoracic pressure: abrupt elevation of intracavitary pressure may rupture air- or fluid-filled structures. Alveolar, oesophageal and diaphragmatic rupture cause pneumothorax, mediastinitis and herniation of abdominal contents into the thoracic cavity respectively (Figure 73c).

3 Shear stress: intrathoracic structures are tethered to adjacent tissues. The shear forces produced by differential organ motion cause visceral or vascular tears including aortic rupture (Figure 73d), tracheobronchial disruption and pulmonary haematoma.

Specific injuries (Figure 73c)

Lung, tracheobronchial and diaphragmatic injuries

- **Pneumothorax/haemothorax** are common and require drainage (Chapter 43).
- **Pulmonary contusions** present as ill-defined infiltrates at the site of trauma on chest radiograph (CXR). Haemoptysis and hypoxaemia are due to localized bleeding, oedema and ventilation/perfusion (V/Q) mismatch.
- **Flail chest** occurs when multiple fractures, usually at two sites, result in a 'free' section of chest wall or sternum. 'Paradoxical' movement of the 'flail segment' (i.e. moves in during inspiration, out during expiration) causes hypoventilation and atelectasis in the underlying lung. Discomfort also impedes ventilation, cough and secretion clearance and requires effective analgesia. Thoracic epidural is most effective. If respiratory failure develops, MV (±tracheostomy) may be required for ~7–14 days to restore normal inspiratory/expiratory movement of the flail segment. External chest wall stabilization (e.g. fixation) is of no benefit.

- **Tracheobronchial tears** should be suspected if the first or second ribs are fractured and with bilateral pneumothoraces, haemoptysis, mediastinal/subcutaneous emphysema and persistent air leaks. Typically, longitudinal tears occur in the posterior membranous portion of the lower trachea (~15%) and spiral tears in the main bronchi (~80%). Bronchoscopy confirms the diagnosis and early surgical repair prevents atelectasis, infection and later development of bronchial stenosis (±bronchiectasis). Occasionally, a main bronchus is completely severed. The 'drop' lung is easily recognized and surgical repair is associated with no long-term complications.
- **Diaphragmatic injuries** occur in ~7%, mostly on the left (~80%) because the right diaphragm is protected by the liver. Mortality is high due to associated splenic or hepatic rupture.
- **Lung torsion** (i.e. rotation on the hilar axis) is rare.

Heart and great vessel injuries

- **Cardiac contusion** causes microvascular haemorrhage and oedema at the site of cardiac impact resulting in myocardial ischaemia, arrhythmias, heart block and ventricular failure. Cardiac enzymes, electrocardiogram, echocardiography and occasionally angiography establish the diagnosis. Treatment is non-specific including management of arrhythmias and circulatory failure (Chapters 8, 32, 34).
- **Aortic tears and dissection** are due to shear stresses associated with abrupt deceleration accidents (Figure 73d). Most cases are fatal at the scene of the accident. Clinically, there may be no evidence of external trauma and rib fractures are not always present. Tears are most common just distal to *ligamentum arteriosum* (~80%). Aortic root tears (~15%) occasionally damage the valve or coronary arteries. Figure 73f illustrates CXR features of aortic rupture. Aortography or contrast CT scans confirm the diagnosis.
- **Pericardial tamponade** may be due to aortic root disruption, coronary artery laceration or rupture of the free ventricular wall. It usually requires surgical drainage.
- **Traumatic damage** may involve the heart, valves (aortic ~60%, mitral ~30%) or papillary muscles. Transmural rupture is rapidly fatal in >80% of cases. Early surgery is required.

Other injuries

- **Oesophageal rupture** is suspected if haematemesis or subcutaneous emphysema occurs with post-traumatic pleural effusion, pneumothorax or mediastinitis. Aspirated pleural fluid reveals food particles and a raised amylase. A gastrografin 'swallow' confirms the diagnosis whereas endoscopy and CT scans are often unhelpful. Mortality is high without immediate surgical repair.
- **Fat embolism syndrome** occurs 1–72 hours after multiple long-bone or pelvic fractures. Lipases liberate unsaturated fatty acids that cause lung toxicity and coagulopathy (e.g. disseminated intravascular coagulation). Small fat emboli also pass through pulmonary capillaries to occlude retinal, skin and central nervous system vessels. The characteristic clinical triad includes **confusion, pulmonary dysfunction** (e.g. cough, dyspnoea, pleurisy, acute respiratory distress syndrome) and a **petechial skin rash** over the upper torso. Investigations reveal hypoxaemia, a normal CXR, and lipase and fat globules in urine and serum.

Pearl of wisdom

Beware blunt chest injury: despite few external signs, it can be associated with severe occult internal injuries like cardiac contusion and aortic rupture

 **Acute abdominal emergencies**

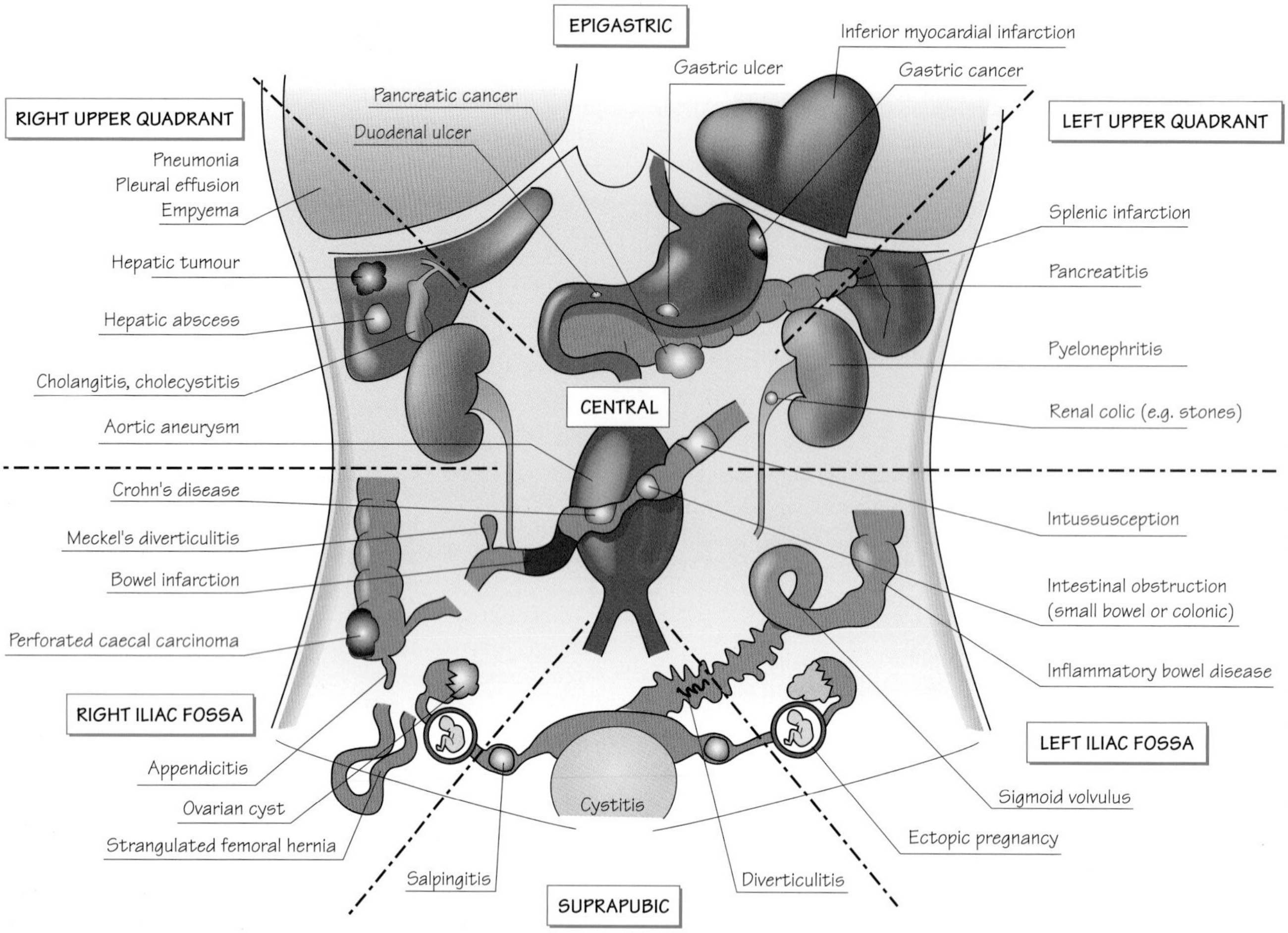

Figure 74a Causes of acute abdominal pain and abdominal emergencies

EPIGASTRIC

Inferior myocardial infarction

Gastric ulcer

Gastric cancer

RIGHT UPPER QUADRANT

Pancreatic cancer

Duodenal ulcer

LEFT UPPER QUADRANT

Pneumonia
Pleural effusion
Empyema

Splenic infarction

Pancreatitis

Hepatic tumour

Hepatic abscess

Pyelonephritis

Cholangitis, cholecystitis

Renal colic (e.g. stones)

Aortic aneurysm

CENTRAL

Crohn's disease

Intussusception

Meckel's diverticulitis

Bowel infarction

Intestinal obstruction
(small bowel or colonic)

Perforated caecal carcinoma

Inflammatory bowel disease

RIGHT ILIAC FOSSA

LEFT ILIAC FOSSA

Appendicitis

Ovarian cyst

Cystitis

Sigmoid volvulus

Strangulated femoral hernia

Ectopic pregnancy

Salpingitis

Diverticulitis

SUPRAPUBIC

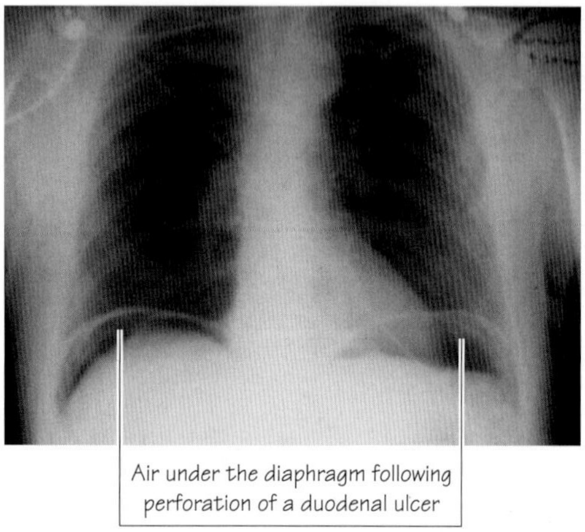

Figure 74b Air under the diaphragm

Air under the diaphragm following
perforation of a duodenal ulcer

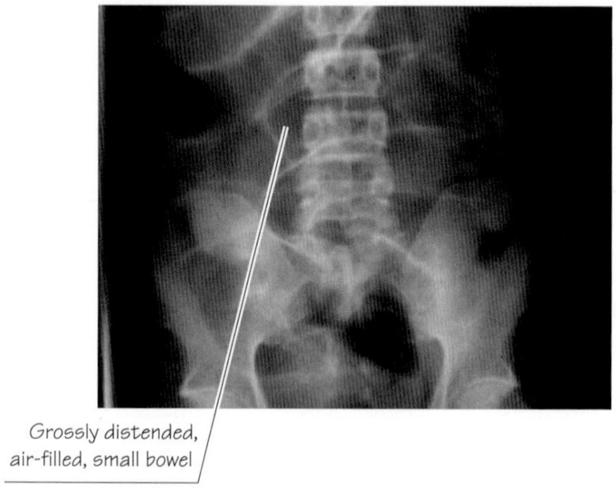

Figure 74c Small bowel obstruction

Grossly distended,
air-filled, small bowel

Critical Care Medicine at a Glance, Third Edition. Richard Leach. © 2014 John Wiley & Sons, Ltd. Published 2014 by John Wiley & Sons, Ltd.

In the intensive care setting setting, abdominal emergencies (Figure 74a) rarely present with typical symptoms and signs because characteristic features (e.g. peritonitis) are masked by coma, spinal injury or drugs (e.g. analgesics). Relatively minor features including diarrhoea, vague discomfort or feeding intolerance may be the only indicators of pathology. Early diagnosis requires a high index of suspicion, vital sign monitoring (e.g. temperature, blood pressure [BP]), repeated examination and timely investigation (e.g. amylase). CT scans provide the best images but ultrasound scans (USSs) are portable and readily detect liver, renal and pelvic disease. If surgery is likely to be required, limit analgesia, withhold feeding and involve the surgeons early. Always exclude non-abdominal pathology (e.g. inferior myocardial infarction [MI] causes epigastric pain). Peritonitis, bacteraemia and subsequent multiple-organ failure complicate many abdominal emergencies (Chapter 25).

Peptic ulceration and perforation

Duodenal (5–10%) rather than gastric (<1%) ulcers are most likely to perforate. There may be no previous history of peptic ulcer disease. Perforation occurs at any age but is most common in 20–40 year-old patients. It usually presents with sudden, severe mid-abdominal pain. Patients appear ill, lie still and take shallow breaths to minimize pain. Examination reveals a rigid, 'board-like' abdomen and absent bowel sounds. Peritonitis may be absent in older or critically ill patients, and those on steroids or non-steroidal anti-inflammatory drugs (NSAIDs). An erect chest radiograph (CXR) (Figure 74b) or left lateral decubitus abdominal radiograph (AXR) detects free air in the abdominal cavity (~80%).

Management includes fluid resuscitation, antibiotics and nasogastric (NG) tube drainage. In unstable patients, duodenal ulcers are oversewn whereas resection and vagotomy are performed in stable patients. Whenever possible, gastric ulcers are resected because of associated cancer risk.

Intestinal obstruction

Small bowel obstruction (SBO; Chapter 56) presents with nausea, vomiting, cramping abdominal pain, distension and high-pitched ('tinkling') bowel sounds. The most common causes are adhesions from previous surgery (~75%), incarcerated hernias, malignancy and volvulus (~25%). AXR demonstrates dilated small bowel (>3 cm) with or without air/fluid levels (Figure 74c).

Management involves fluid/electrolyte resuscitation and gastric decompression with NG tube suction. **Surgery** is indicated if symptoms persist or the clinical condition fails to improve after 24–48 hours.

Large bowel (colonic) obstruction (LBO; Chapter 56) presents with acute abdominal pain, vomiting (~50%), constipation (~50%) and distension. Common causes are colonic cancer, diverticular disease, sigmoid volvulus and faecal impaction. Pseudo-obstruction (i.e. ileus) is usually due to electrolyte imbalance or drugs. Toxic megacolon (±perforation) occurs in severe ulcerative colitis (UC). Plain AXR shows colonic distension: a caecal diameter > 9 m suggests imminent perforation.

Management includes stopping sedative or narcotic drugs, fluid/electrolyte correction and colonic decompression by rectal tube or colonoscopy. **Surgery**: imminent caecal perforation requires decompressive caecostomy. A limited right hemicolectomy, ileostomy and mucous fistula are recommended after perforation.

Inflammatory bowel disease

Crohn's disease and UC are idiopathic, relapsing, chronic inflammatory bowel diseases that cause bloody diarrhoea, colicky abdominal pain, malaise, fever, weight loss and extra-intestinal manifestations (e.g. sacroiliitis, uveitis). In UC, bowel inflammation is limited to mucosa but Crohn's disease affects the entire bowel wall. Crohn's disease affects both large and small bowel and may cause bowel strictures, perforation and fistulae. UC involves the large bowel and rectum. If severe, it causes life-threatening toxic megacolon (±perforation). Eventually ~30% of cases need a total colectomy.

Acute bowel ischaemia (ABI)

Mesenteric ischaemia affects older people with heart and vascular disease. Mortality is ~70%. Superior mesenteric artery (SMA) occlusion causes ~50% of ABI. It presents with severe abdominal pain and leucocytosis but few physical signs. Inferior mesenteric artery (IMA) thrombosis causes ~25% of ABI and presentation is subtle. Proximal SMA or IMA occlusion is usually due to atherosclerosis. Presentation is acute or gradual (i.e. with pain after meals). Embolic occlusion occurs in atrial fibrillation or post-MI mural thrombosis. Vasculitis and mesenteric venous thrombosis are uncommon causes of occlusive ischaemia. Hypotension, cardiac failure and vasopressor drugs are increasingly recognized as non-occlusive causes. Initially, ABI produces mucosal injury with bleeding and/or bloody diarrhoea (~50%). Mucosal sloughing, bowel necrosis, perforation, peritonitis, sepsis, shock and death follow. Refractory metabolic (lactic) acidosis with hyperkalaemia is characteristic.

Management includes fluid resuscitation, electrolyte correction and antibiotics. In selected cases, angiography confirms the diagnosis, allows vasodilator infusion (e.g. nitroglycerin) and aids surgical revascularization. **Surgery** initially resects gangrenous bowel. Re-exploration at 24–36 hours allows demarcation and further resection of non-viable tissue. Unfortunately, delayed diagnosis or extensive infarction often renders the situation hopeless.

Cholecystitis and cholangitis

Gallstone obstruction of the cystic duct causes ~90% of cholecystitis and cholangitis. Acalculous cholecystitis is common in seriously ill patients due to cholestasis or biliary reflux but is often unrecognized as the cause of associated sepsis. The classical triad of fever, rigors and right upper quadrant (RUQ) pain occurs in ~70%. Vomiting, RUQ mass (~20%) and elevated white cell count (WCC; ~70%), bilirubin, alkaline phosphatase and amylase (without pancreatitis) are also typical. Ultrasonography and CT scans detect biliary tract dilation. A distended gallbladder (>5 cm), thickened wall (>3 mm), sediment and pericholecystic fluid collections suggest acalculous cholecystitis. Common infective organisms are *E. coli*, *Klebsiella*, *Streptococcus faecalis* and anaerobes.

Management includes resuscitation, analgesics, broad-spectrum antibiotics and, until the patient is stable, T-tube drainage of the biliary tract. Cholecystectomy may be required later. Consider percutaneous drainage in high-risk patients but potentially lethal bile peritonitis can occur.

Other acute abdominal emergencies

Pancreatitis (Chapter 55), ruptured aortic aneurysms, pelvic disease in females (e.g. pelvic inflammatory disease, ectopic pregnancy, ovarian torsion), appendicitis, retroperitoneal haematoma (e.g. renal trauma) and renal calculi all present as acute abdominal emergencies.

Pearl of wisdom

Severe refractory lactic acidosis (±hyperkalaemia) without an obvious cause should raise the possibility of occult bowel ischaemia

75 Obstetric emergencies

Figure 75a Causes of maternal deaths

Medical condition	Rate/million pregnancies	Deaths/year un UK
Thromboembolism	21.8	~48
Intracranial bleeding (e.g. SAH)	10.9	~25
Pregnancy-induced hypertension	9.1	~20
Amniotic fluid embolism	7.7	~17
Obstetric haemorrhage (e.g. APH)	5.5	~12
Eclampsia/HELLP syndrome	0.1	~1

Figure 75c Amniotic fluid embolism

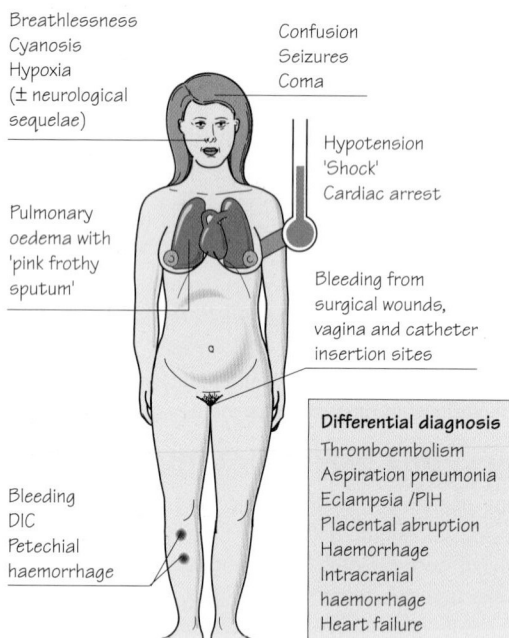

Breathlessness
Cyanosis
Hypoxia
(± neurological sequelae)

Confusion
Seizures
Coma

Pulmonary oedema with 'pink frothy sputum'

Hypotension
'Shock'
Cardiac arrest

Bleeding from surgical wounds, vagina and catheter insertion sites

Bleeding
DIC
Petechial haemorrhage

Differential diagnosis
Thromboembolism
Aspiration pneumonia
Eclampsia /PIH
Placental abruption
Haemorrhage
Intracranial haemorrhage
Heart failure

Figure 75b Features used to define pre-eclampsia and severe pre-eclampsia (American College of Obstetricians and Gynecologists)

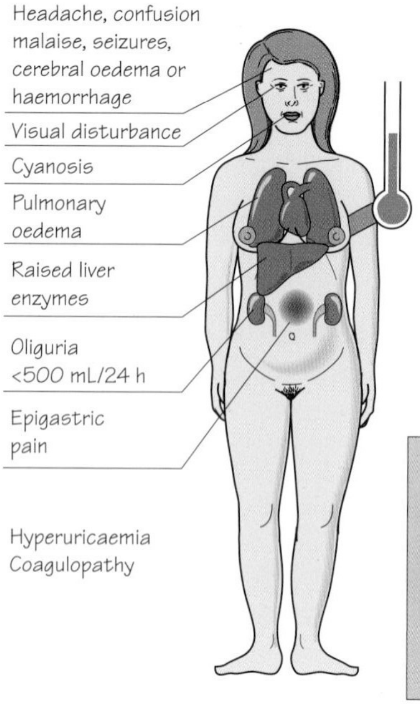

Headache, confusion malaise, seizures, cerebral oedema or haemorrhage

Visual disturbance

Cyanosis

Pulmonary oedema

Raised liver enzymes

Oliguria <500 mL/24 h

Epigastric pain

Hyperuricaemia
Coagulopathy

Pre-eclampsia
1. Blood pressure
• Systolic >140 mmHg
• Diastolic >90 mmHg
2. Renal proteinuria 300mg/24hrs

Severe pre-eclampsia
1. Blood pressure
• Systolic >160 mmHg
• Diastolic >110 mmHg
2. Renal proteinuria >2g/24 hrs +3/+4 on dipstick testing

HELLP syndrome*
A form of severe pre-eclampsia characterised by the triad of:
• Haemolysis
• Elevated Liver enzymes
• Low Platelets
* Not all patients have high BP or proteinuria

Figure 75e Types of placenta praevia

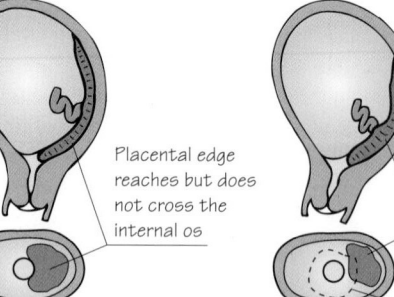

Complete placenta praevia (European classification grade 4)

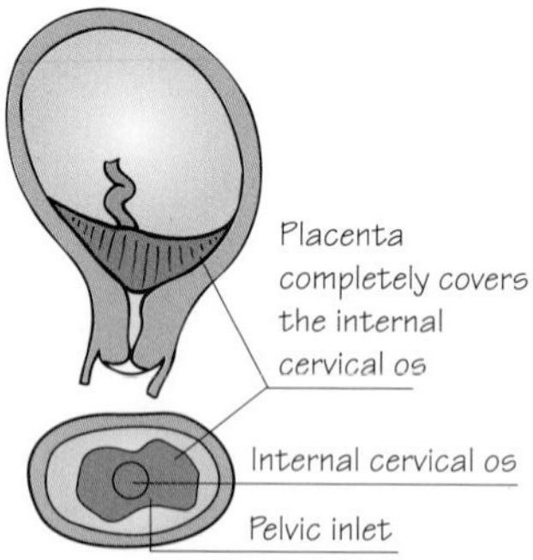

Placenta completely covers the internal cervical os

Internal cervical os

Pelvic inlet

Partial placenta praevia (grade 3)

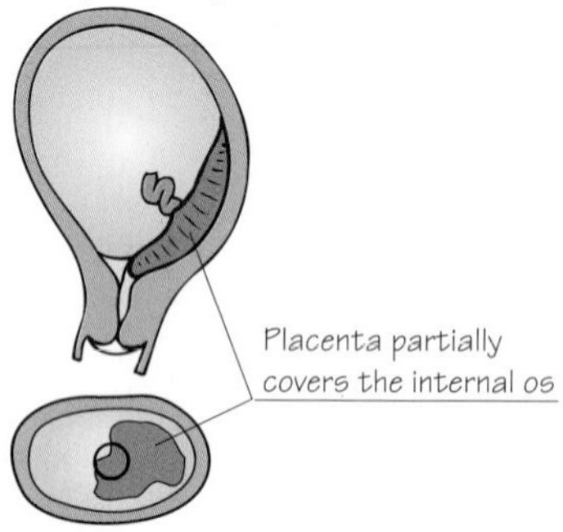

Placenta partially covers the internal os

Marginal placenta praevia (grade 2)

Placental edge reaches but does not cross the internal os

Low-lying placenta (grade 1)

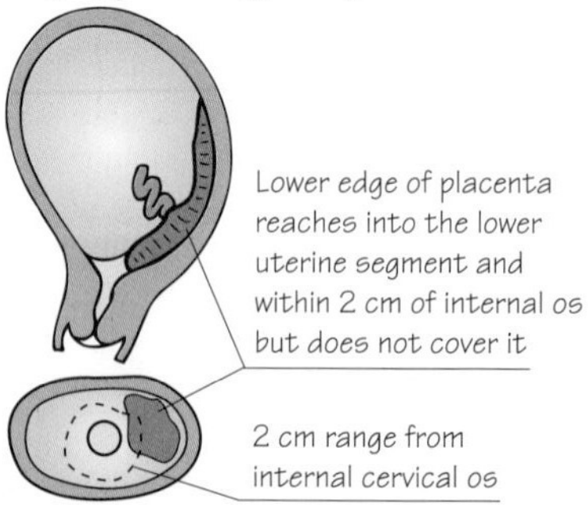

Lower edge of placenta reaches into the lower uterine segment and within 2 cm of internal os but does not cover it

2 cm range from internal cervical os

Figure 75d Risk factors and causes of postpartum haemorrhage (PPH)

Risk factors	Causes
Placenta praevia	Retained products of conception
Placental abruption	Uterine atony
Pre-eclampsia	Trauma
HELLP syndrome	Uterine rupture
Operative delivery	Bi rth canal lacerations
Caesarian section	DIC
Previous PPH	Bleeding diathesis
Obesity	
Chorioamnionitis	

Critical Care Medicine at a Glance, Third Edition. Richard Leach. © 2014 John Wiley & Sons, Ltd. Published 2014 by John Wiley & Sons, Ltd.

Life-threatening obstetric emergencies occur antepartum and postpartum. In developed countries, maternal and foetal mortality is decreasing but avoidable deaths still occur. Figure 75a reports the causes and associated death rates.

Pre-eclampsia or pregnancy-induced hypertension (PIH)

PIH is 'gestational hypertension with proteinuria developing during pregnancy or labour'. It affects ∼2–10% of pregnancies, at ∼32–38 weeks' gestation and resolves 2–3 days after delivery. Figure 75b illustrates the features of pre-eclampsia. Grand mal convulsions define the onset of eclampsia. The main causes of maternal death are cerebral or pulmonary oedema, intracranial haemorrhage and liver damage.

Management aims to control blood pressure (BP), prevent seizures (±end-organ damage) and maintain uterine perfusion (i.e. nurse in a semi-lateral position); but only delivery is curative. Monitor urine output, proteinuria, liver function, platelet count and urate.

• **Antihypertensive therapy** (e.g. nifedipine, labetalol) reduces BP without impairing uterine perfusion.

• **Fluid balance** is difficult because pulmonary oedema is a risk despite intravascular depletion. Initially give crystalloid at ∼75–100 ml/h. Central venous pressure (CVP) is unreliable; consider invasive monitoring if oliguria persists.

• **Magnesium sulphate** is the drug of choice to prevent (or treat) convulsions due to its central nervous system (CNS) depressant, cerebral vasodilator and antihypertensive actions. In overdose, it causes muscle weakness, respiratory paralysis and heart block but can be inhibited by calcium gluconate.

• **Early foetal delivery** may be required. If the pregnancy is <34 weeks, dexamethasone aids foetal lung maturation with best results if delivery can be delayed for 48 hours.

Amniotic fluid embolism (AFE)

AFE causes 5–10% of maternal deaths and affects 1 in 20–80 000 pregnancies. It occurs when amniotic fluid (±foetal matter, meconium) enters the maternal circulation. Figure 75c illustrates clinical features. Classically, AFE presents with severe dyspnoea, cyanosis and hypotension (±cardiac arrest) in older, multiparous mothers with large babies during oxytocin-driven labour. However, it can occur throughout pregnancy (e.g. amniocentesis, termination, membrane rupture). Initial survivors develop seizures (∼20%), disseminated intravascular coagulation (DIC) with bleeding (∼40%) and pulmonary oedema (∼75%). Management is symptomatic (e.g. oxygen) and supportive (e.g. ventilation). Mortality is >80% with ∼50% dying within an hour.

Severe obstetric haemorrhage (SOH)

Peripartum haemorrhage causes 15% (25% with ectopic pregnancies) of maternal deaths. Blood loss >40% is life-threatening and requires prompt resuscitation with fluids, blood and clotting factors (Chapters 7, 10, 69). Compression of the aorta against the vertebral column (pressure above the umbilicus) temporarily impedes blood loss. Obstetric intervention depends on the cause.

Antepartum haemorrhage (APH)

Bleeding after >20 weeks of pregnancy puts the foetus at risk. The main causes are placental abruption (∼25%), placenta praevia (∼20%), uterine rupture and placental abnormalities (e.g. vasa praevia). Ultrasound scan determines the cause.

• **Placental abruption (PA)** occurs when a normally implanted placenta separates from the uterine wall. Precipitating factors include hypertension, trauma or sudden changes in uterine size but often there is no obvious cause. It affects ∼1.5% of pregnancies and is more common in smokers and older, multiparous women. Perinatal mortality is high (∼50%). Bleeding may be concealed or revealed and with increasing placental separation there is abdominal pain and tenderness. Retroplacental bleeding >500 ml can cause foetal death and >1 L results in serious maternal sequelae with shock and DIC.

• **Placenta praevia (PP)** affects ∼1% of pregnancies. It is due to placental encroachment on the lower uterine segment (LUS); the more severe, the higher maternal mortality (Figure 75e). The LUS endometrium is less well developed and placental attachment to underlying muscle (PP accreta) impairs separation during third stage delivery. It classically presents with painless vaginal bleeding in late pregnancy. Significant APH may require hospitalization but management is conservative to allow foetal maturation. Delivery by caesarian section (CS) is usually required.

Primary postpartum haemorrhage (PPH)

This refers to >500 ml blood loss within 24 hours of delivery. It is severe if >1 L/24 h. Risk factors and causes are listed in Figure 75d.

• **Retained products of conception (RPC)** complicate 4% of deliveries and require uterine evacuation. Severe haemorrhage may entail embolization, iliac artery ligation or hysterectomy.

• **Uterine rupture** occurs in multiparous women with foetal malpresentations, operative trauma, breech delivery, PP accreta or oxytocic use.

• **Uterine atony** may be due to drugs (e.g. beta-blockers), uterine sepsis, bladder distension, multiparity or long labour. It is uncommon since the advent of oxytocic drugs. Treatments include uterine massage, bimanual compression, oxytocin, uterine packing or intramyometrial prostaglandin.

• **Coagulation defects** follow PA, PIH, AFE, intrauterine death or sepsis.

Secondary PPH

Secondary PPH is severe bleeding >24 hours post-partum until the end of the puerperium. It is often due to infected RPC and treated with antibiotics.

Sheehan's syndrome is panhypopituitarism following pituitary hypoperfusion during SOH. Failure of lactation and amenorrhoea are early features. Adrenal and thyroid gland failure follow (Chapter 51).

Medical emergencies in pregnancy

Cardiac arrest affects 1 in 30 000 pregnancies. Advanced life support (ALS) guidelines are followed (Chapter 6). Early intubation prevents hypoxaemia due to diaphragmatic splinting and increased oxygen consumption. Chest compressions are performed with a wedge below the right hip or manual uterine displacement to prevent caval compression that impairs venous return. Immediate foetal delivery by CS is required if resuscitation is unsuccessful. ALS is continued until after delivery. Gastric compression makes aspiration a risk.

Pulmonary embolism (PE; Chapter 36) causes ∼20% of maternal deaths and affects ∼1 in 2000 pregnancies. Caval compression by the gravid uterus and pregnancy-induced hypercoagulability predispose to antepartum lower limb and pelvic vein thrombosis. Mobilization after delivery may precipitate PE. Low molecular weight heparin is the treatment and prophylaxis of choice.

Intracranial bleeds cause ∼10% of maternal deaths and are primary or due to subarachnoid haemorrhage.

Pearl of wisdom

Venous thromboembolism is the most common cause of maternal death in pregnancy; investigate new, sudden-onset chest symptoms as normal; there is no justification for withholding imaging (e.g. CT pulmonary angiogram [CTPA])

76 Burns, toxic inhalation and electrical injuries

Figure 76a Classification of burns

First-degree (superficial) burn

Epidermis
Dermis
Muscle + bone

Confined to epidermis
Skin red and painful (without blisters)
Heals spontaneously within 7 days

Second-degree (partial thickness) burn

Blister

Involves epidermis + dermis
Skin red, painful, blistered and oedematous
- If upper dermis involved heals spontaneously within 7 days
- If deep dermis affected, excision and grafting required and healing may take ~4 weeks

Third-degree (full thickness) burn

Destroys all layers of skin + some underlying tissue (Fourth-degree burn involves muscle and bone)

Burn is white (or charred), painless (anaesthetic), indurated and firm.

Even after skin grafting there is functional limitation and scarring

Figure 76b Criteria for hospital admission

Second-degree burn (SDB) >20-25% BSA
Third-degree burn (TDB) >5-10% BSA
Any SDB or TDB if >60 or <5 years old
Hand, feet, face, eye or perineal burns
Burns affecting major joints
Circumferential burns
Inhalational or airways burn injury
Chemical or electrical burns

Figure 76c Symptoms in carbon monoxide poisoning

CO-Hb level	Symptoms
<15%	None
15-20%	Headache, confusion
20-40%	Disorientation, nausea, visual impairment
40-60%	Hallucinations, coma, shock
>60%	Death

Figure 76d Assessment of BSA 'Wallace's Rule of 9s'

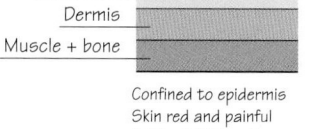

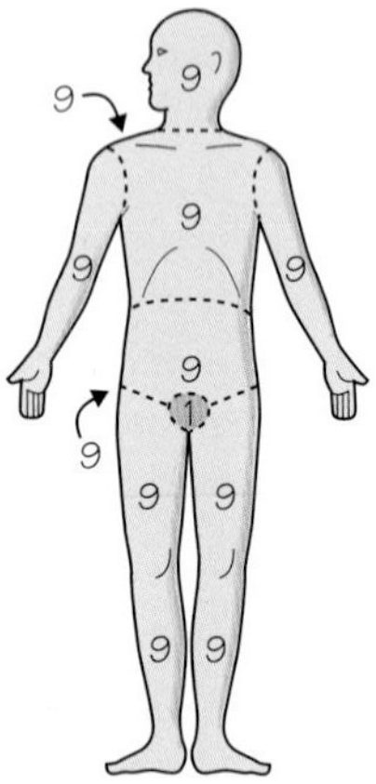

Numbers correspond to
% BSA affected 9 x 11 = 99%

Figure 76e Fluid replacement

First 24h:
- 3-4mL/kg/% BSA burn of Hartmann's solution
- Replace 50% of deficit in first 8 h
- Replace remainder over 16 h

After 24 h:
- Tailor crystalloid / colloid support
- Supplemental water (5% dextrose) and correct electrolytes

Aims:
- Adequate central venous pressure
- Adequate blood pressure + cardiac output
- Urine output 0.5-1.0mL/kg/h

Figure 76f Burns complications and treatment

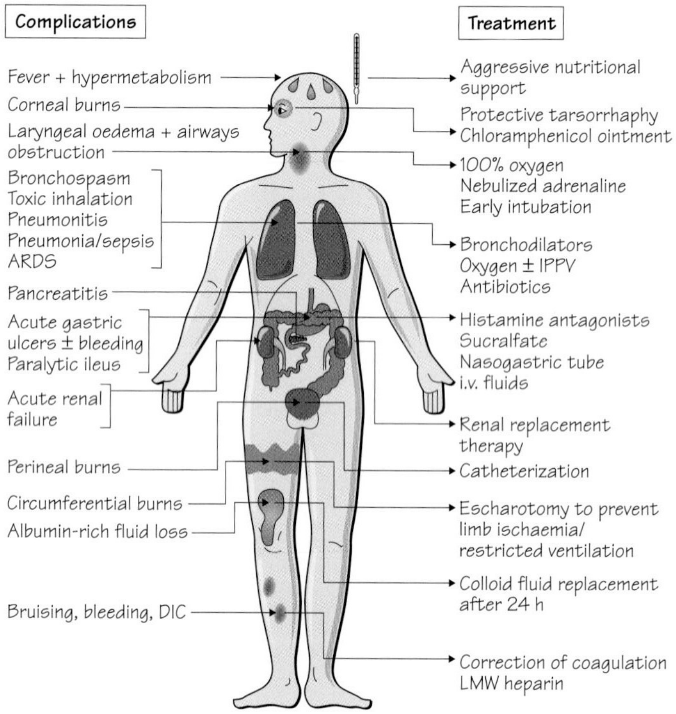

| Complications | | Treatment |

Fever + hypermetabolism — Aggressive nutritional support

Corneal burns — Protective tarsorrhaphy / Chloramphenicol ointment

Laryngeal oedema + airways obstruction — 100% oxygen / Nebulized adrenaline / Early intubation

Bronchospasm / Toxic inhalation / Pneumonitis / Pneumonia/sepsis / ARDS — Bronchodilators / Oxygen ± IPPV / Antibiotics

Pancreatitis

Acute gastric ulcers ± bleeding / Paralytic ileus — Histamine antagonists / Sucralfate / Nasogastric tube / i.v. fluids

Acute renal failure — Renal replacement therapy

Perineal burns — Catheterization

Circumferential burns — Escharotomy to prevent limb ischaemia/ restricted ventilation

Albumin-rich fluid loss — Colloid fluid replacement after 24 h

Bruising, bleeding, DIC — Correction of coagulation / LMW heparin

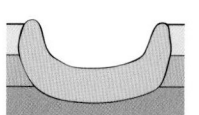
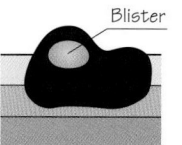

ARDS = acute respiratory distress syndrome;
IPPV = intermittent positive pressure ventilation;
LMW = low molecular weight

Figure 76g Toxic components of smoke and toxic inhalational injury

Material	Product	Effect
Plastic	Phosgene, chlorine, hydrochloric acid	Acute lung injury Airways irritation
Wood/Paper	Acrolein, acetaldehyde Formaldehyde, acetic acid	Bronchospasm, airways irritation, mucosal sloughing
Synthetic materials (e.g. nylon)	Nitrogen oxides (e.g. NO_2) Hydrogen cyanide	Cyanide poisoning, tissue hypoxia, pulmonary oedema
All the above	Carbon monoxide	Tissue hypoxia (see Figure 76c)

Critical Care Medicine at a Glance, Third Edition. Richard Leach. © 2014 John Wiley & Sons, Ltd. Published 2014 by John Wiley & Sons, Ltd.

In the UK, serious burns account for ~10 000 admissions/year and ~500 die. Management in specialized units has improved outcome, and patients may survive burns to >80% of body surface area (BSA). Burns are classified (Figure 76a) by the skin layers affected, appearance and healing, as **first degree** (superficial), **second degree** (partial thickness) or **third degree** (full thickness) burns.

Assessment of burns

- **Depth** determines healing time, scarring and therapy options (e.g. grafting). The crucial, often difficult, decision is whether a burn is full or partial thickness (Figure 76a).
- **Size**, estimated from the 'rule of nines' in adults (Figure 76d), aids assessment of fluid loss and inflammatory response.
- **Cause**: dry (e.g. flame), moist (e.g. hot liquids), blast, electrical or chemical.
- **Time**: replace fluid from the time of the burn, not admission.
- **Site affected**: face (e.g. eyelids), perineum, hands, feet; circumferential burns require specialist attention.
- **Smoke inhalation**: increases mortality.

Management of major burns

Figure 76b lists criteria for hospital admission and/or referral to specialist burns centres. Figure 76f illustrates complications.

1 Resuscitation: burns activate an inflammatory response with vasodilation and increased vascular permeability. Fluid redistribution (i.e. intravascular to extravascular) and exudative 'surface' loss cause hypovolaemia (±shock). Burns >15% BSA (>10% with smoke inhalation) require fluid replacement to restore perfusion, maintain organ function and preserve skin tissue.

- **First 24 hours**: use crystalloid-only regimes as neither colloid nor hypertonic solutions improve outcome. The Parkland formula recommends 4 ml/kg/%BSA burn/day of Hartmann's solution, with 50% given in the first 8 hours (Figure 76e). Clinical response (e.g. urine output) should also guide fluid therapy. Excessive fluid can be harmful; but only specialists should use hypertonic solutions to reduce tissue oedema.
- **After 24 hours**: sodium requirements and vessel permeability decrease and low sodium solutions (±colloids) maintain circulating volume and electrolyte balance.
- **Vasoactive agents** may be required (e.g. sepsis). Avoid α-adrenergic agonists (e.g. norepinephrine), which impair injured skin blood flow.

2 Airway and inhalational complications often cause early death. Facial or neck burns, oropharyngeal swelling, cough, carbonaceous sputum, respiratory distress or stridor suggest smoke inhalation and upper airways damage.

- **Airways obstruction**: hot gases (e.g. steam) and toxic chemicals in smoke cause rapid upper airways obstruction. Early intubation is recommended with second or third degree facial burns, because it may be impossible later due to oedema. If intubation is not required, monitor lung function and give humidified oxygen and nebulized bronchodilators (±ephedrine). Steroids do not reduce oedema and increase infection risks.
- **Toxic inhalational injury (TII)**: highly soluble gases (e.g. SO_2, Cl) dissolve in upper airway secretions forming potent acids that cause mucosal inflammation, ulceration and bronchospasm (Figure 76g). Low solubility toxins (e.g. NO_2, phosgene) penetrate to the lower respiratory tract causing alveolar damage, pulmonary oedema and ventilation/perfusion (V/Q) mismatch. In severe TII, mucosa sloughs at ~72 hours and requires 7–14 days to regenerate. Secondary infection is common.

- **Carbon monoxide (CO) poisoning** causes 75% of fire deaths. Affinity of CO for haemoglobin (Hb) is ~250 times that of oxygen. Low CO concentrations (e.g. 0.1%) readily displace oxygen to produce non-functional carboxyhaemoglobin (CO-Hb). Symptoms of CO poisoning are those of tissue hypoxia and correlate with CO-Hb levels (Figure 76c). Co-oximeters with multi-wavelength spectroscopy differentiate between CO-Hb and oxyhaemoglobin; pulse oximeters cannot do this and record inappropriately high saturations. Treatment with 100% oxygen decreases Hb-CO half-life from 240 to 40 min and is continued until CO-Hb is <10%. If CO-Hb levels are >30%, hyperbaric oxygen therapy reduces neuropsychiatric sequelae but practical issues often outweigh benefits.
- **Cyanide (CN) poisoning** causes histotoxic hypoxia. Mild poisoning is treated with oxygen and inhaled amyl nitrite, more severe poisoning with sodium thiosulphite (i.e. speeds metabolism) or hydroxycobalamin (i.e. forms inactive complexes).

3 Metabolism and nutrition: increased basal metabolic rate, reflected by fever (~38.5 °C) and hypercapnia, peaks at ~7 days and is proportional to burn size (and infection). High environmental humidity and temperatures (e.g. ~32 °C) reduce heat and water loss. Calculate nutritional requirements from burn size and start early enteral feeding and stress ulcer prophylaxis.

4 Burn wound care and skin grafts: initially cover burns with saline gauze (±cling film). Protect partial thickness burns with biological or synthetic (e.g. Duoderm) dressings. Early excision and split-skin grafting of full thickness burns improves outcome (i.e. survival, infection, pain, healing). Consider transplant or biosynthetic skins for burns >60% BSA. Topical antibiotics (e.g. silver sulphadiazine) reduce early staphylococcal and later pseudomonal colonization.

5 General management issues include:

- **Infection**: the most common cause of death after severe burns (e.g. due to skin barrier loss). Isolation, microbiological surveillance and judicious antibiotic use improve outcome.
- **Analgesia**: intravenous opioids (e.g. morphine) are required initially. Ketamine provides good analgesia for dressing changes when combined with a benzodiazepine. Monitor drug levels because renal and hepatic clearance are altered.
- **Complications** (Figure 76f): circumferential contraction of neck, chest or limb burns can cause ventilatory failure and distal limb ischaemia requiring early escharotomy.

Chemical and electrical burns

- **Chemical burns**: copiously irrigate with water and then treat like thermal burns. In acid or alkali burns, avoid neutralizing solutions because exothermic reactions may cause further thermal damage.
- **Electrical burns** (e.g. lightning, high voltage) produce extensive internal tissue damage and rhabdomyolysis with little external evidence of injury. Exit wounds (e.g. hands, feet) are often overlooked. Monitor for arrhythmias and myocardial injury.

Pearl of wisdom

Beware occult carbon monoxide (CO) poisoning in all burns patients but especially those subject to smoke inhalation in enclosed spaces

Case studies and questions

Case 1

A 68-year-old woman with a history of type II diabetes mellitus, nephropathy and mild renal impairment (creatinine ~130 μmol/L) and recurrent urinary tract infections is admitted to the accident and emergency (A+E) department as an emergency. She has a 24-hour history of fever, dysuria and urinary frequency and her husband reports that she has become progressively more confused during the hours before hospital admission. At admission she is obtunded, flushed, febrile (38.5°C), tachycardic (heart rate 140/min), tachypnoeic (respiratory rate 30/min) and hypotensive with a blood pressure (BP) of 90/50 mmHg and a dilated, hyperdynamic (bounding) circulation. She is tender suprapubically but examination is otherwise unremarkable. A central line is inserted and a 250-ml fluid challenge is given. The central venous pressure (CVP) response is measured (Case Figure 1a).

1 *What initial investigations would you perform?*
2 *How would you resuscitate this patient and what is the relevance of the fluid challenges in Case Figure 1a and the later response in Case Figure 1b?*
3 *When would you start antibiotic therapy?*

This patient is given 4 L of normal saline during her 2 hours in the A+E department, which partially restores her BP to 105/60 mmHg. However, after transfer to HDU, her BP falls to 80/40 mmHg and urine output to <20 ml/h. Further investigation reveals a haemoglobin of 100 g/L, P_aO_2 13 kPa, S_aO_2 98%, $S_{cv}O_2$ 65%, lactate 4 mmol/l and creatinine 190 μmol/L. Her cardiac output by thermodilution measurement is 8.5 L/min and she has a dilated circulation with a low systemic vascular resistance. Despite a further 2 L of gelofusin, the BP remains low but a repeat 250-ml fluid challenge produces the response in Case Figure 1b.

4 *How would you maintain the BP in this patient and what other therapies would you consider?*
5 *What is the oxygen delivery in this patient at the time of admission to HDU and why is the lactate raised?*
6 *The patient is found to have a persisting acidosis and a low urine output despite restoration of normal BP after recovery. How can this be explained?*

Case Figure 1a and Case Figure 1b

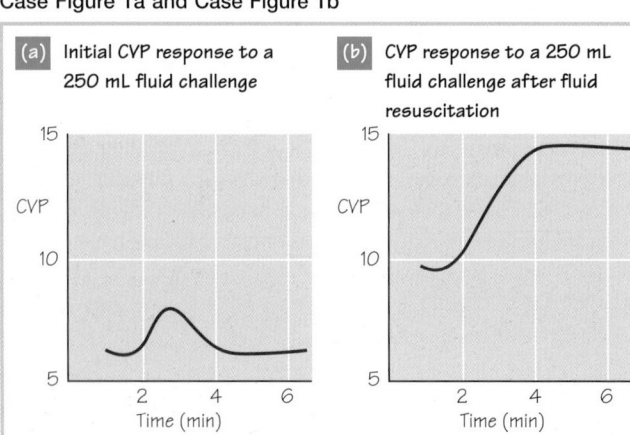

(a) Initial CVP response to a 250 mL fluid challenge

(b) CVP response to a 250 mL fluid challenge after fluid resuscitation

Case 2

Four men have been admitted to HDU with progressive breathlessness and all four have an initial arterial P_aO_2 of 6.6 kPa when breathing air. The first patient is grossly obese, is complaining of a sore throat and an upper respiratory tract infection but has a normal chest radiograph (CXR). Investigation has excluded pulmonary embolism. The second patient with non-specific interstitial pneumonitis has a reduced gas transfer (i.e. mainly diffusion defect), is *on* treatment with steroids and has developed a mild lower respiratory tract infection. The third patient has a true right to left shunt as a result of a long-standing atrial septal defect and, apart from a slightly enlarged heart, has a normal CXR. The fourth patient, a welder who inhaled NO_2 while at work, has developed acute lung injury with widespread alveolar shadowing on CXR. Each patient is to be treated with oxygen. You are the attending physician.

1 *Why is each patient hypoxaemic and what will happen when the F_iO_2 is raised to 1.0 (i.e. 100% oxygen therapy)? Precise answers cannot be calculated but assume reasonable values for unknown data.*
2 *How will you ensure improved oxygenation in each patient?*

Case 3

A 55-year-old man, who is normally healthy but slightly overweight, smokes 15 cigarettes a day and has untreated borderline hypertension, presents to the A+E department with severe epigastric and lower chest pain, nausea, vomiting and profuse sweating. He is currently breathless and reports dizziness. He has been having recurrent indigestion over the last 2 weeks, usually while walking to work but lasting for increasingly long periods before settling spontaneously. Over the past 2 days, he has experienced similar but increasingly severe pain at rest. He takes regular oral antacids with no relief of the pain. The past medical history and review of systems are unremarkable. In particular, he has no history of peptic ulceration, cholecystitis, pancreatitis or diarrhoea. His father had a myocardial infarction (MI) at 65 years old and his brother suffers with angina. On examination, he is in pain, pale and sweaty. He has a heart rate of 55/min and BP of 95/55 mmHg. The heart sounds are normal. The chest is normal with no crepitations. There is no chest wall tenderness or evidence of calf deep venous thrombosis (DVT). Abdominal examination is unremarkable; in particular, there is minimal epigastric tenderness, normal bowel sounds and no melaena on rectal examination.

1 *What is the most likely diagnosis and what is your differential diagnosis?*
2 *What will you do immediately?*
3 *Is pain always a feature of this condition?*
4 *What investigations would you perform to establish the diagnosis in this case?*

The initial electrocardiogram (ECG) demonstrates sinus rhythm with Q-waves, T-wave inversion and ST-elevation in leads II, III and aVF. Subsequent ECGs show intermittent Mobitz I second-

Critical Care Medicine at a Glance, Third Edition. Richard Leach. © 2014 John Wiley & Sons, Ltd. Published 2014 by John Wiley & Sons, Ltd.

degree heart block (Wenckebach phenomenon). The CXR is normal. Troponin T and cardiac enzymes are raised. An echocardiogram shows inferior left ventricular hypokinesia with a reduced ejection fraction.

5 *How would you treat this patient?*

6 *What are the complications of this condition? Does this patient have any and how would you manage them? What is the significance of the hypotension?*

7 *After recovery from the acute condition, what advice and follow-up management is required?*

Case 4

A 65-year-old man presents with severe wheeze and breathlessness after a minor upper respiratory tract infection. He is a long-standing smoker of 20 cigarettes a day and is known to have moderate chronic obstructive pulmonary disease (COPD) (FEV_1 1.2 L, FVC 2.7 L) treated with salbutamol and ipratropium bromide inhalers. In the past, he has had an MI and has echocardiographic evidence of left ventricular impairment with an ejection fraction of 35–40% requiring treatment with cardioselective beta-blockers, angiotensin-converting enzyme (ACE) inhibitors and a small dose of diuretic. He has mild ankle oedema and occasional orthopnoea but the review of systems is otherwise unremarkable. He can normally climb two flights of stairs and is a recently retired porter. On examination he is afebrile, breathless, cyanosed and sweaty. His respiratory rate is 28/min. He has a heart rate of 120/min and BP of 135/90 mmHg. The jugular venous pressure (JVP) is slightly raised at 2–3 cm, the heart sounds are inaudible because of wheeze and there is mild ankle oedema. The chest examination reveals poor air entry bilaterally with widespread wheeze and coarse basal crepitations. His haemoglobin is 160 g/L, white cell count 12×10^{-9}/L, urea 8 mmol/L and creatinine 135 µmol/L. Electrolytes, liver function tests, troponin T and d-dimers are all normal. The ECG shows changes of an old anterior MI. Arterial blood gases (ABGs) on air are pH 7.29, P_aO_2 7.0 kPa, P_aCO_2 8.5 kPa and HCO_3 34 mmol/L. The chest radiograph shows hyperinflation, a large heart, enlarged hila with infiltrative changes in both lower lobes.

1 *What are the two most likely diagnoses and how would you differentiate between them?*

2 *What is the A–a gradient in this patient and what is its relevance?*

3 *How would you manage this case? In particular, discuss oxygen dose, target saturation, ABG frequency, respiratory support and indications for intubation.*

4 *What factors are associated with success or failure of non-invasive ventilation (NIV) and when should NIV be considered to have failed?*

5 *How would you adjust NIV if the P_aCO_2 remained elevated, the P_aO_2 was persistently low or patient ventilator synchronization was poor?*

6 *When would you consider use of continuous positive airways pressure (CPAP) ventilation?*

Case 5

A 58-year-old lady is referred to A+E with a suspected chest infection. After her return from holiday in New Zealand 3 weeks before, she had developed a flu-like illness associated with fever, sore throat and cough that had lasted for a week. Initially she appeared to recover but 3 days ago the fever and cough recurred. Over the past 48 hours, she has developed increasing breathlessness and has deteriorated despite starting antibiotics 24 hours ago. She has no significant past medical history. On arrival in A+E, she is unwell and breathless with a temperature of 37.9 °C, heart rate 120 beats/min, BP 110/65 mmHg, respiratory rate 31/min and S_aO_2 85% on air. Chest examination reveals left-sided upper and lower lobe and occasional right-sided basal coarse crepitations but there is no wheeze. The white cell count is elevated at 15×10^{-9}/L, urea 7.5 mmol/L, creatinine 124 µmol/L and the C-reactive protein (CRP) 94 mg/L at admission, rising to 235 mg/L the following day. The P_aO_2 is 6.6 kPa and P_aCO_2 3.2 kPa on air. An ECG is normal and serology for atypical pneumonias (legionella, mycoplasma) is negative. The CXR at admission (Case Figure 5a[i]) and after 24 hours (Case Figure 5a[ii]) are illustrated. You are the admitting SHO for HDU and are reviewing the patient in A+E.

1 *What is the most likely diagnosis and would you admit this patient to HDU?*

Case Figure 5a CXR at admission (i) and after 24 hours (ii)

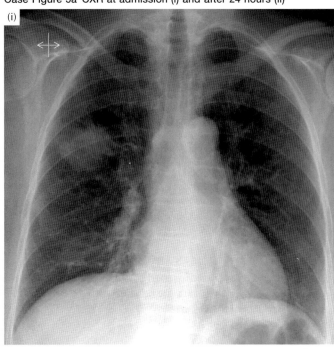
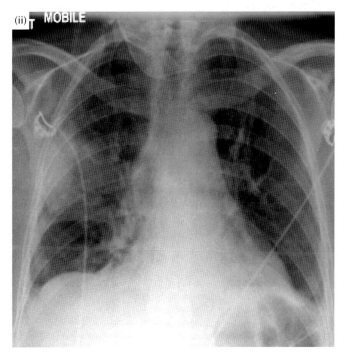

2 *What was the admission A–a gradient in this patient?*

3 *How would you manage this patient and what immediate treatment would you recommend?*

On arrival in HDU, the S_aO_2 is 95% on 60% oxygen therapy but desaturates to 75% when the mask is removed. Overnight, the patient has episodes of confusion and the on-call doctor diagnoses an acute confusional state secondary to pneumonia and treats her with small doses of haloperidol. The confusion resolves and the patient appears to recover. Over the next 48 hours, the patient deteriorates with persisting breathlessness, tachycardia, 'grumbling' fever and hypoxaemia. The nurses report further episodes of confusion and difficulty maintaining S_aO_2 >90% and P_aO_2 >8 kPa despite high-dose oxygen.

4 *Is this patient's severe hypoxaemia consistent with pneumonia and how could this be explained?*

5 *What investigations will help establish the diagnosis?*

6 *In what other ways can this condition present?*

7 *What immediate treatment would you recommend?*

Immediately after her CT scan (Case Figure 5b), the patient deteriorates. She is cold, clammy, cyanosed and confused. The pulse is 'thready', she is hypotensive (BP 90/40 mmHg) and the JVP is raised. She is intubated and transferred to ICU. After initial stabilization, her S_aO_2 is 95% on 100% oxygen, $S_{cv}O_2$ is 65% (right atrial blood sample) and her haemoglobin is 100 g/L. On air the S_aO_2 is 70% and her S_vO_2 40%. Shortly after admission to ICU, she suddenly arrests.

8 *What is the degree of venous admixture (ventilation/perfusion [V/Q] mismatch) and true shunt in this patient after ICU admission?*

9 *What is the likely cause of the arrest and what immediate management would you institute while awaiting the arrest team?*

10 *Would you consider thrombolytic therapy in this patient?*

Case 6

Two young boys (~16 years old) are found collapsed outside a night club at 3.00am in the morning. Both have lacerations to their foreheads, have been drinking alcohol and are confused, agitated

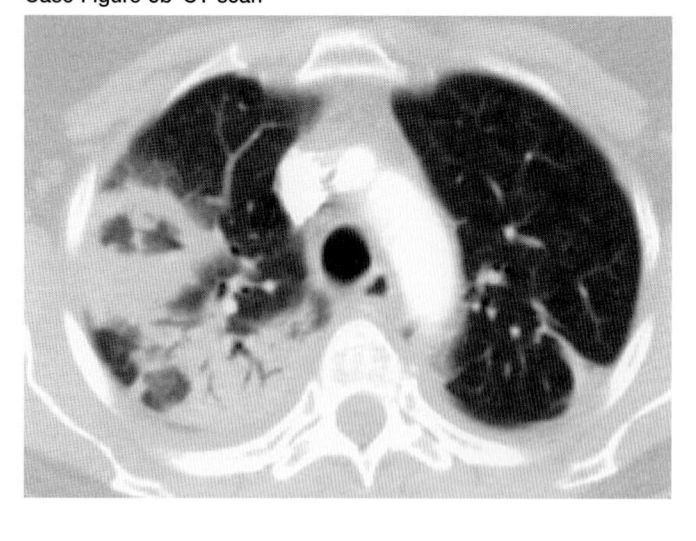

and unresponsive except to painful stimuli. On arrival in A+E, both are tachycardic (120 beats/min), have BPs of 95/50 mmHg and are breathing through unobstructed airways. The first has a respiratory rate of 15 breaths/min, the second 35 breaths/min. Neither has any means of identification.

1 *What test would you perform immediately in both patients?*

2 *In the first patient the result of this test is low. How would you treat him?*

3 *In the second patient the result of this test is high. Why is he hyperventilating and what additional tests would you perform to confirm the diagnosis?*

4 *Having established the diagnosis, how would you treat the second patient and, in particular, what 'pitfalls of management' would you be sure to avoid?*

5 *What are the likely precipitating causes in both patients and what additional tests might you perform?*

6 *What other causes of unconsciousness should be considered in these boys?*

Case studies answers

Case 1: Sepsis with shock

1 Investigation aims to identify the source and cause of the infection (Chapters 24, 25). Routine blood tests, C-reactive protein, coagulation profile, arterial blood gases (ABGs), dipstick urinalysis, electrocardiogram (ECG) and chest radiograph (CXR) should all be performed at admission. Tests that the **sepsis guidelines** recommend, but which are often forgotten, include plasma lactate and central venous (superior vena cava/right atrial) S_aO_2 ($S_{cv}O_2$, e.g. from an internal jugular vein central line), which are measures of global oxygen delivery (Chapter 6). Appropriate cultures including blood, sputum, urine, cerebrospinal fluid (CSF) and wound pus *must* be taken before starting antibiotics, providing this does not delay therapy. At least two blood cultures (≥ 1 drawn percutaneously and one through each vascular access device >48 hours old) are required. Specific investigations including lumbar puncture, ultrasonography and CT scans depend on the likely cause and the patient's condition. In this case, urine dipstick testing revealed haematuria and an elevated nitrite level, and a mid-stream urine examination confirmed an *E.coli* infection.

2 Fluid resuscitation is started *immediately* in patients with hypoperfusion (i.e. lactate >4 mmol/L, raised $S_{cv}O_2$) or hypotension. At the time of admission to HDU, the small transient central venous pressure (CVP) response to the fluid challenge (Case Figure 1a, p. 154, see chapters 3 and 8; figures 3c and 8c) confirms that the patient is still hypovolaemic (Chapter 8). The sepsis guidelines (Chapter 25) recommend crystalloid (1 L) or colloid (0.5 L) fluid challenges aiming to achieve a CVP ≥ 8 mmHg (≥ 12 if ventilated); MAP ≥ 65 mmHg; urine output ≥ 0.5 ml/kg/h; and $S_{cv}O_2$ $\geq 70\%$. If the target $S_{cv}O_2$ is not achieved, consider packed red cell transfusion to a haemocrit $\geq 30\%$ or a dobutamine infusion (max 20 µg/kg/min) to increase oxygen delivery and hence $S_{cv}O_2$. Reduce fluid administration if CVP increases without haemodynamic improvement. In this case, the sustained increase in the CVP to a fluid challenge in Case Figure 1b (p. 154, see chapters 3 and 8; figures 3c and 8c) suggests that the heart is operating at optimal (or even hypervolaemic) filling pressures and is unlikely to benefit from further fluid administration.

3 Antibiotic therapy is started as early as possible in severe sepsis and always within the first hour. It is initially *empiric*, using broad-spectrum agents active against the most likely causative pathogens, and depends on the clinical features, whether community or hospital acquired, the site of primary infection and local antibiotic resistance patterns. Combination therapy is recommended in neutropenic patients and those infected with *Pseudomonas*. Ongoing therapy is modified according to microbiology results and unnecessary antibiotics stopped.

4 In early sepsis, widespread vasodilation (i.e. low systemic vascular resistance [SVR]) causes hypotension and relative hypovolaemia that may respond to fluid administration alone. However, once optimal cardiac filling pressures have been achieved (Case Figure 1b), further fluid resuscitation risks pulmonary oedema. At this stage, norepinephrine (noradrenaline), a vasopressor agent with α-receptor agonist properties, increases SVR and blood pressure (BP). In late sepsis, because toxic myocarditis impairs cardiac contractility, an inotropic agent like dobutamine, often used in combination with norepinephrine, increases both cardiac output and BP (Chapter 12). If hypotension is refractory to fluid and vasopressor support, the possibility of relative adrenocortical insufficiency should be considered. In these patients, low dose steroid therapy (i.e. hydrocortisone 8 mg/h) can be beneficial. In septic shock, activated protein C may improve outcome by modifying microcirculatory thrombosis and preventing organ ischaemia.

5 Oxygen delivery (Do_2; Chapter 5) is calculated from:
  (i) $Do_2 = QT \times C_aO_2 =$ normally ~ 1000 ml/min
where: QT = cardiac output; C_aO_2 = arterial oxygen content.
  (ii) $C_aO_2 = [Hb \times S_aO_2 \times k + (P_aO_2 \times 0.023)] =$ normally ~ 200 mlO$_2$/L
where: Hb = haemoglobin (g/L); k = coefficient of Hb oxygen binding capacity (1.36 ml O_2/g Hb); $P_aO_2 \times 0.023$ = oxygen dissolved in plasma.
In this case:
  (i) $C_aO_2 = 100 \times 0.98 \times 1.36 + (13 \times 0.023) = 133.5$ ml O_2/L
  (ii) $Do_2 = 8.5 \times 133.5 = 1135$ ml/min
Although the Do_2 is greater than normal in this patient at 1135 ml/min, the hypotension, relative hypovolaemia and associated inappropriate distribution of cardiac output can cause regional (i.e. splanchnic, renal, skeletal) ischaemia resulting in raised lactate and in some cases low $S_{cv}O_2$. Inadequate hepatic lactate clearance in liver dysfunction or failure of oxygen utilization due to mitochondrial dysfunction in sepsis are also causes of a raised lactate.

6 This patient was initially resuscitated with large volumes of normal saline to correct sepsis-induced hypotension. She had previous chronic renal impairment due to diabetic nephropathy, and a degree of 'hypotension-induced pre-renal' acute kidney injury (Chapter 45) indicated by the reduced urine output and the increasing creatinine (190 µmol/L) on this occasion. A litre of normal saline contains 154 mmol NaCl or 308 (154 mmol Na^+ + 154 mmol Cl^-) mosmol of solute; so 4 L of normal saline will contain 1232 mosmol of solute. Normal kidneys can achieve a maximum urine concentration of 1000 mosmol/L but much less in renal impairment (i.e. 500 mosmol/L). Consequently, this large solute load (e.g. sodium, chloride) would be difficult to excrete (Chapters 9, 11), particularly with the reduced urine production. This causes hyperchloraemic acidosis (HCA) due to the high chloride (Cl^-) level and may have explained the persisting acidosis in this case. In this situation, the preferred fluid is a physiologically balanced solution (PBS) with low Cl^- content like Hartmann's. This is inexpensive and, compared with normal saline, causes less HCA and associated nausea, confusion and oliguria.

Case 2: Oxygenation and oxygen therapy
Patient 1

1 This patient has a mild upper respiratory tract infection and no significant low respiratory tract pathology. However, he is probably hypoventilating because of gross obesity restricting normal respiratory movement. Assuming his gas transfer and ventilation/

Critical Care Medicine at a Glance, Third Edition. Richard Leach. © 2014 John Wiley & Sons, Ltd. Published 2014 by John Wiley & Sons, Ltd.

perfusion (V/Q) matching are normal, his $P_a\text{CO}_2$ can be calculated from the alveolar gas equation (Chapter 13):

$$P_A\text{O}_2 = P_I\text{O}_2 - (1.25 \times P_a\text{CO}_2)$$

where: $P_I\text{O}_2 = F_I\text{O}_2 \times$ (barometric – water vapour pressure) = $P_I\text{O}_2 = 0.21 \times (101 - 6.2) = 19.9\,\text{kPa}$ breathing air

Note: $1.25 \times P_a\text{CO}_2$ is a simplified expression of $P_a\text{CO}_2/R$ where R is the respiratory quotient ($V_{\text{CO}_2}/V_{\text{O}_2} = \sim 0.75$).

In this case $P_a\text{CO}_2$ must be 10.6 kPa if $P_a\text{O}_2$ is 6.6 kPa on air (and thus $P_A\text{O}_2$ 6.6 kPa):

i.e. $P_A\text{O}_2 = 6.6 = 19.9 - (P_a\text{CO}_2 \times 1.25)$ thus $P_a\text{CO}_2 = 10.6$ kPa.

Therefore, this patient has Type 2 respiratory failure with a raised $P_a\text{CO}_2$ (Chapter 14).

On 100% O_2 ($F_I\text{O}_2$ 1.0):

$P_I\text{O}_2 = F_I\text{O}_2 \times$ (barometric pressure – water vapour pressure)

$= 1 \times (101 - 6.2)$

$= 95\,\text{kPa}.$

$$P_A\text{O}_2 = P_I\text{O}_2 - (1.25 \times P_a\text{CO}_2)$$
$$P_A\text{O}_2 = 95 - (1.25 \times 10.6) = 95 - 13 = 82\,\text{kPa}$$

Thus $P_a\text{O}_2$ will be about 81 kPa.

2 This patient has Type 2 respiratory failure (i.e. hypoxaemia drives ventilation not $P_a\text{CO}_2$). As $P_a\text{O}_2$ rises with increasing oxygen therapy, the drive to breathe decreases and $P_a\text{CO}_2$ increases causing progressive respiratory acidosis, confusion, coma and death. Consequently, this patient should be managed with low dose (24–28%) oxygen therapy aiming for a saturation of 88–92% and regular measurement of ABGs (Chapters 14, 41). The optimal treatment to improve both oxygenation and to reduce hypercarbia in this patient would be non-invasive ventilation (NIV) to improve ventilation and alveolar gas exchange (Chapter 16).

Patient 2

1 This patient has a diffusion defect due to the interstitial lung disease (ILD) although usually there is a significant contribution of V/Q mismatch to the hypoxaemia in these patients. The substantial increase in alveolar partial pressure ($P_A\text{O}_2 = P_I\text{O}_2$) – $(1.25 \times P_a\text{CO}_2)$; $P_A\text{O}_2 = 95 - (1.25 \times 4) = 90$ kPa) when this patient is given 100% oxygen ($F_I\text{O}_2$ 1.0), this will more than overcome the partial diffusion defect associated with the ILD, and if this were a pure diffusion defect the $P_a\text{O}_2$ would approach 90 kPa. Even allowing for a wider than normal range of V/Q ratios in this patient, there would still be a substantial increase in $P_a\text{O}_2$ on 100% oxygen.

2 In this patient, simply increasing the inspired oxygen concentration ($F_I\text{O}_2$ $\sim$0.4–0.6) will correct the hypoxaemia. This patient probably has Type 1 respiratory failure because carbon dioxide (CO_2) diffuses 20 times better than oxygen and consequently the diffusion defect does not impair CO_2 clearance. The hypoxaemia will cause hyperventilation and the associated increase in minute ventilation ensures a low $P_a\text{CO}_2$ ($P_a\text{CO}_2 \propto$ 1/alveolar ventilation). Consequently, there is little risk of hypercapnia during use of high oxygen concentrations in this patient.

Patient 3

1 This patient is hypoxaemic due to right to left shunting causing admixture of venous blood to systemic blood. As in the second case, the $P_A\text{O}_2$ will be 90 kPa with an $F_I\text{O}_2$ of 1.0. However, the saturation is already 100% in oxygenated blood passing through the lungs and oxygen content will not be substantially increased by the high $P_A\text{O}_2$ apart from the small quantity of oxygen dissolved in blood (90×0.023 ml). The blood shunted from right to left through the atrial septal defect remains unaffected by the increased $P_A\text{O}_2$ and acts as venous admixture lowering oxygenation in the

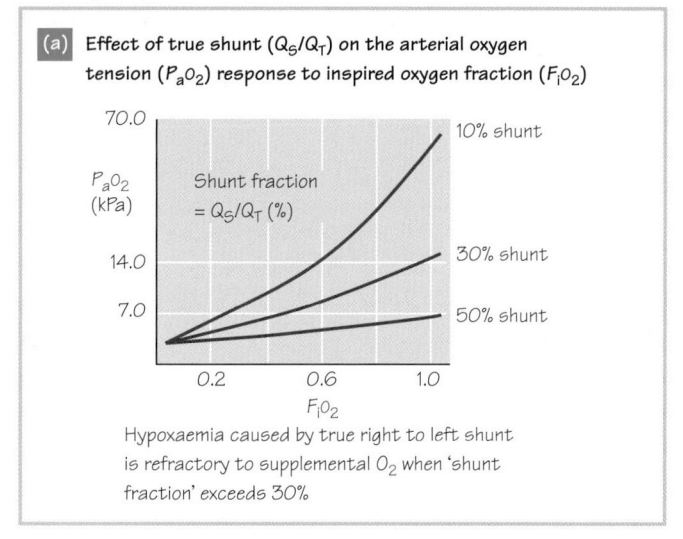

(a) Effect of true shunt (Q_S/Q_T) on the arterial oxygen tension ($P_a\text{O}_2$) response to inspired oxygen fraction ($F_I\text{O}_2$)

Hypoxaemia caused by true right to left shunt is refractory to supplemental O_2 when 'shunt fraction' exceeds 30%

systemic circulation. Consequently, an $F_I\text{O}_2$ of 1.0 only fractionally increases systemic $P_a\text{O}_2$ perhaps to $\sim$7.5 kPa in this case.

2 Only patient 3 will not show a substantial increase in $P_a\text{O}_2$ when given 100% O_2. In this case, oxygenation will only be improved by decreasing the shunt fraction and reducing left-sided venous admixture. Case Figure 2a illustrates the effect of true shunt on the response to increasing $F_I\text{O}_2$.

Patient 4

1 This patient has acute lung injury with alveolar oedema due to alveolar epithelial damage and atelectasis caused by loss of surfactant. A wider than normal range of V/Q ratios will be present throughout the lungs and the resulting V/Q mismatch causes hypoxaemia. Nevertheless the $F_I\text{O}_2$ of 1.0 will ensure a sufficiently high $P_A\text{O}_2$ even in low V/Q units to substantially increase $P_a\text{O}_2$. However, true shunt and units with a very low V/Q ratio cause hypoxaemia that is resistant to correction with increased $F_I\text{O}_2$.

2 In this patient, an increase in inspired oxygen concentration ($F_I\text{O}_2$ $\sim$0.4–0.6) will improve arterial oxygenation. However, there are a number of other strategies that may improve oxygenation in this case. First, NIV with continuous positive airways pressure (CPAP; Chapter 16) will reinflate collapsed (atelectatic) alveoli, reducing V/Q mismatch which improves oxygenation. Second, reducing alveolar oedema by avoiding excessive fluid administration ($\pm$gentle diuresis, $\pm$lowering pulmonary circulation hydrostatic pressure) will improve alveolar ventilation, reduce V/Q match and increase arterial oxygenation. Third, prone positioning may improve oxygenation in severe acute lung injury because oedema and perfusion are greatest in dependent lung. Turning the patient prone ensures perfusion of ventilated non-dependent lung that is now dependent (Chapter 42). Finally, inhaled nitric oxide dilates capillaries supplying ventilated alveoli (but not unventilated alveoli), tending to improve V/Q matching. However, although nitric oxide improves oxygenation in the short term, it can form toxic oxygen radicals that may eventually cause further damage to alveolar epithelium with increasing alveolar oedema. There is no evidence that nitric oxide improves outcome in severe acute lung injury (Chapter 42).

Case 3: Inferior myocardial infarction (MI)

1 The sudden onset of severe pain, nausea, bradycardia, reduced cardiac output (i.e. pale, sweaty and hypotensive) and absence of melaena and abdominal tenderness suggests that the most likely cause of this patient's symptoms is cardiac. Although the pain is epigastric (i.e. referred abdominal discomfort), this is often the case with inferior myocardial ischaemia and may be misinterpreted as abdominal pathology. The patient is a smoker with borderline hypertension and a family history of ischaemic heart disease (IHD) and the most likely diagnosis is myocardial ischaemia or MI. However, other causes of chest or epigastric pain that mimic myocardial ischaemia include reflux oesophagitis, peptic ulceration, oesophageal spasm, cholecystitis, costochondritis, anterior pleurisy, pericarditis and pulmonary embolism. A careful history and examination will often, but not always, differentiate the potential causes and further investigation may be required. In this case, a bleeding peptic ulcer with hypovolaemia and shock should have been considered, although a tachycardia would have been expected. Bradycardia (heart rate 55/min) is a common feature of inferior myocardial ischaemia because the atrioventricular node is usually supplied by the right coronary artery.

2 If a diagnosis of myocardial ischaemia or MI is suspected, the patient should be given aspirin 300 mg immediately. Within 15 minutes of chewing a non-enteric aspirin tablet, irreversible cyclo-oxygenase inhibition prevents platelet aggregation, and in unstable angina reduces deaths from MI by 50%. Antiplatelet agents that inhibit glycoprotein IIb/IIIa are useful in patients with aspirin allergy but the onset of action is slow. Ideally, the aspirin should be given before transfer to hospital.

3 Myocardial ischaemia normally causes 'crushing' or heavy substernal chest pain radiating to the neck and medial aspect of the left arm. However, pain associated with myocardial ischaemia may be atypical (i.e. burning), localized (i.e. jaw, left arm or epigastric only) or completely absent in ~20% of patients (e.g. diabetics). MI is characterized by an abrupt onset of severe, prolonged pain, autonomic symptoms, dyspnoea and anxiety. Angina (i.e. reversible myocardial ischaemia) is usually precipitated by exercise or anxiety, is short-lived and relieved by rest or sublingual nitrates. In this case the indigestion while walking to work was suggestive of angina. This was followed by unstable angina, which refers to anginal pain occurring at rest, more frequently and for longer periods (>15 minutes). It is characterized by 'altered angina pattern' (i.e. with less exercise), 'a change in the character of previous anginal pain', autonomic manifestations (e.g. nausea, sweating) and radiation to new sites (e.g. jaw, arm). However, unstable angina only precedes MI in ~25% of cases (Chapters 30, 31).

4 Serial ECGs and cardiac enzymes usually establish the diagnosis of myocardial ischaemia. A raised cardiac troponin T (CTT) is particularly useful and confirms MI after surgery or when the ECG is non-specific (i.e. >40% of MI are non-Q wave). In non-MI acute coronary syndromes (e.g. unstable angina), a raised CTT indicates an increased risk of subsequent MI (Chapter 31). A CXR will exclude other causes of chest pain and detect pulmonary oedema due to left ventricular failure following an MI. Echocardiography, although not often required immediately, establishes the degree of cardiac muscle impairment (i.e. ejection fraction) and excludes potential complications (e.g. papillary muscle rupture). The need for immediate angiography and percutaneous coronary angioplasty is discussed below.

5 This patient has had an inferior MI as confirmed by the raised troponin T and the ECG findings in leads II, III and aVF. The development of Mobitz type I, second-degree heart block suggests atrioventricular node (AVN) ischaemia.

Immediate management aims to reperfuse ischaemic tissue and minimize MI size, which reduces hospital mortality from 13%

to <10%. Initial management includes bed rest, pain relief, cardiac monitoring (~48 hours) and >60% oxygen. Aspirin prevents further platelet aggregation. Opiates (e.g. diamorphine) relieve anxiety and chest pain. They also improve cardiac output and reduce or prevent pulmonary oedema by reducing preload. Sublingual nitrates reduce chest pain and preload but often aggravate hypotension. Early beta-blockade (e.g. bisoprolol) limit infarct size, arrhythmias and mortality but contraindications include asthma, heart failure and bradycardia.

Revascularization with reperfusion of ischaemic myocardium limits tissue damage and reduces future complications (e.g. heart failure, arrhythmias).

(i) ***Percutaneous coronary intervention*** (PCI) within ≤90 minutes of presentation is the preferred method of revascularization following MI if the facilities are available. Primary PCI within 6 hours reopens >90% of occluded coronary arteries with few complications and has the best outcomes. Rescue PCI is considered if thrombolytic therapy fails but has a relatively high mortality (~40%) if unsuccessful.

(ii) **Thrombolytic therapy** (TT) clears coronary artery clot and reduces mortality by more than 25% if therapy occurs within 12 hours but it is more effective within 3 hours. Reperfusion occurs in 50–75% of cases. TT accelerates conversion of plasminogen to plasmin, an enzyme that attacks fibrin. Consequently it increases the risk of haemorrhage and contraindications (e.g. peptic ulceration, stroke) prevent use in many cases. The thrombolytic agent streptokinase is allergenic and can only be used once. About 2% of patients have reactions (e.g. hypotension, pruritus) with the first use. Tissue plasminogen activator (TPA) is more expensive but only activates plasminogen bound to fibrin (i.e. better targeted at thrombus). If given within 3 hours, it is more effective than streptokinase but surprisingly causes more strokes. TPA is given if streptokinase has been used previously. Intravenous heparin is required for 48–72 hours after TPA because of its short half-life and fibrin specificity.

Angiotensin-converting enzyme (ACE) inhibitors, orally, should be started 24 hours after admission and reduce heart failure in high-risk patients. Unless contraindicated, prophylactic subcutaneous heparin prevents thromboembolic complications. Prophylactic antiarrhythmic therapy is not recommended but arrhythmias must be treated as required (see heart block later). Inotropic support may be required in patients with cardiogenic shock.

6 Complications after MI include arrhythmias (e.g. atrial fibrillation, ventricular tachycardia), papillary muscle or free wall rupture, pericarditis, cardiac aneurysms and ventricular septal defects. Heart failure can occur when >20% of the left ventricle is damaged and is characterized by breathlessness and pulmonary oedema on CXR. Cardiac auscultation often reveals a fourth heart sound and gallop rhythm. Hypotension (systolic BP <90 mmHg), particularly with anterior ischaemia, suggests a large MI (i.e. >40% left ventricular damage) and heralds cardiogenic shock and the need for resuscitation (±inotropic support). Prophylactic anticoagulation is required in immobile patients who are at risk of DVT and in patients with large infarcts who are at risk of developing intracardiac thrombus and embolic sequela (e.g. stroke) in areas of akinetic cardiac muscle.

Bradycardia (±heart block) is more frequent after inferior MI. This is because the right coronary artery supplies the AVN and surrounding conducting tissue, as well as the inferior part of the heart. Although bradycardia and heart block are common after inferior MI, they are usually transient and rarely require intervention. By contrast, tachycardia usually accompanies anterior MI, and heart block in these patients suggests a particularly large infarct and requires early pacemaker insertion. In this case, second-degree heart block followed the MI. This occurs when some atrial beats are not conducted to the ventricles. *Mobitz 1 AVN block* (Wenkebach) causes progressive PR interval lengthening, culminating in failure of transmission of an atrial impulse. This sequence is repetitive. Treatment is rarely required. *Mobitz II block* originates below the AVN in the His–Purkinje system. Every second or third atrial impulse initiates ventricular contraction (2:1; 3:1 block). In this situation, pacemaker insertion may be required (e.g. following an anterior MI) because symptoms or complete heart block may follow (Chapter 33).

7 Risk factors must be reduced following recovery from the initial MI. Hypertension, hypercholesterolaemia and diabetes mellitus are treated and smoking cessation is strongly encouraged. The family history of IHD in this patient suggests the possibility of familial hypercholesterolaemia and cholesterol levels should be checked and followed up in other family members. Patients with IHD should be treated with lipid-lowering drugs (e.g. statins) to reduce the risk of future ischaemic episodes. Patients with unstable angina or at high risk of MI on exercise testing should be referred for angiography and early revascularization procedures (e.g. angioplasty, surgical coronary artery bypass grafting). Warfarin is administered for 3-months after a large, usually anterior MI, to prevent mural clot forming on akinetic heart wall and embolizing into the systemic circulation causing strokes, ischaemic legs or bowel. Aspirin should be continued indefinitely but beta-blockers and ACE inhibitors may be discontinued after 6–52 weeks in low-risk patients (Chapter 31).

Case 4: COPD and Type 2 respiratory failure

1 Clinically the history and examination suggest an infective exacerbation of chronic obstructive pulmonary disease (COPD) with Type 2 respiratory failure. The raised bicarbonate on ABG analysis suggests an acute on chronic increase in P_aCO_2. Peak expiratory flow rate (PEFR) and lung function testing will aid the diagnosis of COPD. However, this patient also has a previous history of left ventricular failure (LVF) and the clinical features of pulmonary oedema can be surprisingly difficult to differentiate from COPD (Chapter 34). **B-type natriuretic peptide (BNP)** has been particularly useful in detecting heart failure in patients with lung disease, especially when combined with echocardiography (Chapter 34). Most BNP is released from the ventricular myocardium. The serum BNP level, and its breakdown product NT-BNP, increases during myocardial wall stress and major studies demonstrate a high sensitivity (73–99%) and specificity (60–97%) for heart failure. Occasionally, invasive measurements of pulmonary artery wedge pressure and cardiac output may be required to confirm the diagnosis of heart failure (Chapter 3). Alternatively, a trial of therapy (e.g. diuretic) is less invasive and often the most effective means to establish or exclude the presence of pulmonary oedema.

2 The alveolar–arterial (A–a) gradient is calculated from the difference between the alveolar oxygen partial pressure and the arterial blood oxygen partial pressure (Chapter 13).

Alveolar oxygen tension (P_AO_2) is calculated from the simplified alveolar gas equation:

$$P_AO_2 = P_IO_2 - (1.25 \times P_aCO_2)$$

where P_IO_2 is the inspired oxygen partial pressure corrected for barometric pressure and water vapour pressure:

$$P_IO_2 = F_iO_2 \times (\text{barometric pressure (kPa)} -$$
$$\text{water vapour pressure (kPa)})$$

Thus: breathing air:

$$P_IO_2 = 0.21 \times (101 - 6.2) = 19.9 \text{ kPa}$$

Thus:

$$P_AO_2 (\text{breathing air}) = 19.9 - (1.25 \times 8.5)$$
$$= 19.9 - 10.63 = 9.3 \text{ kPa}$$

The alveolar — arterial oxygen tension difference is

$$P_{(A-a)}O_2 = P_AO_2 - P_aO_2 = 9.3 - 7.5 = 1.8 \text{ kPa}$$

The A–a gradient determines efficiency of gas exchange. By incorporating P_ACO_2 into the alveolar gas equation, it is possible to determine when hypoventilation or hypercapnia are the cause of hypoxaemia (i.e. a high P_ACO_2 lowers P_AO_2). Shunts, V/Q mismatch and diffusion impairment increase the A–a gradient. The normal A–a gradient is ~0.2–0.4 kPa but increases with age and F_iO_2. In this case, although the P_aO_2 is 7.5 kPa, the A–a gradient is only 1.8 kPa, indicating that a large component of the hypoxaemia is due to hypercapnia or hypoventilation rather than V/Q mismatch or shunt, and suggests that improving alveolar ventilation (i.e. bronchodilation, use of NIV) is important.

3 In patients with Type 2 respiratory failure, low-dose oxygen therapy should be delivered through fixed performance, Venturi masks aiming for a target saturation of 88–92% (Chapters 13, 14). A higher S_aO_2 has no advantages, but, in chronically hypoxaemic patients dependent on hypoxic ventilatory drive, it can instigate hypoventilation, further hypercapnia and respiratory acidosis. Recheck ABG at 1 hour after starting oxygen therapy and at regular intervals while on oxygen, particularly after oxygen dose changes. In the absence of an air compressor, nebulizers are driven with oxygen but only for 6 minutes to limit the risk of further hypercapnic respiratory failure. NIV should be considered in hypercapnic ($P_aCO_2 > 6$ kPa) patients with acidosis (pH < 7.35), especially if the acidosis has persisted for over 30 minutes despite appropriate treatment (Chapter 16). Venturi masks can be changed to nasal cannulae at low flow rates 1–2 L/min when the patient is stable. High-dose, aerosolized beta-agonists and anticholinergic bronchodilators and short courses of oral corticosteroids (i.e. 30 mg/ day for 10 days) improve symptoms, gas exchange, lung function and aid recovery. Antibiotic therapy is directed at likely organisms (e.g. *H. influenzae*) and adjusted according to microbiological results (Chapter 41). Indications for intubation include a RR >35/min, $P_aO_2 < 8$ kPa on >50% F_iO_2; $P_aCO_2 > 7.5$ kPa, pH < 7.25, decreased conscious level (Glasgow Coma Scale [GCS] <8), inadequate secretion clearance, exhaustion and failure to improve within 1–4 hours with NIV (Chapters 13, 16).

4 Factors associated with successful NIV include a high P_aCO_2, pH 7.3-7.35, improvement in pH, low A–a gradient, reducing P_aCO_2 and respiratory rate within 1 hour of NIV, and good conscious level. Factors associated with failure of NIV include pneumonia on CXR, pH < 7.25-7.3, poor nutritional status, impaired consciousness, copious secretions and poor mask fit. Benefit from NIV is usually evident at 1 hour and certainly after 4–6 hours of NIV. The point at which treatment is considered to have failed and should be withdrawn depends on severity of respiratory failure, patient's wishes and whether other factors (e.g. secretions) could be better managed following intubation (Chapter 16).

5 If the P_aCO_2 remains elevated on NIV, the inspiratory positive airways pressure (IPAP) should be increased or expiratory positive airways pressure (EPAP) decreased (Chapter 41), both of which will raise inspiratory pressure support, increasing tidal volume and alveolar minute ventilation with improved CO_2 clearance ($P_aCO_2 \propto$ 1/alveolar ventilation). A persistently low P_aO_2 on NIV can be corrected by raising F_iO_2 or by increasing either IPAP or EPAP, both

of which will encourage alveolar recruitment and improve ventilation (Chapter 41). Patient–ventilator synchronization can be optimized by ensuring a good mask fit, adjusting the trigger sensitivity and setting EPAP to overcome auto-PEEP, thus reducing the effort of triggering the ventilator (Chapter 41, Figure 41d[iii]).

6 CPAP primarily encourages alveolar recruitment, reduces V/Q mismatch and improves oxygenation. Consequently, it is most effective in those conditions associated with alveolar atelectasis or oedema including cardiogenic pulmonary oedema and acute lung injury (Chapter 16). CPAP does not assist inspiration (i.e. ventilation), although by preventing alveolar collapse and increasing the functional residual capacity it may reduce the work of breathing by making the lungs easier to inflate (i.e. the steep upstroke of the lung pressure–volume relationship). In obstructive sleep apnoea, it can prevent upper airways collapse.

Case 5: Community-acquired pneumonia and pulmonary embolism

1 On the basis of the past history of an upper respiratory tract infection with subsequent fever, cough, crepitations on chest examination, raised white cell count and C-reactive protein (CRP) and consolidation on the CXR, the most likely diagnosis appears to be community-acquired pneumonia (CAP). The relatively normal CXR in comparison to the clinical findings at admission is sometimes seen with atypical pneumonias but this was subsequently excluded in this case. The most likely infecting organism is *Streptococcus pneumoniae*, although secondary staphylococcal chest infections often follow influenza (Chapter 38). On the basis of the vital signs alone, the 'Patient at Risk' (PAR) score in this patient is >6 (at least 9), indicating the need for management in a high dependency area (Chapter 1). The CURB-65 score for assessing CAP severity was 2 (respiratory rate >30, urea >7 mmol/L), suggesting the need for hospital admission but not necessarily HDU. However, in this case the hypoxaemia, raised white cell count and multilobar involvement on clinical examination would alert the clinician to the potential severity of the CAP (Chapter 38).

2 The A–a gradient is calculated from the difference between the alveolar oxygen partial pressure and the arterial blood oxygen partial pressure (Chapter 13).

Alveolar oxygen tension ($P_A O_2$) is calculated from the simplified alveolar gas equation:

$$P_A O_2 = P_I O_2 - (1.25 \times P_a CO_2)$$

where $P_I O_2$ is the inspired oxygen partial pressure corrected for barometric pressure and water vapour pressure:

$$P_I O_2 = F_I O_2 \times (\text{barometric pressure (kPa)}$$
$$- \text{water vapour pressure (kPa)})$$

Thus: breathing air:

$$P_I O_2 = 0.21 \times (101 - 6.2) = 19.9 \text{ kPa}$$

Thus:

$$P_A O_2 \text{(breathing air)} = 19.9 - (1.25 \times 5.3) = \sim 13.5 \text{ kPa}$$

The alveolar − arterial oxygen tension difference is:

$$P_{(A-a)} O_2 = P_A O_2 - P_a O_2$$

(in this case $P_a O_2$ is 6.6 kPa at admission on air)

$$= \sim 13.5 - 6.6 = 6.9 \text{ kPa}$$

The A–a gradient differentiates between hypoxaemia due to: (i) hypoventilation and alveolar hypercapnia (i.e. a high $P_A co_2$ lowers $P_A O_2$); and (ii) V/Q mismatch, shunt or diffusion impairment (Chapter 13). In this case, the A–a gradient is 6.9 kPa (normally <1 kPa) indicating that V/Q mismatch, shunt or diffusion impair-

ment are the principal causes of the hypoxaemia, and treatment must be aimed at these defects rather than improving ventilation.

3 This patient was admitted to the HDU with high flow oxygen therapy and physiotherapy to aid expectoration (Chapters 14, 19). As recommended by the British Thoracic Society guidelines for the management of CAP (Chapter 38), the patient was treated with high-dose intravenous antibiotics to cover *Streptococcus pneumoniae* (e.g. cefuroxime) and atypical organisms (e.g. clarithromycin). As the patient was immobile, prophylactic low molecular weight heparin (LMWH) was started as prophylaxis against venous thromboembolism. Although NIV can be used in patients with pneumonia, it is less effective than when used in acute hypercapnic failure and some studies suggest it may be associated with a worse outcome than early mechanical ventilation (Chapter 16).

4 Although severe hypoxaemia due to V/Q mismatch can occur with pneumonia, in this case the severity of the hypoxaemia and respiratory failure appeared disproportionate to the presenting clinical features (e.g. CXR). Similarly, the failure to improve with high-dose antibiotics over the first 48 hours raised the possibility of alternative diagnoses like pulmonary embolism (PE), heart failure and acute lung injury. PE should be considered in all hypoxaemic patients with a normal or near normal CXR. The air travel from New Zealand and the intermittent episodes of increased hypoxaemia and confusion also suggest PE (Chapter 36) in this case.

5 ABG abnormalities are common after PE including hypoxaemia with widening of the A–a gradient, hypoxaemia and hypocapnia (despite increased dead space). In the majority of patients, the ECG is not helpful and shows non-specific ST segment changes. However, ~30% of patients with large PE develop a right ventricular strain pattern with the classical changes of an S wave in lead I and a Q wave and T wave inversion in lead III ($S_1 Q_3 T_3$ pattern), right axis deviation and right bundle branch block. Most patients have non-specific abnormalities on CXR including atelectasis due to reduced surfactant production in areas of poorly perfused lung. The presence of a lower limb deep venous thrombosis (DVT) should be sought with a Doppler ultrasound scan (or impedance plethysmography). Echocardiography may show right ventricular dysfunction and pulmonary hypertension. A transoesophageal echocardiograph may detect PE in the main pulmonary arteries but not in lobar or segmental arteries.

Spiral CT pulmonary angiograms (CTPAs) are increasingly the initial investigation of choice, particularly in patients with CXR abnormalities (as in this case). They have a sensitivity for PE of 70–95% (higher for more proximal emboli) and a specificity >90%. They also allow visualization of parenchymal abnormalities and are useful in patients with COPD or extensive CXR abnormalities when V/Q scanning will be indeterminate (Chapter 36). In less severe cases with a normal CXR, a V/Q scan may be the initial diagnostic investigation. A negative perfusion scan rules out a PE whereas a 'high probability' scan (i.e. multiple segmental perfusion defects and associated normal ventilation) has a >85% probability of a PE. With a high clinical suspicion, a high probability V/Q scan has a positive predictive value >95%. Unfortunately, most V/Q scans are not diagnostic or are indeterminate with a 15–50% likelihood of PE, necessitating further imaging. Absence of a DVT combined with a low probability V/Q scan permits withholding treatment whereas a negative Doppler ultrasound scan with an intermediate probability V/Q scan (or underlying cardiac or pulmonary disease) necessitates further imaging. Pulmonary angiography remains the diagnostic standard but is invasive.

6 Patients with PE may present with pleuritic pain and haemoptysis in about 65% of cases, isolated dyspnoea in about 25% and circulatory collapse in ~10% of cases. Dyspnoea is not present in ~30% of patients with confirmed PE. Other non-specific features include apprehension, tachypnoea, tachycardia, cough, sweating and syncope. Following a large PE, features of right ventricular failure (e.g. hypotension, jugular venous distension) may occur.

7 Anticoagulation stops propagation of existing lower limb thrombus and allows organization of the remaining clot, which reduces the risk of further PE. Immediate therapy in patients with a high suspicion of a PE prevents further life-threatening emboli. Unfractionated heparin (UFH) or low molecular weight heparin (LMWH) for 5–7 days, is followed by warfarin for 4–6 weeks when temporary risk factors (air travel in this case) are the cause and 3–6 months in idiopathic cases. UFH and warfarin must be monitored, because subtherapeutic levels increase the risk of recurrent PE. LMWH is more bioavailable and does not require monitoring. About 20% of patients with thromboembolic disease have inherited or acquired hypercoagulation problems (e.g. antithrombin III deficiency, protein C deficiency, lupus anticoagulant) and may require lifelong therapy. If contraindications prevent anticoagulation (e.g. recent surgery, haemorrhagic stroke, central nervous system metastases) or PE occurs while on therapeutic anticoagulation, an inferior vena cava filter may prevent further PE.

8 Venous admixture (Q_S/Q_T) can be calculated from the S_aO_2 (70% or 0.7) and S_vO_2 (40% or 0.4) on air and the haemoglobin concentration as illustrated in Chapter 13.

$$Q_S/Q_T = (C_cO_2 - C_aO_2)/(C_cO_2 - C_VO_2)$$

$$\text{when } C_{c,a,v}O_2 = [(Hb \times S_aO_2 \times k) + (P_aO_2 \times 0.023)]$$

C denotes oxygen content and c, a and v denote end capillary, arterial and venous (note that end capillary and calculated alveolar oxygen tensions are assumed to be equivalent; thus on air end capillary S_aO_2 is expected to be 0.98); Hb = haemoglobin (g/L); k = coefficient of Hb oxygen binding capacity (1.36 ml O_2/g Hb); $P_aO_2 \times 0.023$ = oxygen dissolved in plasma (usually so small as to be insignificant).

Thus:

$$Q_S/Q_T = ([100 \times 0.98 \times 1.36] - [100 \times 0.70 \times 1.36])/$$

$$([100 \times 0.98 \times 1.36] - [100 \times 0.4 \times 1.36])$$

$$= (133 - 95)/(133 - 54) = 38/79 = 0.48$$

$$= \textbf{48\% venous admixture}$$

'True shunt' (i.e. corrected for partial V/Q mismatch) is calculated from the S_aO_2 (95%) and S_vO_2 (65%) when on 100% oxygen (i.e. F_iO_2 1.0). (Note that end capillary S_aO_2 would be expected to be 100% or 1.0 on 100% oxygen).

Thus:

$$Q_S/Q_T = ([100 \times 1 \times 1.36] - [100 \times 0.95 \times 1.36])/$$

$$([100 \times 1 \times 1.36] - [100 \times 0.65 \times 1.36])$$

$$= (136 - 129)/(136 - 88) = 7/48 = 0.15$$

$$= \textbf{15\% true shunt}$$

9 The CT scan in Case Figure 1b, (p. 156) demonstrates consolidation consistent with pneumonia and also shows a cavitating wedge infarct following a PE in a left segmental pulmonary artery. A single, sudden, large PE with marked obstruction of pulmonary blood flow is the likely cause of the cardiac arrest. In general, circulatory collapse occurs with >50% obstruction of the pulmonary arterial bed. Smaller emboli may be fatal when pre-existing lung or heart disease co-exist. Cardiopulmonary resuscitation must be started immediately. The cardiac massage may help break up a large clot into smaller segments that travel distally and reduce the degree of pulmonary bed occlusion. Following intubation high-dose oxygen must be administered. Immediate plasma expanders and inotropic support are often given in an attempt to increase right ventricular pressure and to displace clot distally, but risk severe right ventricular distension and subsequent myocardial damage.

10 Thrombolytic therapy is recommended in severe life-threatening massive PE with cardiovascular collapse. Thrombolytics hasten resolution of perfusion defects and correct right ventricular dysfunction but there is limited evidence of survival benefit. Nevertheless, thrombolytic therapy would be appropriate in this patient with life-threatening cardiovascular collapse. In patients without massive PE, there is no survival benefit with thrombolysis and there is a substantial increase in bleeding complications, including a 0.3–1.5% risk of intracerebral haemorrhage. Consequently thrombolysis is not recommended in these patients. This patient was thrombolysed and survived.

Case 6: Diabetic emergencies

1 A bedside blood sugar (BS) level must be checked at admission in every confused, agitated or unconscious patient. The brain is dependent on glucose for its metabolism and severe hypoglycaemia results in permanent brain damage within a matter of minutes. Every year hypoglycaemic patients fail to be recognized despite protocols, education and the legal consequences.

2 The first patient is hypoglycaemic. If he were able to swallow safely, he would be given a glucose drink or 'carbohydrate snack'. However, as his conscious level is severely depressed, intravenous glucose (e.g. 50 ml 20% dextrose) is given. Provided the glucose has been given before significant cerebral damage has occurred, the patient will often 'wake up' within a few minutes. Glucagon (1 mg i.v./i.m.) or hydrocortisone therapy is occasionally required in severe or refractory hypoglycaemia, as in sulphonylurea overdoses. These patients should be admitted for blood sugar monitoring (± glucose infusions). If BS measurement is not available (e.g. sudden onset of confusion in a diabetic while out hill walking), glucose should be given empirically as a sugary drink. Supplemental thiamine prevents Wernicke's encephalopathy (i.e. eye movement paralysis, ataxia, confusion) in hypoglycaemic malnourished patients, especially alcoholics.

3 The second patient is hyperglycaemic. An ABG test will establish that he is acidotic (in this case the ABG was pH 6.95, P_aO_2 14 kPa, P_aco_2 3.2 kPa, bicarbonate 3 mmol/L and base excess −21), a biochemical profile confirms he is dehydrated and hyperkalaemic (urea 20 mmol/L, creatinine 140 μmol/L and K^+ 6.9 mmol/L) and a urine dipstix will demonstrate the presence of ketones. This patient is hyperventilating to blow off carbon dioxide in an attempt to correct the metabolic acidosis; consequently his P_aco_2 is low. Similarly, the bicarbonate buffer has been depleted and the base excess is high.

4 The diagnosis is diabetic ketoacidosis (DKA). The immediate threats to this patient's life are the dehydration, acidosis and rapid ion fluxes that cause haemodynamic instability, with hypotension due to hypovolaemia, and reduced myocardial contractility and cardiac arrest due to hyper- or hypo-kalaemia. Rapid fluid replacement with ~3–5 L normal saline (NS) in <6 hours (i.e. 1 L in 30 minutes, then 1 L over 1 hour) rapidly corrects hypovolaemia and restores initial cardiovascular stability. Total fluid deficits of ~5–10 L and sodium losses of ~400 mmol are replaced over 48 hours. Monitor CVP if pulmonary oedema is a risk. The acidosis is corrected with insulin, which enables intracellular glucose uptake and metabolism. This stops intracellular lipolysis, hepatic metabolism of released fatty acids, ketone production (e.g.

β-hydroxybutyrate) and reverses the metabolic acidosis (Chapter 50). Insulin is given as an initial bolus (6–10 U i.v.), followed by an infusion (~6 U/h). Hyperglycaemia is often corrected before the acidosis but insulin must be continued until the acidosis has resolved by replacing the NS with a 10% dextrose infusion to maintain BS (monitored hourly) at 6–10 mmol/L. The use of sodium bicarbonate to correct the acidosis is controversial. It may reduce oxygen delivery and cause hypokalaemia. However, in severe acidosis (pH < 7.1) with myocardial depression, treatment may be unavoidable.

Potassium ion (K^+) fluxes can cause cardiac arrest during initial treatment of DKA. Initial serum K^+ levels are high due to acidosis-induced K^+ movement out of cells. Insulin therapy stimulates cellular K^+ uptake with a rapid fall in serum K^+. Hourly monitoring and K^+ supplements correct the K^+ depletion and prevent profound hypokalaemia (±cardiac arrest). Potassium supplementation before the onset of insulin therapy may cause hyperkalaemic VF/VT arrest. Hypomagnesaemia is corrected to prevent insulin resistance and arrhythmias. Phosphate supplementation maintains tissue oxygenation.

5 Hypoglycaemia is usually related to diabetic therapy including inadequate food intake, excessive exercise, accidental or deliberate overdose of diabetic drugs (e.g. sulphonylureas), prolonged drug effect (e.g. long-acting oral hypoglycaemics) and poor clearance in renal failure (e.g. insulin). Other causes include starvation, alcohol, renal and liver disease, systemic diseases (e.g. sepsis, hypothermia), endocrine disease (e.g. hypopituitarism), poisoning or drug therapy (e.g. salicylate) and rare insulin-secreting tumours (e.g. insulinomas). The first patient, a known insulin dependent diabetic, had taken his normal dose of evening insulin with his supper. The exercise of dancing at the night club had resulted in a low sugar level and faintness. He had left the nightclub for some fresh air where he had collapsed sustaining a forehead laceration during the fall.

DKA occurs in type 1 diabetes mellitus (DM) due to severe insulin deficiency. Precipitants include infection (~30%), myocardial infarction, surgery, pancreatitis and non-compliance. No cause is found in ~25%. The second patient was not known to be a diabetic but had been experiencing increasing thirst, dehydration and polyuria for several weeks following a viral illness. While dancing at the night club, he had felt faint and had gone outside for fresh air where he had collapsed, injuring his head during the fall. About 10% of type 1 DM presents as DKA.

6 Alternative causes of unconsciousness in a young patient include alcohol intoxication, drugs, trauma, non-convulsive epilepsy and post-ictal states, and infective causes including meningitis and encephalitis. Less likely causes include cerebrovascular, metabolic (e.g. hyponatraemia), endocrine (e.g. hypopituitarism) and cardiac problems (e.g. arrhythmias).

Appendix I: Classification of antiarrhythmic drugs (based on Vaughan Williams classification)

Class/examples	Mechanisms of action	Use
Class I:	All block Na^+ channels slowing depolarization + raising threshold for triggering impulses (AP). Drug dissociation rates from Na^+ channels vary; Class Ia ~5 s, Ib ~500 ms, Ic ~10–20 s	Slows conduction, suppresses re-entry + automaticity
Ia: disopyramide, quinidine	↑AP duration, ↑QT interval = ↑automaticity AVN conduction = ↑HR in AF	SVT + VT but must block AVN (e.g. digoxin) in AF
Ib: lidocaine (lignocaine), mexiletine	↓AP duration + greatly ↓conduction	VT especially after MI
Ic: flecainide	Greatly ↓ conduction, no effect on AP duration but ↓contractility may cause hypotension	VT + some SVT (e.g. WPW syndrome)
Class II atenolol, metoprolol	Beta-blockers act mainly on SAN: ↓spontaneous depolarization = ↓HR + ↓sympathetic drive (e.g. MI, stress) = ↓automaticity (↓latent pacemakers)	SVT + VT especially after MI
Class III amiodarone, sotalol	Block K^+ channels. ↑AP duration by ↓ repolarization. ↑QT interval risks automaticity (e.g. torsades de pointes). Also has class Ia, II + VI actions	SVT + VT. Most effective in re-entry tachycardias
Class VI verapamil, diltiazem	Block Ca^{2+} slow channels, ↓nodal conduction + automaticity. Also ↓contractility + risks hypotension	SVT especially AVN re-entrant tachycardias
Other classes adenosine, digoxin	Adenosine acts on A_1 receptors + ↓Ca^{2+}/↑K^+ currents to ↓AVN conduction. Digoxin ↓AVN conduction by vagal stimulation	Adenosine rapidly terminates + digoxin slows (± cardioverts) SVT

Critical Care Medicine at a Glance, Third Edition. Richard Leach. © 2014 John Wiley & Sons, Ltd. Published 2014 by John Wiley & Sons, Ltd.

Appendix II: Pacemaker types and classifications

Pacemakers may be either:

- Single chamber, with an electrode in either the right atrium or ventricle
- Dual chamber, with electrodes in both to pace the ventricle synchronously after sensing each atrial p wave (i.e. HR determined by SAN rate)

Pacemaker classification:

- The first letter identifies the paced chamber (i.e. V = ventricle, A = atrium; D = both)
- The second letter reports the chamber paced (V, A, D or 0 for none)
- The third letter indicates the response to electrical activity detection (i.e. I = inhibited, T = triggered, D = both)
- The fourth letter shows rate responsiveness (i.e. R) during activity

Thus, VVI-R indicates single chamber ventricular pacing in the inhibited mode and rate responsive.

Critical Care Medicine at a Glance, Third Edition. Richard Leach. © 2014 John Wiley & Sons, Ltd. Published 2014 by John Wiley & Sons, Ltd.

Appendix III: Acute injury network staging system 2008 for acute kidney injury (AKI)

AKI stage	Serum creatinine (SCr) criteria	Urine output (UO)criteria
1	SCr increase $\geq$26.4 µmol/L (0.3 mg/dl) or SCr increase $\geq$150–200% (1.5–2 fold) from baseline	<0.5 ml/kg/h for >6 h
2	SCr increase >200–300% (2–3 fold) from baseline	<0.5 ml/kg/h for >12 h
3	SCr increase $\geq$354 µmol/L (4.0 mg/dl) with an acute rise of $\geq$44 µmol/L in $\leq$24 h or SCr increase $\geq$300% (3-fold) from baseline or Initiated on RRT (irrespective of stage at time of initiation)	<0.3 ml/kg/h for >24 h or anuria for 12 h

Notes: RRT = renal replacement therapy, SCr = serum creatinine, UO = urine output. Only one criterion (SCr or UO) need be fulfilled to qualify for a stage. Changes in SCr or UO should occur within <48 h.

Critical Care Medicine at a Glance, Third Edition. Richard Leach. © 2014 John Wiley & Sons, Ltd. Published 2014 by John Wiley & Sons, Ltd.

Appendix IV: Rockall risk-scoring system for GI bleeds

	Score			
	0	1	2	3
Age	<60 yr	60–79 yr	>80 yr	
Shock	SBP > 100 mmHg	SBP > 100 mmHg	SBP < 100 mmHg	
	Pulse < 100/min	Pulse > 100/min		
Co-morbidity	None	CF, IHD	Renal/liver failure	Metastases
Diagnosis	No lesion, Mallory–Weiss tear	All other diagnoses	Upper GI malignancy	
Signs of recent bleeding on OGD	None or dark-red spot		Blood in upper GI tract; adherent clot; visible vessel	

Notes: Rockall score assists prediction of rebleeding risk and death after upper GI bleeding. A score >6 suggests surgery may be required, but the decision is rarely taken on the basis of the Rockall score alone.
CF = cardiac failure, GI = gastrointestinal, IHD = ischaemic heart disease, OGD = oesophagogastroduodenoscopy, SBP = systolic blood pressure.

Critical Care Medicine at a Glance, Third Edition. Richard Leach. © 2014 John Wiley & Sons, Ltd. Published 2014 by John Wiley & Sons, Ltd.

Appendix V: Child–Pugh grading: A = 5–6; B = 7–9; C = 10–15. Risk of variceal bleeding increases ≥8

	1 point	2 points	3 points
Bilirubin (μmol/L)	<34	34–51	>51
Albumin (g/L)	>35	28–35	<28
Prothrombin ratio (s >normal)	1–3	4–6	>6
Ascites	None	Minor	>Moderate
Encephalopathy (grade)	None	1–2	3–4

Critical Care Medicine at a Glance, Third Edition. Richard Leach. © 2014 John Wiley & Sons, Ltd. Published 2014 by John Wiley & Sons, Ltd.

Appendix VI: Typical criteria for liver transplantation

Paracetamol poisoning	Other pathologies (e.g. drugs, viruses)
pH < 7.3, 24 h after ingestion or INR > 6.5 Creatinine > 300 µmol/L Hepatic encephalopathy (grade 3–4)	INR > 6.5 or any 3 of: Drug or non-A, non-B virus aetiology Age < 10 or >40 years old Jaundice for >7 days before encephalopathy INR > 3.5 Bilirubin > 300 µmol/L

Critical Care Medicine at a Glance, Third Edition. Richard Leach. © 2014 John Wiley & Sons, Ltd. Published 2014 by John Wiley & Sons, Ltd.

Appendix VII: Royal College of Physicians' top nutrition tips

Royal College of Physicians' 'Ten Top Tips' for oral nutrition

1. NUTRITION IS IMPORTANT: it improves healthcare morbidity and mortality.
2. The Malnutrition Universal Screening Tool (MUST) should be used to identify malnourished or 'at risk' patients at admission to any healthcare facility.
3. Nutritional status should be assessed regularly in all healthcare settings.
4. Refer malnourished or 'at risk' patients to the dietician for specialist dietary advice.
5. Record food intake in malnourished or 'at risk' patients while in hospital or care homes.
6. Check that the swallowing reflex is safe to avoid aspiration (e.g. following strokes).
7. Occupational therapy assessment may be required in disabled or elderly patients (e.g. feeding aids, such as large-handle cutlery).
8. 'Red trays', 'protected' mealtimes and eating assistance improve food intake in vulnerable patients.
9. Consider oral nutritional supplements (e.g. 'high calorie drinks') if normal oral food intake remains inadequate (e.g. poor appetite).
10. Ensure community follow-up in nutritionally 'at risk' patients discharged from inpatient facilities.

Royal College of Physicians' 'Ten Top Tips' for nasogastric tube feeding

1. Consider nasogastric tube (NGT) feeding if a patient has a functional gut but poor oral intake or unsafe swallow.
2. Assessment, calculation of requirements and feed choice need appropriate advice (e.g. dietician).
3. NGT placement must be performed by trained, experienced staff using radio-opaque tubes with external length markings.
4. Use pH testing with CE marked indicator paper to assess NGT tip position. A pH between 1 and 5.5 is safe.
5. Keep the NGT clean and flush regularly with water using a 50 ml syringe (e.g. before/after feeding, between medications and 4–6 hourly if used continuously).
6. Position patients at 30–45 degrees to the horizontal during NGT feeding or hydration and keep raised for ≥1 hour after feeding.
7. Document refeeding risk in the medical notes and follow appropriate refeeding guidelines (e.g. NICE CG32).
8. Review medications to be administered via an NGT with a pharmacist or the nutrition support team.
9. Gastrointestinal disturbances: (i) Diarrhoea (e.g. infection, malabsorption, drug causes, constipation with overflow diarrhoea): consider reducing feed osmolality, remove fibre and decrease feed rate; (ii) Nausea/vomiting requires exclusion of obstruction/ileus: correct electrolyte imbalances, review drug prescriptions and consider pro-motility agents or post-pyloric feeding; reduce feeding rate.
10. Tube difficulties: (i) Blocked tubes: flush (i.e. push/pause technique) with warm water using 50 ml syringe; (ii) Repeated NGT displacement: consider NGT bridle/bolus feeding/early gastrostomy.

Royal College of Physicians' 'Ten Top Tips' for intravenous fluid administration

1. Determine whether intravenous (IV) fluid administration is required (e.g. coma). When possible, oral (or nasogastric) fluid is preferable.
2. IV fluid administration should follow clinical assessment including biochemical and fluid balance review (e.g. input/output measurement, weight).
3. IV fluid and/or electrolyte administration should be supervised by a senior clinician because inadequate or excessive therapy is associated with excess morbidity and mortality.
4. The three main IV fluid regimens are: (a) resuscitation; (b) maintenance; or (c) maintenance with correction for ongoing losses, redistribution or fluid/electrolyte imbalance.
5. Fluid resuscitation regimens aim to restore haemodynamic stability and maintain tissue perfusion following excessive fluid losses (e.g. haemorrhage) or critical illness (e.g. sepsis).
6. Maintenance fluid regimens aim to replace normal daily fluid and electrolyte losses (i.e. 2 L of water and 1 mmol/kg NaCl and KCl).
7. Fluid regimes that address ongoing fluid/electrolyte losses or correct previous fluid/electrolyte imbalance are determined from measured fluid inputs/outputs and biochemical assessment of serum or 'lost' fluids. Correct the normal fluid maintenance regime for the additional (or reduced) fluid/electrolyte requirements.
8. Large volume IV fluid resuscitation may be associated with excess electrolyte administration and has physiological consequences (e.g. hyperchloraemic acidosis) or causes complications (e.g. pulmonary oedema).
9. Resuscitation to haemodynamic stability may be achieved with slightly lower volumes of colloid, compared with crystalloid fluids; but has no clear morbidity or mortality benefits.
10. Stop IV fluids when oral (or nasogastric) intake is possible, or when the patient is haemodynamically stable, to reduce associated complications (e.g. line sepsis).

Royal College of Physicians' 'Ten Top Tips' for parenteral nutrition

1. Parenteral nutrition (PN) is most safely given through a dedicated single lumen catheter.
2. When feeding through a central vein the catheter tip should be at the vena cava/right atrial junction.
3. Before starting PN there should be an assessment of the risk of re-feeding problems.
4. PN is not an emergency treatment and should be started electively with clear aims.
5. PN should always include vitamins and trace elements.
6. The volume of PN must be included on fluid balance charts.
7. Patients having PN in hospital should be clinically monitored every day (especially fluid balance).
8. Catheter-related sepsis (CRS) usually originates from the hub connection so surgical aseptic non-touch techniques are needed for all procedures that access the catheter*.
9. SVC thrombosis is an emergency that needs treatment to re-establish venous patency.
10. Abnormal LFTs on PN more commonly relate to pre-existing liver disease, drugs or sepsis than to the parenteral nutrition solutions.

Critical Care Medicine at a Glance, Third Edition. Richard Leach. © 2014 John Wiley & Sons, Ltd. Published 2014 by John Wiley & Sons, Ltd.

Index

Page numbers in *italics* denote figures, those in **bold** denote tables.

Critical Care Medicine at a Glance, Third Edition. Richard Leach. © 2014 John Wiley & Sons, Ltd. Published 2014 by John Wiley & Sons, Ltd.